The Psychology of Sport Injury and Rehabilitation

Written by internationally known experts *The Psychology of Sport Injury and Rehabilitation* draws on the latest research in sport psychology and sports medicine. Using case studies to augment the reader's experience, this new edition emphasizes the importance of a holistic, interprofessional approach to sport injury management and care. By doing so, the book provides injured individuals, their families, and healthcare professionals a thorough overview of how psychology plays a role in sport injury prevention, rehabilitation, and return to participation process.

Athletes routinely use psychological skills and interventions for performance enhancement but, perhaps surprisingly, not always to assist in recovery from injury. This book demonstrates the ways in which athletes and practitioners can transfer psychological skills to an injury and rehabilitation setting to enhance recovery and the well-being of the athlete.

Psychology of injury is an integral part of sport injury prevention, rehabilitation, and return to participation process. The second edition of *The Psychology of Sport Injury and Rehabilitation* is a comprehensive text grounded in biopsychosocial theory and scientific evidence.

The fully revised second edition is an important resource for students, academic scholars, and applied practitioners working in sport psychology, sports medicine, sports coaching, and other related healthcare professions.

Monna Arvinen-Barrow is Associate Professor in the School of Rehabilitation Sciences and Technology at the University of Wisconsin–Milwaukee, USA; an online contributing faculty at the University of St. Augustine for Health Sciences, USA; and the Establishing Editor-in-Chief of the *Journal for Advancing Sport Psychology in Research*. She is a Chartered Psychologist (CPsychol) and an associate fellow (AFBPsS) of the British Psychological Society, a Certified Mental Performance Consultant (CMPC®), and a fellow (FAASP) of the Association for Applied Sport Psychology, and a Certified Mental Performance Coach and Exercise Practitioner (UPV sert.) of the Finnish Psychological Association. Monna is the lead editor of two textbooks: *The Psychology of Sport Injury and Rehabilitation* (2013) and *The Psychology of Sport and Performance Injury: An Interprofessional Case-Based Approach* (2019).

Damien Clement is Associate Dean of the Honors College and a professor of sport, exercise, and performance psychology at West Virginia University, USA. He is a certified athletic trainer, a national certified counsellor, and a Certified Mental Performance Consultant (CMPC®) and fellow (FAASP) of the Association for Applied Sport Psychology. In 2014, Damien was the recipient of the Dorothy V. Harris Award by the Association for Applied Sport Psychology for his distinguished contributions in the field of sport and exercise psychology as a scholar/practitioner. He is the co-editor of the 2019 book *The Psychology of Sport and Performance Injury: An Interprofessional Case-Based Approach*.

The Psychology of Sport Injury and Rehabilitation

Second Edition

**Edited by Monna Arvinen-Barrow
and Damien Clement**

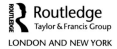

LONDON AND NEW YORK

Designed cover image: PeopleImages / Getty Images

Second edition published 2024
by Routledge
4 Park Square, Milton Park, Abingdon, Oxon, OX14 4RN

and by Routledge
605 Third Avenue, New York, NY 10158

Routledge is an imprint of the Taylor & Francis Group, an informa business

First edition published by Routledge 2013

ISBN: 978-1-032-28204-6 (hbk)
ISBN: 978-1-032-28203-9 (pbk)
ISBN: 978-1-003-29570-9 (ebk)

DOI: 10.4324/9781003295709

Typeset in Times New Roman
by Apex CoVantage, LLC

Äidin aikuiselle enkelille, Amielle (to mom's grown-up angel, Amie), and in memory of Pörrö-Neilikka, whose unconditional emotional support was unmatched.

Monna

Family is everything, and without you all, I am nothing. This book is a testament and direct reflection of your unwavering support of me and my career goals.

Damien

Contents

Figures

Tables

About the Contributors

Kylee J. Ault-Baker, PhD, CMPC, completed her doctoral degree at Michigan State University (USA) studying psychosocial aspects of sport and physical activity. She received her undergraduate degree from the Ohio State University in sport industry while being a member of the cheerleading team. Kylee continued her schooling with a master's degree in sport psychology and motor behavior from the University of Tennessee before coming to MSU. Kylee's research primarily focuses on life skill and mental skill development of youth and high school student-athletes. She is also a Certified Mental Performance Consultant (CMPC®) and is continuing her career as a Postdoctoral Scholar at The Ohio State University.

Monna Arvinen-Barrow, PhD, is Associate Professor in Sport and Performance Psychology at the University of Wisconsin–Milwaukee, USA, and an online contributing faculty at the University of St. Augustine, Florida, USA. Monna is a Chartered Psychologist (CPsychol.) and an associate fellow (AFBPsS) of the British Psychological Society, a Certified Mental Performance Consultant (CMPC®) and a fellow (FAASP) of the Association for Applied Sport Psychology, and a certified mental performance coach and exercise practitioner (UPV sert.) of the Finnish Psychological Association. She is the lead editor of three textbooks on psychology of sport injury and has authored 40+ book chapters, 60+ journal articles, and 200+ workshops, seminars, symposia, podcasts, webinars, and conference presentations, published in English, Finnish, Korean, and French. Monna serves the professional sport community as the Establishing Editor-in-Chief of the *Journal for Advancing Sport Psychology in Research* and as the USA Swimming Safe Sport Chair for Wisconsin Swimming LLC. She provides sport and performance psychology consultancy services for youth, collegiate, and professional athletes in various sports. A fun fact: Monna is a double high school graduate (Riverside, California, and Vantaa, Finland), and her first higher degree is in technical fashion designing, which she completed while working as a full-time figure and synchronized skating coach.

Amie Barrow is an undergraduate student in the Program in Liberal Medical Education (BS/MD) at Brown University, RI, USA. Amie is also a member of the Brown Women's Swimming and Diving Team. Born in the United Kingdom to Finnish and Gambian immigrant parents, Amie grew up in Wisconsin, USA. In her free time, Amie enjoys designing and sewing clothes, photography, and video editing.

Britton W. Brewer, PhD, is Professor Emeritus of Psychology at Springfield College in Springfield, Massachusetts, USA.

Megan M. Byrd, PhD, CMPC® (she/her), is Assistant Professor in Sport and Exercise Psychology at Georgia Southern University, USA, where she teaches graduate and undergraduate classes. Megan serves on numerous committees for the Association for Applied Sport Psychology and on the executive board for the American Psychological Association Division 47. As part of her role at the university, Megan supervises graduate students in their sport psychology internships and is a member of the Mental Performance team, delivering sport psychology services to collegiate athletes. She is also the co-director of Mental Performance at South Georgia Tormenta FC. Originally from Florence, Kentucky, Megan received her undergraduate degree from Eastern Kentucky University, a master's degree from Miami University, and a master's and PhD from West Virginia University. In addition to consulting work, Megan's research is focused on emotional and behavioral responses to concussion, perfectionism, and professional issues related to ethics and training. She has authored many research articles and book chapters and presented at international and national conferences. Prior to entering the field of sport psychology, Megan was a staff sportswriter at her college newspaper.

Hailey A. Chatterton is a graduate student in the athletic counseling master's program at Springfield College, MA, USA. Born and raised in California, she earned her BA in psychology from the University of California–Davis. Hailey is currently a teaching and research support fellow in the Department of Psychology, and she provides counseling and mental performance services to student-athletes and teams. Her research interests and current projects center on pre-competitive anxiety, clinical anxiety, and eating disorders in student-athletes.

Damien Clement, PhD, is Professor in Sport, Exercise, and Performance Psychology at West Virginia University. Damien is a Certified Mental Performance Consultant (CMPC®), a fellow (FAASP) of the Association for Applied Sport Psychology, a certified athletic trainer (ATC), and a national certified counselor (NCC). He is currently the Associate Dean of the Honors College at West Virginia University, USA. Damien was born and raised in Trinidad and Tobago and pursued his undergraduate and graduate studies in the USA at the University of Charleston (WV) and West Virginia University, respectively.

Melissa Day, PhD, is Reader in Sport and Exercise Psychology at the University of Chichester, United Kingdom. She is a UK Health and Care Professions Council (HCPC) practitioner psychologist and is British Association of Sport and Exercise Sciences (BASES) accredited. Her research interests are in the psychology of injury and rehabilitation, focusing specifically on traumatic injury and vicarious trauma. Melissa is a passionate qualitative researcher and chaired the 2014 International Conference for Qualitative Research in Sport and Exercise, held at the University of Chichester.

Ciara Everard is a PhD student at St. Mary's University and a sport and exercise psychology lecturer at Roehampton University, United Kingdom. She is a UK Health and Care Professions Council (HCPC) Physiotherapist. Her research interests are in the psychology of injury and rehabilitation, qualitative research, and narrative inquiry.

Jessica L. Ford, PhD, is Assistant Professor of Kinesiology at McDaniel College (Westminster, MD, USA), where she teaches courses in areas related to sport, exercise, and performance psychology. As part of her responsibilities at the college, she also serves as an academic advisor and senior capstone (undergraduate thesis) sponsor for many cross-disciplinary independent research projects. Outside of the classroom, Jessica provides performance consulting services to local athletes and performing artists. Her more recent publications, workshops, and presentations involve the application of sport psychology to domains outside of athletics, primarily among musicians. A musician herself, Jessica has taken over a decade of voice lessons and can play the guitar. Over the years, she has performed at some fun locations, such as Summerfest (Milwaukee, WI, USA; one of the largest music festivals in the USA) and the Stone Pony (Asbury Park, NJ, USA) with Jon Bon Jovi as a part of a benefit concert. Jessica recently decided to go back to school to earn an additional master's degree in clinical mental health counseling to complement her sport psychology/kinesiology degrees.

John J. Fraser, DPT, PhD, FACSM is a board-certified orthopedic physical therapist, scientist, and leader in the United States Navy, currently serving as the Deputy Director for Operational Readiness and Health at the Naval Health Research Center, San Diego, CA, USA. John is a graduate of the physical therapy program at the College of Staten Island, City University of New York, in 2002 and the post-professional DPT program at the University of St. Augustine for Health Sciences. He was conferred the PhD in education, kinesiology (sports medicine), from the University of Virginia in 2017, where he studied the role of the foot in lateral ankle sprains and chronic ankle instability. John's specialized clinical experience include the prevention, primary care, and rehabilitation of tactical, collegiate, and recreational athletes with neuromusculoskeletal injuries, in both traditional clinical settings and austere expeditionary environments. His research interests and scholarship include the study of ankle-foot neuromusculoskeletal function, rehabilitation, and public health of military tactical athletes. John's experience includes leadership of interdisciplinary teams, clinical practice and research development, medical and operational planning, and teaching in graduate professional and medical education.

Samantha Glynn is a PhD student at the University of Limerick, Ireland. Her research interests are in the psychology of injury and mental health, qualitative research, and narrative inquiry.

Michael A. Hansen is a PhD student at the University of Wisconsin–Milwaukee, USA. His research interests are in sport and performance psychology, coping mechanisms, and military/veteran populations. Prior to his baccalaureate and graduate education, Michael was a member of the US military for ten years, serving in military intelligence and cybersecurity roles. Outside of academia, Michael enjoys climbing, backpacking, and providing inclusive firearms safety training to historically underrepresented communities in shooting sports.

Brandonn S. Harris, PhD, CMPC®, LPC, NCC (he/him), is the Graduate Program Director and Professor of Sport and Exercise Psychology at Georgia Southern University, USA. He is a Certified Mental Performance Consultant CMPC®, licensed professional counselor, national certified counselor, AASP fellow and is listed on the United States Olympic and Paralympic Committee Sport Psychology Registry. His professional service has included serving as President for Division 47 of the American Psychological Association, as well as Chair of the Certification Council and Ethics Committee for the Association for Applied Sport Psychology. He teaches courses in the areas of ethical issues in sport psychology, psychological aspects of peak performance, and supervises graduate students' practicums and internships in sport and exercise psychology. As a practitioner working within primarily collegiate and professional sport, he utilizes an integrational approach to therapy and mental skills training, drawing from various frameworks to ensure his clients receive the care and support that best suit their interests and needs. Brandonn also maintains an active research agenda that has resulted in several articles, book chapters, and (inter)national presentations in the areas of ethics and professional issues in sport psychology, burnout, and youth sport. He obtained his bachelor's degree in exercise science with a sport psychology specialization from Truman State University in Kirksville, Missouri. He holds two master's degrees in sport and exercise psychology and counseling, both from West Virginia University, USA. His PhD in sport and exercise psychology was also completed at West Virginia University.

Caroline Heaney, PhD, is Senior Lecturer in Sport and Fitness at the Open University, UK. She is a British Association of Sport and Exercise Sciences (BASES) and Health and Care Professions Council (HCPC) registered Sport and Exercise Psychologist. Caroline specializes in the psychological aspects of sport injury and has extensive applied, teaching, and research experience in this field. Her research and applied work focus on educating athletes and those supporting them (e.g., physiotherapists, sport therapists, athletic trainers, coaches) about the psychological impact of injury and developing supportive environments for injured athletes. Her interest in this field grew from her own injury experiences as a track-and-field athlete and an observation that those around the injured athlete had a limited understanding of the psychological aspects of injury but a willingness to learn more.

John Heil, Doctor of Arts, is born in the American city of Philadelphia and is a product of its sport culture. He is a clinical and sport psychologist with Psychological Health Roanoke. John authored the original edition of the *Psychology of Sport Injury* and has published widely in professional and popular sources, as diverse as Tehran's *Hamshahri Daily News* and *American Police Beat*. He continues to work to extend the scope of sport and performance injury with partners, including simulated performance with injury in tactical populations (Roanoke City Police Department), sport hazing (Society for Sport, Exercise, and Performance Psychology and the Gordie Center of University of Virginia), on-field sport violence (Roanoke College), and critical incident and mass casualty response (Virginia Tech Carilion School of Medicine). John has consulted at three Olympic Games. He served as Chair of Sports Medicine and Science for USA Fencing, as Director of Sports Medicine for the Commonwealth State Games of Virginia, and is a board member of Virginia Amateur Sports and the International Swim Coaches Organization. John is a Certified Mental Performance Consultant, Emeritus (CMPC®-E), and a fellow in the American Psychological Association and the Association of Applied Sport Psychology. He is the past President of the Society for Sport, Exercise, and Performance Psychology.

Brian Hemmings, PhD, is Senior Lecturer in Applied Sport Psychology at the University of Winchester, UK. Brian is a registered Sport and Exercise Psychologist with the Health and Care Professions Council (HCPC), a chartered psychologist with the British Psychological Society (BPS), and a fellow of the British Association of Sport and Exercise Sciences (BASES). He has published extensively in applied sport psychology, including co-authoring 5 books, 17 book chapters, and over 50 peer-reviewed research articles. He has worked in sport psychology combining academic, supervisory, and applied roles since 1993, having 30 years of experience as a consultant psychologist in golf, cricket, motorsport, and boxing in a variety of training and competition environments. He has presented extensively worldwide to a variety of audiences, including coaches, athletes, students, and psychologists. Brian has three daughters, is a lifelong Chelsea supporter, and is a big fan of Quentin Tarantino films.

Joanne Hudson, PhD, is Professor in exercise and sport psychology at Swansea University. She is a UK Health and Care Professions Council (HCPC) Practitioner Psychologist, a British Psychological Society (BPS) Chartered Psychologist, and is British Association of Sport and Exercise Sciences (BASES) accredited. She is an associate fellow of the BPS and a fellow of BASES and the Royal Society of the Arts. Joanne has published over 60 peer-reviewed research articles and has edited and written six books. She is a past chair of the BPS Division of Sport and Exercise Psychology and convened its inaugural conference and several international and national conferences since. Joanne has an extensive record of PhD and research master's supervision and is passionate about helping others achieve their potential. Outside of academia, she is an endurance runner who competes as a Welsh Masters athlete.

Ken Ildefonso, PhD, LAT, is Associate Athletic Trainer assisting with football at Miami University in Oxford, Ohio, USA. Originally from North Haven, Connecticut, Ken is a first-generation college graduate with a BS in athletic training from Southern Connecticut State University, USA; MA in sport and exercise psychology from Minnesota State University, Mankato, USA; and PhD in kinesiology with an emphasis in sport and performance psychology from the University of Wisconsin–Milwaukee, USA. Ken has athletic training experience in Alabama, Connecticut, Minnesota, Ohio, Virginia, and Wisconsin in various sports. In addition to various athletic training clinic positions, Ken has also worked as a graduate assistant athletic trainer for cross-country, track-and-field, at Minnesota State University, Mankato; a seasonal athletic trainer for football, swim/dive, and water polo at the Virginia Military Institute; and a head athletic trainer for the Philadelphia Stars in the United States Football League. Ken has completed five Ironman triathlons and multiple ultramarathons.

Andreas Ivarsson, PhD, is Professor in Psychology at Halmstad University, Sweden. He is also a scientific adviser for the Swedish Ice Hockey Federation, the Swedish Soccer Federation, and a research fellow at Arsenal Football Club, UK. Andreas also works as a sport psychology consultant, mainly focusing on soccer. Andreas has authored over 110 scientific journal articles and has given 200+ workshops, seminars, symposia for different audiences. Andreas is Senior Section Editor at the *Scandinavian Journal of Medicine and Science in Sport* and is Associate Editor for three journals: *Psychology of Sport and Exercise, International Journal of Sport and Exercise Psychology*, and *Science and Medicine in Football.* His research interests and current projects center on sustainable participation in sports.

Kaytlyn Johnson (she/her) is a graduate student in the sport and exercise psychology master's program at Georgia Southern University, USA. She received her bachelor's degree from Anderson University in Indiana, where she also played collegiate softball. Kaytlyn is currently a graduate research assistant under the direction of Dr. Megan M. Byrd, assisting in several research projects on topics such as perfectionism, the yips, and other professional issues in sport psychology. She has co-authored many research articles and presented at both regional and national conferences. As a student, Kaytlyn utilizes a humanistic approach to provide mental performance services to both adolescent and collegiate athletes. Her research interests include perfectionism, the yips, mental health and well-being in sport, youth and international sport, and developing psychologically safe sport environments. Outside of the professional arena, Kaytlyn enjoys hiking, traveling, and spending time with loved ones.

Urban Johnson, PhD, is Professor in Sport and Exercise Psychology at Halmstad University, Sweden. He has a previous background working full-time as a coach in handball, and his main research focus is about the psychological aspects of sports injury, prevention, rehabilitation, and intervention. He also conducts research in areas such as health psychology and exercise science. Dr. Johnson has vast experience in working with applied sport psychology, especially for team sport athletes in elite contexts such as soccer, handball, and volleyball.

Jonathan Katz, PhD, is a consultant psychologist. His applied psychology experience of 37 years and counting crosses several delivery domains working in a clinical psychology department of a psychiatric hospital, support provision to stakeholders (athletes, coaches, managers, sport scientists, and medics) in high-performance (Olympic, Paralympic, and professional) sport. Jonathan continues to be involved in fencing as an athlete (now retired) and remains active as both a coach and a coach developer. At its core, his applied work focuses on blending and balancing the performance-focused drivers of "the athlete" with the mental health and well-being needs of "the person." He also engages in training, supervising, and mentoring practitioners across the stages of professional development and career-long growth. A career-long passion for Jonathan has been his "lifting the cover" on the "how" to provide applied psychology support across the range of contexts he's involved with. Jonathan is dual British Psychological Society (BPS) chartered and Health and Care Professions Council (HCPC) registered as a counseling psychologist and sport and exercise psychologist, British Association of Sport and Exercise Sciences (BASES) High Performance Sports Accredited (HPSA), and fellow of BASES (FBASES).

Georgia K. Kundrat (she/her/hers) is an undergraduate student at the University of Wisconsin–Madison studying psychology and gender and women's studies and planning to graduate in 2024. Georgia is passionate about developing and utilizing inclusive and affirming education techniques. Georgia has been involved with several organizations, such as Easterseals, the Central Iowa Center for Independent Living, the Autism Society of Southeastern Wisconsin, and Girls Inc. of Greater Madison, to develop accessible education and training materials. In her leisure time, Georgia enjoys playing music, hiking, and spending time with friends and family.

Annamari Maaranen, PsyD, is Operational Psychologist at the United States Air Force, Special Warfare Human Performance Squadron, where she provides assessment and selection, sport and performance psychology, and mental health services to special warfare trainees and staff, with a focus on supporting trainees rehabilitating from an injury or illness. She is a licensed psychologist and has worked extensively in medical, rehabilitation, and military settings. Dr. Maaranen completed a postdoctoral fellowship in clinical health psychology at the Brooke Army Medical Center, where she specialized in the treatment of neurological disorders and orthopedic injuries. She earned her PsyD in counseling psychology with a concentration in athletic counseling and MS in athletic counseling from Springfield College, MA, USA, and her BA in psychology from the University of Denver, CO, USA. Dr. Maaranen's primary interests include functional neurological and headache disorders, injury and rehabilitation, and mental blocks in artistic sports.

Karen Menard, PhD, OT, is the Academic Program Director for the Post-Professional Doctor of Occupational Therapy Program at the University of St. Augustine for Health Sciences in St. Augustine, FL, USA. Her academic leadership focus is related to program and curriculum development/assessment, instructional management, capstone and dissertation advisement, as well as contributions to international cross-cultural projects and interprofessional education and collaboration (IPE/IPC) course development. Karen is a licensed occupational therapist and brings more than 35 years of managerial and clinical experience in a variety of settings specializing in orthopedic, neurological, cognitive, and emotional disorders. She completed her PhD from Walden University in 2014 with a concentration in education, MS in health sciences with a concentration in education from University of Central Florida in 1992, and a BS in occupational therapy from Florida International University in 1985. She is a member of professional organizations, including the World Federation of Occupational Therapy, American Occupational Therapy Association, Florida Occupational Therapy Association, and NexusIPE. Karen is an international scholar, presenting at conferences in the United States, Switzerland, France, and Greece. Published works on interprofessional education, occupational therapy clinical practice and education, and biopsychosocial intervention occupational therapy model are found in journals focused on occupational therapy, interprofessional education and collaboration, mental health, and health sciences.

Peter Olusoga, PhD, CPsychol, is a British Nigerian Geordie living in Sheffield in the UK. Pete is a husband and father and a senior lecturer in psychology at Sheffield Hallam University. His PhD thesis, completed in 2012, focused on stress and coping in elite sports coaching, and his current research focuses on coach burnout and well-being in high-performance sports environments. Pete has authored a whole bunch of research papers, book chapters, conference presentations, workshops, webinars, and such and is an associate editor for *The Psychologist* (British Psychological Society magazine) and for the *Journal of Applied Sport Psychology*. In addition, Pete is a BPS chartered psychologist (CPsychol), an experienced consultant, and a producer/host of the award-winning sport and performance psychology podcast *Eighty Percent Mental*.

Stephen Pack, PhD, is a Senior Lecturer in Sport and Exercise Psychology at the University of Hertfordshire, UK. Stephen is a British Psychological Society chartered psychologist and associate fellow (CPsychol, AFBPsS) and is registered with the Health and Care Professions Council (HCPC) as a practitioner psychologist. Alongside teaching undergraduate students, Stephen also supervises MSc and PhD students, is currently supervising clinical psychology trainee/students, and has contributed to a range of degree programs within life and medical sciences at the university in various capacities. Stephen's research has focused largely on professional practice processes/issues within sport psychology support. He has also provided extensive sport psychology support within a range of sports and to a number of polar explorers. Stephen has a growing interest in nature-based exercise and nature connection, and he recently qualified as a forest therapy guide and is currently leading several associated research projects.

Leslie Podlog, PhD, is Professor in the School of Kinesiology and Physical Activity Sciences at the Université de Montréal and CHU Sainte-Justine Research Centre in Montreal, Canada. He has held faculty positions at the University of Utah, Texas Tech University, Charles Sturt University (Australia), and the German Sport University, Cologne. He completed his doctoral studies in sport and exercise psychology at the University of Western Australia, in Perth, Australia. He has published extensively on the psychological aspects of return to sport from injury. Outside of work, he enjoys spending time with his two kids, hiking, and traveling.

Judi Schack-Dugré PT, DPT, MBA, EdD, FNAP, is Director of Clinical Education in the Doctor of Physical Therapy Program at the University of Florida, with a top five ranking of public universities in the USA. She has two doctoral degrees, one in physical therapy and the other in education, with an emphasis on online teaching of health professionals. She also has earned a master's in business administration for executives, with an emphasis in global business. Her bachelor's degree is in physical therapy. She is a national leader in academic physical therapy. She is a member of the American Council of Academic Physical Therapy and holds a seat on its Leadership Oversight Committee. She has over 35 years of experience that crosses over academic and clinical settings. She was the sole owner of a multilocation clinical practice for nearly two decades. She is a distinguished scholar fellow of the National Academies of Practice. Her research in interprofessional education has led to multiple international and national presentations. She also received the designation of State of the Art most likely to change practice at the World Confederation for Physical Therapy. She continues to pursue a research agenda that intersects clinical education and practitioner competency and efficacy of online learning strategies that include competency-linked academic progression.

Travis R. Scheadler, MSW, MS, LSW, is a PhD student in the College of Social Work at the Ohio State University. He also is a licensed social worker in Ohio, a junior associate editor of the *Journal for Advancing Sport Psychology in Research*, and an openly gay emerging scholar. His research and practice interests emphasize LGBTQ+ rights, antiracism, advocacy, and community belonging both in- and outside sport contexts. Travis regularly engages in Stonewall Columbus Sports and leads volunteer efforts in the community. He plans to complete his PhD in 2025.

J. Jordan Utley, PhD, LAT, ATC, FNAP, is Corporate Education Director for Pima Medical Institute, based in Tucson, Arizona, USA. Jordan is a research fellow of the National Academies of Practice and a 30-year member of the National Athletic Trainer's Association. With nearly three decades of higher education administrative experience in health professions education, Jordan has contributed to student success through faculty, program director, department chair, and dean of health science roles and is currently leading health professions education for a 17-campus system across eight states. Jordan believes in educating graduates to be change agents of healthcare, to lead interprofessional patient-centered care teams that are population-focused, are cost-effective, and foster personal and professional well-being. Related to this mission, she collaborates with industry partners to connect federal grant funds to upskill and reskill the healthcare workforce. Her current research agenda includes examining the effectiveness of IPE across systems in higher education to create behavioral change in practicing clinicians. Prior research foci included identifying concussion biomarkers and establishing the effectiveness of post-injury biopsychosocial interventions. Clinically, Jordan has 29 years of experience as a certified athletic trainer (ATC), working with athletes from high school to professional sports, including the men's and women's US soccer teams. She is an international scholar, publishing and presenting her work on interprofessional education (IPE), concussion, and biopsychosocial interventions.

Amanda J. Visek, PhD, is an Association for Applied Sport Psychology (AASP) fellow and Certified Mental Performance Consultant (CMPC®) and United States (US) Centers for Disease Control Physical Activity in Public Health fellow and a trained scientist-practitioner and associate professor in the Department of Exercise and Nutrition Sciences at The George Washington University's Milken Institute School of Public Health in Washington, DC, USA. She has served in leadership positions for both AASP and the American Psychological Association's Division 47 Society for Sport, Exercise, and Performance Psychology, organizations from which she has received career achievement awards for her science and practice contributions. Amanda uses highly translational research approaches to identify and quantify determinants of fun in sport ecosystems using innovative mapping techniques, known broadly as FUN MAPS. Her research, sponsored by federal agencies and national sport governing bodies in the United States and abroad, has been enthusiastically received, worldwide, to guide the delivery of sport programs, inform coach education, and shape policy. Her work has been headlined, globally, across all major media, including television, newspapers, radio, and podcasts. She is an establishing editor of the *Journal for Advancing Sport Psychology in Research*, AASP's only open-access scientific journal. Born and raised in the US Army, Amanda earned five degrees, which coincidentally is the number of times she moved countries or states during her childhood. When not focused on research, she serves as a mental performance provider to Washington, DC, area athletes and teams.

Ross Wadey, PhD (he/him/his), is Professor at St. Mary's University, Twickenham, UK. He is a chartered psychologist with the British Psychological Society and an associate editor for the *Journal of Applied Sport Psychology*. Currently, Ross's research operates at the intersections between disciplines (e.g., sport psychology, sports sociology, sports medicine, sports communication) and aims to co-produce research with external stakeholders across various fields (e.g., sport, military, health, performing arts) to support their craft (i.e., performance, health, well-being) and, where appropriate, to bring about social justice. In addition to teaching and research, Ross is a trustee to the charity LimbPower that aims to engage amputees and individuals with limb impairments in physical activity to improve quality of life and lifelong learning.

Natalie C. Walker, PhD, is a British Psychological Society Chartered/Health and Care Professions Council registered psychologist. She is employed as the Associate Head of the School for Student Experience in Life Sciences at Coventry University, UK, and as an associate lecturer at the Open University. She has written several publications in the field of psychology of sport injuries, examined and supervised postgraduate/doctoral research in the area, and has consulted with injured athletes supporting their return to play. Her interest in this field grew from her own injury experiences in martial arts and football (soccer). Natalie is married to Christina, and both are avid Liverpool FC fans. Their other passion in life is their English show cocker spaniels.

Julie A. Waumsley, PhD, CPsychol, DipCouns, FHEA, PGCHE, MNCS (Snr Accred), AFBPsS, is a Chartered Sport and Exercise Psychologist with the British Psychological Society and associate fellow (CPsychol. AFBPsS) and has worked with many athletes over the years. Julie began professional life as a physical training instructor in the British Army and so has seen human behavior and performance under the most extreme of conditions. Julie has taught sport and exercise psychology in several universities across the UK and specializes in counseling, again passing on her expertise to others in a teaching environment and running CPD courses accordingly. Julie is a senior accredited therapist with the National Counselling Society and is registered with the Professional Standards Authority. She currently works as a psychotherapist in private practice, seeing clients who struggle with many and varied difficulties, including C-PTSD, bulimia nervosa, anxiety, illness and injury, and the huge range of other presentations that affect the human psyche. Julie is particularly interested in neurobiology and the way this impacts our emotions and behavior in any given circumstance. In her free time, she loves walking her dogs along the English Cornish beaches, where she currently lives and works.

Shameema M. Yousuf, MSc, MEd, MBACP, HCPC (she/her/hers) is a UK Health and Care Professions Council (HCPC) Practitioner Psychologist and British Association of Counseling and Psychotherapy (BACP) therapist. She is a member of the Association for Applied Sport Psychology, American Psychological Association, the European Federation of Sport Psychology, and the International Society of Sport Psychology. Her scholarly work and practice are at the intersection of performance, mental health, and culture in sport and the corporate world, with a global presence in her private practice Empower2Perform. Her activities include guest lecturing at several UK and US universities, running webinars, speaking at conferences, and coaching/counseling teams and individuals in their domain. Shameema has published chapters and peer-reviewed journal articles, is the editor of a book project, and her work is featured on media platforms. She serves as an executive leader, being the current Head of Publications and Information on the Executive Board of the Association for Applied Sport Psychology. Educated in Zambia, Zimbabwe, UK, and USA, and given her previous expertise in the corporate financial industry, she draws on her multiple professional identities and cultural experiences to support strong processes, effect policy change, and impact belonging in the spaces that she operates. Her small frame would never have you thinking she was an elite field hockey player who maintains that competitive spirit on a tennis court.

Luca Ziegler (he/him) is a graduate student in the sport and exercise psychology master's program at Georgia Southern University. Luca was born and raised in Germany and received his bachelor of science in psychology from Presbyterian College in South Carolina, USA. Luca currently instructs undergraduate physical activity courses as a graduate teaching assistant. As a student, he provides mental performance services to collegiate student-athletes as he pursues his Certified Mental Performance Consultant (CMPC®) credential. Luca has presented at both regional and national conferences. His research interests include elite performance, mindfulness, personality in sport, and emotional regulation, with a particular focus on implicit beliefs and competitive anxiety in student-athletes.

Derek M. Zike, MS (he/him/his), is a wheelchair user who identifies as a person with an acquired disability. Born and raised in Fishers, Indiana, Derek sustained a spinal cord injury playing ice hockey at 16 years old. Derek earned both his MS and BS in kinesiology and health from Miami University, USA, and is currently a doctoral candidate in sport and performance psychology at the University of Wisconsin–Milwaukee (UWM), USA, with an anticipated PhD completion in 2023. Derek is a disabled emerging scholar whose research focuses on critical disability studies, with a particular focus on the psychosocial impact of acquired physical disability from sport. Derek serves both the sport psychology and disability community in a number of ways. He is the junior managing editor of the *Journal for Advancing Sport Psychology in Research* and an interim co-chair of the Advocacy Committee of the Association for Applied Sport Psychology. Derek also holds service positions on the UWM campus; he is a leader of the Disability Rights, Education Activism, and Mentoring student organization and an officer of the Sport Psychology and Performance Excellence student organization.

Foreword

As the former Director of the Sport Psychology and Motor Behavior Graduate Program at the University of Tennessee, I've had the pleasure of interacting with many undergraduate and graduate students who wanted to become sport psychology professionals (SPPs). These students – for the most part – wanted to work with "elite-level" performers who were at the "top of their game" and in amazing physical condition; most did not consider the fact that athletes can suffer physical and mental injury and must learn to cope with rehabilitation during their athletic career.

This desire to work with "perfect" athletes is not surprising, given the sport systems we have all worked and competed in. In fact, in most elite-level sport contexts, coaches and athletes themselves believe that athletes should *give 110%, not show weakness*, and *be mentally tough* (Hughes & Coakley, 1991). They promote the notion that a "good" athlete is a "coachable" athlete; as a result, it becomes "normal" for a coach to yell at athletes, control their behaviors – both on and off the field – and in some cases, treat all athletes as if they were the same. Those of us who love and work in sport are still subject to believing these types of majoritarian narratives (Solórzano & Yosso, 2002).

Myself and colleagues (i.e., Schinke & Hanrahan, 2009) have focused in recent years on developing a more cultural sport psychology. We have suggested that it is important to center our analysis of sport on important cultural factors such as sport norms, gender, identity, social structure, power, religion, and to explore the ways that these cultural factors impact individual sport experiences (Fisher & Anders, 2010, 2020), like injury rehabilitation. We believe this type of analysis has real value because we can only understand sport participants' cognitions, behaviors, performance outcomes, well-being, engagements, and identities by also understanding how cultural spaces are infused with relational power dynamics. As sport psychology professionals, we believe it is important to ask ourselves, for example: (a) "To what extent am I privileging athlete performance and performance enhancement ahead of athlete well-being?" (b) "How do I cultivate a commitment to athletes that begins with an awareness of the intersections of their interpersonal and institutional power (or lack thereof) and how I might be deploying my own power against them?" and (c) "How do I practice aligning my values and moral commitments across my personal and professional life?" (Fisher & Anders, 2020).

Learning to see the athlete as a whole person in a specific cultural context with a particular evolving set of cultural identities requires both commitment and action (Fisher & Anders, 2020). What I most appreciate about Arvinen-Barrow and Clement's second edition of *The Psychology of Sport Injury and Rehabilitation* is their attention to socioculturally situated, athlete-centered, and holistic interprofessional approaches to rehabilitation management and sport injury risk. Just like in the first edition, the latest research and theoretical evidence have been presented from the fields of sports medicine and sport psychology; however, this edition incorporates what

I would call cultural sport psychology experiences – in addition to their continued emphasis on a biopsychosocial approach – that impact the psychology of sport injury.

This is a forward-thinking and important book for anyone aspiring to work with athletes. As a sport psychology professional, I couldn't agree more with the holistic approach adopted in this book, and I believe it to be a crucial framework for viewing athlete experience moving forward.

Leslee A. Fisher, PhD, FAASP, CMPC©, NBCC, LLPC
Professor Emerita, University of Tennessee

References

Fisher, L., & Anders, A. D. (2010). Critically engaging with sport psychology ethics through cultural studies. In T. V. Ryba, R. J. Schinke, & G. Tenenbaum (Eds.), *The cultural turn in sport and exercise psychology* (pp. 101–126). Fitness Information Technology.

Fisher, L., & Anders, A. D. (2020). Engaging with cultural sport psychology to explore systemic sexual exploitation in USA Gymnastics: A call to commitments. *Journal of Applied Sport Psychology*, *32*(2), 129–145. https://doi.org/10.1080/10413200.2018.1564944

Hughes, R., & Coakley, J. (1991). Positive deviance among athletes: The implications of over conformity to the sports ethic. *Sociology of Sport Journal*, *8*(4), 307–325. https://doi.org/10.1123/ssj.8.4.307

Schinke, R. J., & Hanrahan, S. J. (Eds.). (2009). *Cultural sport psychology*. Human Kinetics. https://doi.org/doi.org/10.5040/9781492595366.

Solórzano, D., & Yosso, T. J. (2002). Critical race methodology: Counter-storytelling as an analytical framework for education research. *Qualitative Inquiry*, *8*(1), 23–44. https://doi.org/10.1177/107780040200800103

Preface

Ten years ago, Dr. David Lavallee opened his foreword to the first edition of *The Psychology of Sport Injury and Rehabilitation* by stating, "[A] book on the psychology of sport injuries is not groundbreaking. I start with this not as a criticism but as an acknowledgement of how this area of study has advanced in recent years" (Arvinen-Barrow & Walker, 2013, p. xv).

The same holds true today. Over the past decade, the field has seen an exponential growth in the number of books dedicated to the topic (i.e., Arvinen-Barrow & Clement, 2019; Brewer & Redmond, 2017; Gledhill & Forsdyke, 2021; Granquist et al., 2014; Ivarsson & Johnson, 2020; McKay, 2022; Wadey, 2021; Wadey et al., 2020). The wider fields of sport psychology and sports medicine have also increasingly recognized the importance of integrating sport injury psychology within professional competency content, evidenced by an increased number of dedicated chapters in certification exam preparatory materials (e.g., Association for Applied Sport Psychology, 2021b; National Athletic Trainers' Association, see Prentice, 2020). Sport injury psychology has also gained some worldwide attention in non-English print, with a translated version of the first edition of *The Psychology of Sport Injury and Rehabilitation* in Korean (Arvinen-Barrow & Walker, 2019), and related seminal book chapters published in Finnish (Arvinen-Barrow & Kaski, 2021) and in French (Clement et al., 2016).

The first edition of *The Psychology of Sport Injury and Rehabilitation* aimed to "emphasize the importance of a holistic, multi-disciplinary approach to sport injury and rehabilitation" (Arvinen-Barrow & Walker, 2013, book blurb). While this still holds true, the second edition aims to extend the aforementioned. In recent years, a significant shift toward holistic, athlete-centered, and socioculturally situated interprofessional approaches to sport injury risk and rehabilitation management has taken place. By incorporating the latest theoretical and research evidence from sport psychology and sports medicine, the goal of the second edition is to present the reader with representative and contemporary content.

In this second edition, consistent with existing sport injury psychology literature, we consider sport injury to be a biological phenomenon, both affecting and being affected by psychological and sociocultural factors (Arvinen-Barrow & Clement, 2019; Brewer & Redmond, 2017; Wadey, 2021). The book is also underpinned by a philosophy that injury and high performance exist on a continuum representing opposite ends, where "at any given time, a performer is able to operate at a [performance] level somewhere along the continuum, with the goal of moving toward the high performance" (Arvinen-Barrow & Clement, 2019, p. xxiii). We also consider sport injury to be a potential risk factor for individuals' mental health, a crucial component to personal, community, and socio-economic development (World Health Organization, 2022). For the purposes of the book, *mental health* is defined as:

A state of well-being that enables people to cope with the stresses of life, to realize their abilities, to learn well and work well, and to contribute to their communities. Mental health is an integral component of health and well-being and is more than the absence of a mental disorder.

(World Health Organization, 2022, p. 8)

Consistent with both the World Health Organization (2022) and the Association for Applied Sport Psychology (2021a), the book considers mental health to exist on a continuum, ranging from an optimal state of mental *wellness* to a debilitating state of mental *illness*, both of which influence, and are influenced by, injury and high performance.

The book refers to any professional trained to attend to the psychosocial needs of athletes with injuries as a *sport psychology professional (SPP)*. Further, three specific professional titles consistent with the definitions depicted by Jones et al. (2022) are adopted in the book to distinguish variability in professional competencies due to different training backgrounds. *Mental performance consultant (MPC)* refers to professionals who work to enhance psychological *skills* (i.e., mental abilities) and teach how to use psychosocial *strategies* (i.e., methods an athlete can use to rehearse or improve psychological *skills*) that aid mental and emotional preparation for sport performance. *Licensed mental health provider (LMHP)* refers to professionals who are trained to address clinical mental health concerns, including but not limited to anxiety, depression, and eating disorders, but do not have extensive formal training or certification in sport psychology. *Licensed sport psychology professional (LSPP)* refers to professionals who have the licensure to address clinical mental health concerns AND the appropriate training and certification in sport psychology to enhance psychological skills and teach athletes how to use psychosocial strategies for performance enhancement. To expand the applicability of the content across various contexts, collectively, the term *sports medicine professional (SMP)* is used as an overarching title for all medical professionals who may be involved in the care of an injured athlete. This includes, but is not limited to, athletic trainer, chiropractor, occupational therapist, physical therapist, physician, physiotherapist, rehabilitator, sports therapist, and surgeons. The term *sport professional (SP)* is used to acknowledge individuals who interact with athletes with injuries on a regular basis (e.g., sport coach, selected support personnel) but are not sports medicine professionals.

The book is divided into four parts. Part 1, "Biopsychosocial Approach to Sport Injury," introduces key terminology and existing theoretical frameworks developed to explain the biopsychosocial sport injury risk and rehabilitation process. Part 1 also presents the reader with a theoretical and empirical understanding of the psychosocial process in two non-acute injuries with high prevalence with athletes – sport-related concussion and patellofemoral pain. Part 2, "Professional Practice in Sport Injury," extends the original first edition by focusing on several interconnected factors that influence the sport injury rehabilitation and return to participation process. These include introduction to pertinent interprofessional practice models applicable to sport injury, consideration of ethical issues, and the role of counseling skills in sport injury and rehabilitation. Part 2 also provides the reader with guidance on how to make psychosocial assessments and referrals and brings forth multicultural considerations pertinent to sport injury and rehabilitation. Part 3, "Psychosocial Strategies in Sport Injury," introduces the reader to some of the most salient psychosocial strategies used in sport injury rehabilitation by sport psychology and sports medicine professionals. New to the second edition, chapters on *coping with sport injury and rehabilitation* and *patient education in sport injury and rehabilitation* have been added to complement the upgraded original chapters of goal setting, self-talk, relaxation techniques, imagery, and social support. Part 4, "Return to Participation and Transition Out of Sport," focuses on the psychosocial processes that are associated with possible outcomes of the sport injury, including return to participation and retirement from sport due to injury.

Since the publication of the first edition, the world – and sport as a microcosm within it – has also faced multiple global social movements, such as Black Lives Matter and #MeToo. The world has navigated, and continues to navigate, through the COVID-19 pandemic. In addition to insurmountable death toll, the pandemic has unapologetically exposed numerous health disparities within, and across, countries and communities. We have also seen a new rise of both nationalism and the fight for social justice. These significant global events have undoubtedly shaped our personal, social, and sporting worlds. The contents in this book aim to capture elements of this shift – through the addition of new topical content (see Chapters 4–6, 8, 10–13, and 19–20), the revision of original content (see Chapters 2, 3, 7, 9, 14–18), and the presentation of carefully crafted diverse case studies and associated questions in Chapters 2–20.

The list of invited chapter authors is also representative of the changing and diverse global world. While some authors are undoubtedly esteemed scholars and practitioners in their respective fields (e.g., counseling, ethics, sport psychology, sports medicine), several early-career scholars, undergraduate, and graduate students have also been invited to contribute. In doing so, the many authors that have contributed to the book represent diverse intersectional identities across age, disability, national and ethnic origin, race and color, religion, sex, gender, and sexual orientation.

We hope you enjoy the read.

Dr. Monna Arvinen-Barrow
Dr. Damien Clement

References

Arvinen-Barrow, M., & Clement, D. (Eds.). (2019). *The psychology of sport and performance injury: An interprofessional case-based approach*. Routledge.

Arvinen-Barrow, M., & Kaski, S. (2021). Urheilupsykologian merkitys vammojen kuntoutusprosessissa. [Role of sport psychology in injury rehabilitation]. In K. Pasanen, H. Haapasalo, P. Halen, & J. Parkkari (Eds.), *Urheiluvammojen ehkäisy, hoito ja kuntoutus [Sport Injury prevention, treatment and rehabilitation]*. VK-Kustannus Oy.

Arvinen-Barrow, M., & Walker, N. (Eds.). (2013). *The psychology of sport injury and rehabilitation*. Routledge. https://doi.org/10.4324/9780203552407

Arvinen-Barrow, M., & Walker, N. (Eds.). (2019). *Psychology of sport injury and rehabilitation (Korean translation)*. Sungshin Women's University Press.

Association for Applied Sport Psychology. (2021a). *AASP statement on the continuum of mental health & relationship to performance. A response to the conversation supporting Naomi Osaka and Simon Biles*. Retrieved November 13, from https://appliedsportpsych.org/media/news-releases-and-association-updates/aasp-statement-on-the-continuum-of-mental-health-and-relationship-to-performance-a-response-to-the-conversation-supporting/

Association for Applied Sport Psychology (Ed.). (2021b). *The essential guide for mental performance consultants*. Web Textbook. Human Kinetics.

Brewer, B. W., & Redmond, C. J. (2017). *Psychology of sport injury*. Human Kinetics.

Clement, D., Arvinen-Barrow, M., & Van Horn, S. (2016). Lés émotions comme antécédent et conséquences de la blessure en sport. [Emotions as antecedents and consequences of sport injury]. In M. Campo &

B. Louvet (Eds.), *Lés émotions en sport et en EPS: Appretissage, Performance et Santé. [Emotions in sport, exercise and physical education – Learning performance and health]* (pp. 401–415). De Boeck.

Gledhill, A., & Forsdyke, D. (Eds.). (2021). *The psychology of sports injury: From risk to retirement.* Routledge.

Granquist, M., Hamson-Utley, J. J., Kenow, L. J., & Stiller-Ostrowski, J. (2014). *Psychosocial strategies for athletic training.* F. A. Davis Company.

Ivarsson, A., & Johnson, U. (Eds.). (2020). *Psychological bases of sport injuries* (4th ed.). Fitness Information Technology.

Jones, M., Zakrajsek, R., & Eckenrod, M. (2022). Mental performance and mental health services in NCAA D1 athletic departments. *Journal for Advancing Sport Psychology in Research*, *2*(1), 4–18. https://doi.org/10.55743/0000010

McKay, C. D. (Ed.). (2022). *The mental impact of sports injury.* Routledge.

Prentice, W. (Ed.). (2020). *Rehabilitation techniques for sports medicine and athletic training* (7th ed.). SLACK Incorporated.

Wadey, R. (Ed.). (2021). *Sport injury psychology: Cultural, relational, methodological, and applied considerations.* Routledge.

Wadey, R., Day, M., & Howells, K. (Eds.). (2020). *Growth following adversity in sport.* Routledge.

World Health Organization. (2022). *World mental health report: Transforming mental health for all.* Retrieved November 13 from www.who.int/publications/i/item/9789240049338

Acknowledgments

It is with sincere humility that we, as the editors of the second edition of *The Psychology of Sport Injury and Rehabilitation*, look back a decade and thank the original contributors for providing this book a solid foundation, both structurally and in content. Without their immaculate attention to detail, there would not be a second edition.

We are forever indebted to the invaluable efforts of the true pioneers of sport injury psychology. Thank you to Mark Andersen, Britton W. Brewer, Lynne Evans, Frances Flint, Sandy Gordon, Charles Hardy, John Heil, Urban Johnson, Gregory Kolt, David Lavallee, David Pargman, Aynsley Smith, Ron Smith, Frank Smoll, Jim Taylor, Judy Van Raalte, Maureen Weiss, Diane Wiese-Bjornstal, and Jean Williams. Without your meticulous work in developing a solid theoretical and empirical foundation for interprofessional, biopsychosocial sport injury research and applied work, there would not be a need for a second edition.

We are also grateful for the authors of the second edition. Thank you for trusting us and collectively creating a book that reflects what sport injury psychology currently is and provides a vision for what it can become in years to come.

Lastly, there is a need to recognize the impact *sisu* [si-sue] (noun) can have on a Finn. Loosely defined as "a strength of will," *sisu* is more than determination. It drives one forward when grit and perseverance run out. It is the emotional state that one is in, a personality trait that one has and draws strength and energy from at the time of adversity. It is an innate characteristic of oneself, yet it is also a mindset, a cultural norm, often even an internal and/or an external expectation. To put it simply, when all else fails, a Finn will dig deeper and find sisu. This book is a tangible testament to how one's roots and cultural heritage can be of great benefit when in need.

Monna and Damien

Part 1

Biopsychosocial Approach to Sport Injury

1 Introduction to Sport Injury Psychology

Monna Arvinen-Barrow

Chapter Objectives

- To define sport, sport injury, and sport injury psychology.
- To explain the role of psychology in sport injury and rehabilitation.
- To outline the role of sport psychology professionals, sports medicine professionals, and sport professionals in addressing the psychological aspects of sport injury.

Introduction to Sport and Sport Injury

Dating back to the early 14th century, the term *sport* refers to an "activity that offers amusement or relaxation; entertainment, fun" (Douglas Harper, 2001–2022). The first reference to sport involving *physical activity* dates to the early 16th century, a sentiment that holds true in definitions used today. For example, the term *sport* "means all forms of physical activity which, through casual or organised participation, are aimed at maintaining or improving physical fitness and mental well-being, forming social relationships or obtaining results in competition at all levels" (Enlarged Partial Agreement on Sport (EPAS) and Council of Europe, 2022, p. 12). At its best, sport can provide opportunities for physical, psychological, and economic growth and be a vehicle for fun, exciting, challenging, rewarding, and memorable experiences for all those involved. Despite the aforementioned positive benefits, some experiences gained through sport are in fact the opposite (Brown, 2005). Involvement in sport frequently places the participants under immense physical and psychological stress, which, in turn, has the potential to amplify the likelihood of unwanted outcomes, such as injuries.

In general, the term *sport injury* refers to injuries that occur in active individuals (National Institute of Arthritis and Musculoskeletal and Skin Diseases, 2021). More specific definitions continue to focus on the abstract conceptualization of *what is sport injury* or on the operational understanding of the *properties of sport injury*. For example, *The International Olympic Committee Manual of Sport Injuries* conceptualize sport injury as a "damage to the tissues of the body that occurs as a result of sport or exercise" (Bahr et al., 2012, p. 1). Operational understanding of the properties of sport injury (e.g., location, mechanics of onset, time taken for tissue to become injured, tissue type affected, and injury severity; Granquist et al., 2014) has predominantly focused on physical/biomechanical factors, largely ignoring any psychological factors, such as stress, attentional focus shifts, and/or anxiety (Arvinen-Barrow & Clement, 2019a).

DOI: 10.4324/9781003295709-2

Commonly divided into two overarching categories – *acute and overuse* – sport injuries are part of any sport participation. While worldwide sport injury prevalence statistics do not exist, data from Australia, Finland, United Kingdom (UK), and United States (US) suggest sport and recreation injuries account for approximately 18% to 50% of *all* injuries among children, adolescent, and/or adults (see Finch et al., 1998; Konttinen et al., 2011; Sheu et al., 2016; Uiten-broek, 1996). Existing data from the United States also suggests males (61.3%) and individuals aged 5–24 years (64.9%) account for more than 50% of all sport and recreation injuries (Sheu et al., 2016).

While no known prevalence data on adult overuse injuries exists (Chéron et al., 2017) and data on children and adolescents are largely underreported (DiFiori et al., 2014; Ristolainen et al., 2012), it is known that female athletes experience higher rate of overuse injuries than male athletes (Sheu et al., 2016). Sport-related traumatic brain injuries (sport TBI) are also common among adults and children alike. In the United States alone, it is estimated that 3.8 million adults will experience a sport TBI (Winkler et al., 2016), and that 21% of all TBIs among children and adolescents are caused by sport (Mickalide, 1995). Drawing from the preceding statistics, all athletes, regardless of sport and competitive level, are likely to experience an injury that can temporarily (or permanently) impede any subsequent sport participation (Taylor & Taylor, 1997). Indeed, Brown (2005) has argued that "serious athletes come in two varieties: those who have been injured, and those who have not been injured *yet*" (p. 215).

Sport injuries, particularly at the elite level, can also be costly. It is estimated that professional soccer teams lose an equivalent of 10% to 30% of annual player payroll costs to injuries (Abotel, 2015). Prospective research with athletes participating at the 2018 Olympic Winter Games (Soligard et al., 2019) and at the 2020 Junior Olympic Winter Games (Palmer et al., 2021) reported approximately 12 injuries per 100 athletes during the Games, of which approximately 33% were expected to result in time loss from sport. Research with collegiate student-athletes has shown that 63.8% of sport injuries happen during competitions (as opposed to practice), and 21.9% of all injuries require more than seven days off sport (Kerr et al., 2015). Given the high financial and time loss costs, it is no surprise that much research and resources have been dedicated to identifying solutions to minimize risk of injury (e.g., Aaltonen et al., 2007; Faude et al., 2017; Orchard et al., 2014; Orchard & Powell, 2003; Petushek et al., 2018) and testing alternative treatment modalities (e.g., Arvinen-Barrow et al., 2020) in the hope to facilitate both quick and safe return to participation.

Introduction to Sport Injury Psychology

With the aid of modern medicine, most athletes with injuries have the potential for full recovery. Yet numerous athletes fail to recover back to their pre-injury level of performance, and often this is attributable to psychological and/or sociocultural factors (e.g., Brewer & Redmond, 2017). Interest in understanding the role of psychological (e.g., personality, cognitions, affect) and sociocultural factors (e.g., social support, culture of risk) in sport injury date back five decades – over which sport injury psychology has grown "into a thriving academic field with rich, varied, and ever-expanding scholarly literature on theory, research, and practice pertaining to the topic" (Evans & Brewer, 2022, p. 1011). Some of the early work focused on understanding how selected psychological factors such as personality (e.g., Jackson et al., 1978; Valiant, 1981) and stress (Andersen & Williams, 1988) impact athletes' sport injury onset risk. Over the years, the role of *stress* – broadly defined as the physiological or psychological response to a perceived imbalance between demands and resources (American Psychological Association, 2022; Lazarus & Folkman, 1984) – has been found to be central to the sport injury experience.

Elevated *stress response* has been both theoretically proposed (Andersen & Williams, 1988; Williams & Andersen, 1998) and empirically supported (Ivarsson et al., 2017) as a salient factor affecting sport injury risk and occurrence. Equally, injury itself has also been theoretically proposed (Wiese-Bjornstal et al., 1998) and empirically supported (see Brewer, 2017) as a *stressor*, thus highlighting the central role of stress in rehabilitation and return to participation.

Psychological factors have also been found to influence physical symptoms of injury, most notably pain. Commonly defined as a "distressing experience that is associated with actual or potential tissue damage and which has sensory, emotional, cognitive and social elements" (Williams & Craig, 2016; cited in Ayers & de Visser, 2018, p. 92), *pain* is closely related to both sport performance and sport injury (Brewer & Redmond, 2017). Most sport injuries will cause nociceptive pain, which sends pain messages to the central nervous system, triggering a *sensation* of pain. This *sensation* is *cognitively* interpreted by the person experiencing pain, and the resultant *pain perceptions* are influenced by various personal, cultural, and contextual factors (Ayers & de Visser, 2018).

Despite lacking strong empirical evidence in support (Brewer, 2017), rehabilitation adherence has also been proposed as a significant psychological factor affecting sport injury and rehabilitation outcomes. Defined as "the extent to which an individual completes behaviors as part of a treatment regimen designed to facilitate recovery from injury" (Granquist & Brewer, 2013, p. 42), adherence is considered a desired rehabilitation *behavior* by sports medicine professionals (SMPs). As such, rehabilitation adherence is grounded in the act of *doing* and considered instrumental for the success of many treatment modalities and rehabilitation strategies:

> We as humans *do* things. No activity we *do* (be it physical activity, eating or sleeping for example) will happen without us *do*ing it. And our *do*ing (behavior) is influenced by the ways in which we think (cognition) and feel (emotion) about the activity in question.
>
> (Arvinen-Barrow, 2015, p. 508)

Integrating Sport Injury Psychology into Sports Medicine

While the importance of sport injury psychology is increasingly recognized within sports medicine, its application into real-world injury prevention and rehabilitation is moderate at best. Much of sports medicine research and clinical practice has been, and continue to be, dominated by the biomedical model, where *injury* is defined as a biological defect that *occurs in* active individuals (Engel, 1977). This is contrary to the biopsychosocial framework widely accepted in sport injury psychology, where *injury* is defined as a biological defect that is both *affecting* and *being affected* by a myriad of physical, psychological, sociocultural, and environmental factors (Arvinen-Barrow & Clement, 2019b; Brewer & Redmond, 2017; Wadey, 2020). It is therefore not surprising that many rehabilitation protocols are focused on the physiological phases of sport injury (acute, repair, and remodeling) that closely align with biological healing processes (Prentice & Arnheim, 2014).

To better understand the reciprocal relationship between physical and psychological factors influencing sport injury, Kamphoff et al. (2013) proposed a three-phase framework where psychological responses are aligned with physiological healing phases. It proposes that once injured, an athlete will go through three interconnected phases, namely, *reactions to injury*, *reactions to rehabilitation*, and *reactions to return to participation*. The *reaction to injury* phase is proposed to represent the athlete's initial psychological responses to injury (Hamson-Utley, 2010). Heavily influenced by the physical characteristics of the injury (e.g., type, location, history, severity) and the associated physiological *acute* injury consequences (e.g., swelling, discoloration, muscle spasm, pain, and lack of mobility), typical psychological responses include varying primary and secondary cognitive appraisals and re-appraisals, and emotional and behavioral responses (Arvinen-Barrow & Granquist, 2020; Kamphoff et al., 2013).

The *reaction to rehabilitation* phase starts when the athlete has dealt with the initial impact of the injury. The *reaction to rehabilitation* phase often occurs parallel to the physiological phase of repair, which typically means decreases in physical injury complications, and requires engagement in rehabilitation activities aimed to increase strength, balance, and mobility (Kamphoff et al., 2013). Triggered by new rehabilitation activities and associated physiological responses, this phase is characterized by new cognitive appraisals or re-appraisals, variable rehabilitation enhancing and debilitating emotional responses (e.g., excitement and sadness), and numerous behavioral responses, most notably adherence, under-adherence, or over-adherence to rehabilitation (Arvinen-Barrow & Granquist, 2020; Clement & Arvinen-Barrow, 2020b).

The third and final phase, the *reaction to return to play*, incorporates the cognitive appraisals and emotional and behavioral reactions the athlete is experiencing in relation to their physical and psychological readiness to return to participation (Hamson-Utley, 2010). Associated with the *remodeling* phase, athletes in the *reaction to return to play* phase react to challenges associated with setbacks in the healing process, the process of returning back to performance (Kamphoff et al., 2013), and in some instances, the process of transitioning out of sport. While limited research evidence has explicitly explored the three phases of rehabilitation (e.g., Clement et al., 2015; Ruddock-Hudson et al., 2014), existing theoretical model (Wiese-Bjornstal et al., 1998) and empirical evidence (Clement et al., 2015; Murphy & Sheehan, 2021; Ruddock-Hudson et al., 2014) do support the cyclical and bidirectional nature of varied psychological responses during different phases of rehabilitation.

Delivering Sport Injury Psychology

In an ideal world, all athletes would have access to an interprofessional team of professionals responsible for sport injury management (Arvinen-Barrow & Clement, 2019b), but rarely does this exist in practice (Clement & Arvinen-Barrow, 2020a). At times, this could be due to lack of physical proximity to psychological services (Ayers & de Visser, 2018), limited financial resources allocated to psychological support (Carr & Davidson, 2014), or considerable administration costs (Müller et al., 2014). Sometimes, barriers to an interprofessional team approach are interpersonal in nature, such as poor communication, lack of role clarity, and misunderstandings related to the scope of practice (Kraemer et al., 2019). A scoping review by Fletcher et al. (2017) identified six key interpersonal constructs as influencing interprofessional practice within sports medicine. These include *professionalization* of "newer" healthcare professions; *professional dominance*, particularly when "outside professionals" enter the sports domain; *status imbalances* between different members of the interprofessional team; *interprofessional negotiations* between the athlete and the different members of the interprofessional team; differences in culture of *confidentiality* within competitive sport and sports medicine; and *compromise and competition*, particularly as it relates to making return-to-play decisions (see Fletcher et al., 2017).

In the absence of a widely adopted interprofessional team approach to sport injury management, it is important to consider the role and responsibilities of various key stakeholders in the delivery of sport injury psychology. While sport psychology professionals (SPPs) are likely the most comprehensively[1] educated professionals to address the psychological aspects of sport injuries and to use psychosocial strategies with injured athletes, "only infrequently are SPCs [sport psychology consultants] directly involved in the prevention and treatment of sport injury"

(Evans & Brewer, 2022, p. 1014). Many SPPs also report lack of access to athletes with injuries (Arvinen-Barrow & Clement, 2017), since "gaining entry" to the sports medicine space continues to be difficult. Some of the main barriers of integrating sport psychology into sports medicine include ongoing "stigma" associated with psychological support and potential confusion of the scope of practice for different types of sport psychology and mental health professionals (Carr & Davidson, 2014). In the absence of SPPs providing psychological support to athletes while injured, Evans and Brewer (2022) argue that SMPs, sport coaches, and athletes themselves are likely to share a responsibility of facilitating psychological care during sport injury. It is also likely that other significant individuals (e.g., parents, teammates, and friends) will play important roles in providing psychological support to athletes with injuries.

Traditionally, many sports medicine professionals, such as athletic trainers (Arvinen-Barrow & Clement, 2015; Clement & Arvinen-Barrow, 2019; Clement et al., 2013; Cormier & Zizzi, 2015; Estepp, 2013; Zakrajsek et al., 2017; Zakrajsek et al., 2016), physicians (Mann et al., 2007), and physiotherapists (Arvinen-Barrow, Hemmings et al., 2007; Arvinen-Barrow, Penny et al., 2010; Francis et al., 2000; Gordon et al., 1991; Heaney, 2006; Jevon & Johnston, 2003), have reported feeling underprepared to deliver sport injury psychology during rehabilitation. Recognizing both the increasing need for addressing psychological factors in sport injury and the apparent lack of adequate training and skills in psychological aspects of injuries (e.g., Zakrajsek et al., 2017), some sports medicine professions have embraced integrating psychological content into educational programs and professional competencies.

While sport psychology education has increased athletic trainers' ability to identify symptoms of psychological concerns and making sport psychology and mental health referral decisions, they appear to struggle with selecting appropriate psychosocial strategies to use with athletes (Cormier & Zizzi, 2015). Similar disparities have also been found among physiotherapists who appear to have knowledge of sport psychology content but lack the ability to appropriately apply it into clinical practice (Arvinen-Barrow et al., 2010; Heaney et al., 2017). Since research found that only 41% of the sport psychology education for physiotherapists in the UK contained content focused on relevant theory (Heaney et al., 2012), the preceding findings are not surprising. After all, theories and conceptual models provide an understanding of why and how a given phenomenon occurs – and how different factors can influence/are influencing each other and the outcomes. Consequently, much of sports medicine research and clinical practice continues to struggle with how to integrate psychology into sport injury prevention and rehabilitation. Many SMPs also report lack of access to psychological services (Arvinen-Barrow et al., 2010; Zakrajsek et al., 2018), thus leaving many SMPs feeling they need to either dabble with the psychological aspects of injuries on their own or deliberately ignore the psychological aspects of injuries.

Conclusion

A growing body of evidence exists in support of sport injuries being biopsychosocial in nature, where the injury, that is, a biological defect, is both *affecting and being affected* by a myriad of physical, psychological, sociocultural, and environmental factors (Arvinen-Barrow & Clement, 2019b; Brewer & Redmond, 2017; Wadey, 2020). Existing research has also demonstrated the integral role psychology plays in sport injury risk, sport injury occurrence, biopsychosocial responses to sport injury and rehabilitation, overall sport injury recovery outcomes, potential return to participation, and in some injury cases, transition out of sport. While a strong case for integrating sport injury psychology into sports medicine has been made, ambiguity still exists with regard to which professionals are best qualified and positioned to deliver sport injury psychology to athletes with injuries.

Reflective Questions

1. How do the different definitions of sport injury outlined in this chapter (there are several) align with your views on what is sport injury?
2. Based on your own experiences, in addition to stress, pain, and adherence discussed in this chapter, what other psychological and/or sociocultural factors likely influence sport injury and rehabilitation?
3. How can the three phases of rehabilitation help sport psychology, sports medicine, and sports professionals in conceptualizing sport injury rehabilitation?
4. What is your (future or current) professional role in delivering sport injury psychology to athletes with injuries? Consider the professional core competencies of your discipline or field, and provide two (2) examples of psychological support that are within your (future or current) scope of practice and two (2) examples that would warrant referral.

Note

1 Given that the term *sport psychology professional* in this book refers to various sport psychology– and mental health–trained professionals worldwide, it is acknowledged that not all have the requisite education and formal training that denotes domain-specific theoretical, empirical, and applied knowledge and skills in sport injury psychology.

References

Aaltonen, S., Karjalainen, H., Heinonen, A., Parkkari, J., & Kujala, U. M. (2007). Prevention of sports injuries: Systematic review of randomized controlled trials. *Archives of Internal Medicine, 197*(15), 1585–1592. https://doi.org/10.1001/archinte.167.15.1585

Abotel, K. (2015). The crippling cost of sports injuries. *Forbes*. Retrieved December 20, 2022, from www.forbes.com/sites/sap/2015/08/11/the-crippling-cost-of-sports-injuries/?sh=6d7daf4d1f7a

American Psychological Association. (2022). *APA dictionary of psychology*. https://dictionary.apa.org/

Andersen, M. B., & Williams, J. M. (1988). A model of stress and athletic injury: Prediction and prevention. *Journal of Sport & Exercise Psychology, 10*(3), 294–306. https://doi.org/10.1123/jsep.10.3.294

Arvinen-Barrow, M. (2015). Role of psychology in therapy and rehabilitation: Where does it "fit"? *International Journal of Therapy and Rehabilitation, 22*(11), 508.

Arvinen-Barrow, M., & Clement, D. (2015). A preliminary investigation into athletic trainers' views and experiences of a multidisciplinary team approach to sports injury rehabilitation. *Athletic Training & Sports Health Care, 7*(3), 97–107. https://doi.org/10.3928/19425864-20150422-05

Arvinen-Barrow, M., & Clement, D. (2017). Preliminary investigation into sport and exercise psychology consultants' views and experiences of an interprofessional care team approach to sport injury rehabilitation. *Journal of Interprofessional Care, 31*(1), 66–74. https://doi.org/10.1080/13561820.2016.1235019

Arvinen-Barrow, M., & Clement, D. (2019a). A case for interprofessional care. In M. Arvinen-Barrow & D. Clement (Eds.), *The psychology of sport and performance injury: An interprofessional case-based approach* (pp. 1–9). Routledge. https://doi.org/10.4324/9781351111591

Arvinen-Barrow, M., & Clement, D. (Eds.). (2019b). *The psychology of sport and performance injury: An interprofessional case-based approach*. Routledge.

Arvinen-Barrow, M., & Granquist, M. D. (2020). Psychosocial considerations for rehabilitation of the injured athletic patient. In W. Prentice (Ed.), *Rehabilitation techniques for sports medicine and athletic training* (7th ed., pp. 93–116). SLACK Inc.

Arvinen-Barrow, M., Hemmings, B., Weigand, D. A., Becker, C. A., & Booth, L. (2007). Views of chartered physiotherapists on the psychological content of their practice: A national follow-up survey in the United Kingdom. *Journal of Sport Rehabilitation, 16*(2), 111–121. https://doi.org/10.1123/jsr.16.2.111

Arvinen-Barrow, M., Maresh, N., & Earl-Boehm, J. E. (2020). Functional outcomes and psychological benefits of active video games in the rehabilitation of lateral ankle sprains: A case report. *Journal of Sport Rehabilitation, 29*(2), 213–224. https://doi.org/10.1123/jsr.2017-0135

Arvinen-Barrow, M., Penny, G., Hemmings, B., & Corr, S. (2010). UK chartered physiotherapists' personal experiences in using psychological interventions with injured athletes: An interpretative phenomenological analysis. *Psychology of Sport and Exercise, 11*(1), 58–66. https://doi.org/10.1016/j.psychsport.2009.05.004

Ayers, S., & de Visser, R. (2018). *Psychology for medicine and healthcare* (2nd ed.). Sage Publishing.

Bahr, R., Engebretsen, L., Laprade, R., McCrory, P., & Meeuwisse, W. H. (Eds.). (2012). *The IOC manual of sports injuries: An illustrated guide to the management of injuries in physical activity.* John Wiley & Sons.

Brewer, B. W. (2017). Psychological responses to injury. In *Oxford research encyclopedia of psychology.* Oxford University Press.

Brewer, B. W., & Redmond, C. J. (2017). *Psychology of sport injury.* Human Kinetics.

Brown, C. H. (2005). Injuries: The psychology of recovery and rehab. In S. M. Murphy (Ed.), *The sport psych handbook* (pp. 215–235). Human Kinetics.

Carr, C., & Davidson, J. (2014). The psychologist perspective. In G. T. Brown (Ed.), *Mind, Body, and Sport: Understanding and Supporting Student-Athlete Mental Wellness* (pp. 17–20). National Collegiate Athletic Association. www.ncaapublications.com/productdownloads/MindBodySport.pdf

Chéron, C., Le Scanff, C., & Leboeuf-Yde, C. (2017). Association between sports type and overuse injuries of extremities in adults: A systematic review. *Chiropractic & Manual Therapies, 25*(4).

Clement, D., & Arvinen-Barrow, M. (2019). Athletic trainers' views and experiences of discussing psychosocial and mental health issues with athletes: An exploratory study. *Athletic Training & Sports Health Care, 11*(5), 213–224. https://doi.org/10.3928/19425864-20181002-01

Clement, D., & Arvinen-Barrow, M. (2020a). An investigation into former high school athletes' experiences of a multidisciplinary approach to sport injury rehabilitation. *Journal of Sport Rehabilitation, 30*(4), 619–624. https://doi.org/10.1123/jsr.2020-0094

Clement, D., & Arvinen-Barrow, M. (2020b). Psychosocial strategies for the different phases of sport injury rehabilitation. In A. Ivarsson & U. Johnson (Eds.), *Psychological bases of sport injuries* (4th ed., pp. 297–330). Fitness Information Technology.

Clement, D., Arvinen-Barrow, M., & Fetty, T. (2015). Psychosocial responses during different phases of sport injury rehabilitation: A qualitative study. *Journal of Athletic Training, 50*(1), 95–104. https://doi.org/10.4085/1062-6050-49.3.52

Clement, D., Granquist, M. D., & Arvinen-Barrow, M. (2013). Psychosocial aspects of athletic injuries as perceived by athletic trainers. *Journal of Athletic Training, 48*(4), 512–521. https://doi.org/org/10.4085/1062-6050-48.3.21

Cormier, M. L., & Zizzi, S. J. (2015). Athletic trainers' skills in identifying and managing athletes experiencing psychological distress. *Journal of Athletic Training, 50*(12), 1267–1276.

DiFiori, J. P., Benjamin, H. J., Brenner, J., Gregory, A., Jayanthi, N., Landry, G. L., & Luke, A. (2014). Overuse injuries and burnout in youth sports: A position statement from the American medical society for sports medicine. *Clinical Journal of Sport Medicine, 24*(1), 3–20. https://doi.org/10.1097/JSM.0000000000000060

Douglas Harper. (2001–2022). Sport (v.). In *Online etymology dictionary.* Retrieved December 20, 2022, from www.etymonline.com/search?q=sport

Engel, G. L. (1977). The need for a new medical model: A challenge for biomedicine. *Science, 196*(4286), 129–136. https://doi.org/10.1126/science.847460

Enlarged Partial Agreement on Sport (EPAS), & Council of Europe. (2022). Revised European sports charter. https://edoc.coe.int/en/sport-for-all/11299-revised-european-sports-charter.html#:~:text=The%20European%20Sports%20Charter%20is%20the%20Council%20of,with%20opportunities%20to%20practise%20sport%20under%20well-defined%20conditions.

Estepp, M. K. (2013). *NCAA division I ahtletic trainers' perceptions and use of psychological skills during injury rehabilitation*. University of Tennessee.

Evans, L., & Brewer, B. W. (2022). Applied psychology of sport injury: Getting to – and moving across – The valley of death. *Journal of Applied Sport Psychology*, *34*(5), 1011–1028. https://doi.org/0.1080/10 413200.2021.2015480

Faude, O., Rössler, R., Petushek, E. J., Roth, R., Zahner, L., & Donath, L. (2017). Neuromuscular adaptations to multimodal injury prevention programs in youth sports: A systematic review with meta-analysis of randomized controlled trials. *Frontiers in Physiology*, *8*. https://doi.org/10.3389/fphys.2017.00791

Finch, C. F., Valuri, G., & Ozanne-Smith, J. (1998). Sport and active recreation injuries in Australia: Evidence from emergency department presentations. *British Journal of Sports Medicine*, *32*(3), 220–225. http://bjsm.bmjjournals.com/cgi/content/abstract/32/3/220

Fletcher, S., Breitbach, A. P., & Reeves, S. (2017). Interprofessional collaboration in sports medicine: Findings from a scoping review *Health and Interprofessional Practice*, *3*(2). https://doi. org/10.7710/2159-1253.1128

Francis, S. R., Andersen, M. B., & Maley, B. (2000). Physiotherapists' and male professional athletes' views on psychological skills for rehabilitation. *Journal of Science and Medicine in Sport*, *3*(1), 17–29. https://doi.org/10.1016/S1440-2440(00)80044-4

Gordon, S., Milios, D., & Grove, R. J. (1991). Psychological aspects of the recovery process from sport injury: The perspective of sport physiotherapists. *Australian Journal of Science & Medicine in Sport*, *23*, 53–60.

Granquist, M. D., & Brewer, B. W. (2013). Psychological aspects of rehabilitation adherence. In M. Arvinen-Barrow & N. Walker (Eds.), *The psychology of sport injury and rehabilitation* (pp. 40–53). Routledge.

Granquist, M. D., Hamson-Utley, J. J., Kenow, L. J., & Stiller-Ostrowski, J. (2014). *Psychosocial strategies for athletic training*. F. A. Davis Company.

Hamson-Utley, J. J. (2010). Psychology of sport injury: A holistic approach to rehabilitating the injured athlete. *Chinese Journal of Sports Medicine*, *29*(3), 343–347.

Heaney, C. (2006). Physiotherapists' perceptions of sport psychology intervention in professional soccer. *International Journal of Sport and Exercise Psychology*, *4*(1), 73–86. https://doi.org/10.1080/16121 97X.2006.9671785

Heaney, C., Green, A. J. K., Rostron, C. L., & Walker, N. C. (2012). A qualitative and quantitative investigation of the psychology content of UK physiotherapy education programs. *Journal of Physical Therapy Education*, *26*(3), 24–56.

Heaney, C., Rostron, C. L., Walker, N. C., & Green, A. J. K. (2017). Is there a link between previous exposure to sport injury psychology education and UK sport injury rehabilitation professionals' attitudes and behaviour towards sport psychology? *Physical Therapy in Sport*, *23*(1), 99–104. https://doi. org/10.1016/j.ptsp.2016.08.006

Ivarsson, A., Johnson, U., Andersen, M. B., Tranaeus, U., Stenling, A., & Lindwall, M. (2017). Psychosocial factors and sport injuries: Meta-analyses for prediction and prevention *Sports Medicine*, *47*(2), 353–365. https://doi.org/10.1007/s40279-016-0578-x

Jackson, D. W., Jarrett, H., Barley, D., Kausch, J., Swanson, J. J., & Powell, J. W. (1978). Injury prediction in the young athlete: A preliminary report. *American Journal of Sports Medicine*, *6*(1), 6–14. https://doi. org/10.1177/036354657800600103

Jevon, S. M., & Johnston, L. H. (2003). The perceived knowledge and attitudes of governing body chartered physiotherapists towards the psychological aspects of rehabilitation. *Physical Therapy in Sport*, *4*(2), 74–81. www.sciencedirect.com/science/article/B6WPB-48N2TX1-6/2/862463a5c75a68c4052cab c07a083fe8

Kamphoff, C. S., Thomae, J., & Hamson-Utley, J. J. (2013). Integrating the psychological and physiological aspects of sport injury rehabilitation: Rehabilitation profiling and phases of rehabilitation. In M. Arvinen-Barrow & N. Walker (Eds.), *The psychology of sport injury and rehabilitation* (pp. 134–155). Routledge.

Kerr, Z. Y., Marshall, S. W., Dompier, T. P., Corlette, J., Klossner, D. A., & Gilchrist, J. (2015). College sports-related injuries – United States, 2009–10 through 2013–14 academic years. *Centers for Disease Control and Prevention Morbidity and Mortality Weekly Report*, *64*(48), 1330–1336. www.cdc.gov/mmwr/pdf/wk/mm6448.pdf

Konttinen, N., Mononen, K., Pihlaja, T., Sipari, T., Arvinen-Barrow, M., & Selanne, H. (2011). Urheiluvammojen esiintyminen ja niiden hoito nuorisourheilussa – Kohderyhmänä 1995 syntyneet urheilijat [Sport injury occurence and treatment in youth sports – athletes born in 1995 as a target population]. *KIHUn julkaisusarja nro 25 (PDF-julkaisu)*.

Kraemer, E., Keeley, K., Martin, M., & Breitbach, A. P. (2019). Athletic trainers' perceptions and experiences with interprofessional practice. *Health, Interprofessional Practice & Education*, *3*(4), eP1171; 1171–1115. https://doi.org/10.7710/2159-1253.1171

Lazarus, R. S., & Folkman, S. (1984). *Stress, appraisal, and coping*. Springer Publishing Company.

Mann, B. J., Grana, W. A., Indelicato, P. A., O'Neill, D. F., & George, S. Z. (2007). A survey of sports medicine physicians regarding psychological issues in patient-athletes. *American Journal of Sports Medicine*, *35*, 2140–2147.

Mickalide, A. (1995). The National SAFE KIDS Campaign (USA). *Injury prevention*, *1*(2), 119–121. https://doi.org/10.1136/ip.1.2.119

Müller, C., Zimmermann, L., & Körner, M. (2014). Förderfaktoren und Barrieren interprofessioneller Kooperation in Rehabilitationskliniken – Eine Befragung von Führungskräften [Facilitators and barriers to interprofessional collaboration in rehabilitation clinics – a survey of clinical executive managers] *Die Rehabilitation*, *53*(6), 390–395. https://doi.org/10.1055/s-0034-1375639

Murphy, G. P., & Sheehan, R. B. (2021). A qualitative investigation into the individual injury burden of amateur rugby players. *Physical Therapy in Sport*, *50*, 74–81. https://doi.org/10.1016/j.ptsp.2021.04.003

National Institute of Arthritis and Musculoskeletal and Skin Diseases. (2021, December 20). *Overview of sports injuries*. National Institute of Arthritis and Musculoskeletal and Skin Diseases.

Orchard, J. W., McCrory, P., Makdissi, M., Seward, H., & Finch, C. F. (2014). Use of rule changes to reduce injury in the Australian Football League. *Minerva Ortopedica E Traumatologica*, *65*, 355–364.

Orchard, J. W., & Powell, J. W. (2003). Risk of knee and ankle sprains under various weather conditions in American football. *Medicine and Science in Sports and Exercise*, *35*, 1118–1123.

Palmer, D., Engebretsen, L., Carrard, J., Grek, N., Königstein, K., Maurer, D. J., . . . Soligard, T. (2021). Sports injuries and illnesses at the Lausanne 2020 Youth Olympic Winter games: A prospective study of 1783 athletes from 79 countries. *British Journal of Sports Medicine*, *55*(17), 968–974. https://doi.org/10.1136/bjsports-2020-103514

Petushek, E. J., Sugimoto, D., Stoolmiller, M., Smith, G., & Myer, G. D. (2018). Evidence-based best-practice guidelines for preventing anterior cruciate ligament injuries in young female athletes: A systematic review and meta-analysis. *The American Journal of Sports Medicine*, *47*(7), 1744–1753. https://doi.org/10.1177/0363546518782460

Prentice, W. E., & Arnheim, D. D. (2014). *Principles of athletic training: A competency-based approach* (15th ed.). McGraw-Hill.

Ristolainen, L., Kettunen, J. A., Kujala, U. M., & Heinonen, A. (2012). Sport injuries as the main cause of sport career termination among Finnish top-level athletes. *European Journal of Sport Science*, *12*(3), 274–282. https://doi.org/10.1080/17461391.2011.566365

Ruddock-Hudson, M., O'Halloran, P., & Murphy, G. (2014). The psychological impact of long-term injury on Australian football league players. *Journal of Applied Sport Psychology*, *26*(4), 377–394. https://doi.org/10.1080/10413200.2014.897269

Sheu, Y., Chen, L. H., & Hedegaard, H. (2016). Sports- and recreation-related injury episodes in the United States, 2011–2014. *National Health Statistics Reports*. www.cdc.gov/nchs/data/nhsr/nhsr099.pdf

Soligard, T., Palmer, D., Steffen, K., Lopes, A. D., Grant, M. E., Kim, D., . . . Engebretsen, L. (2019). Sports injury and illness incidence in the PyeongChang 2018 Olympic Winter games: A prospective study of 2914 athletes from 92 countries. *British Journal of Sports Medicine*, *53*(17), 1085–1092. https://doi.org/10.1136/bjsports-2018-100236

Taylor, J., & Taylor, S. (1997). *Psychological approaches to sports injury rehabilitation*. Aspen.

Uitenbroek, D. G. (1996). Sports, exercise, and other causes of injuries: Results of a population survey. *Research Quarterly for Exercise and Sport*, *67*, 380–385. https://doi.org/10.1080/02701367.1996.1060 7969

Valiant, P. M. (1981). Personality and injury in competitive runners. *Perceptual and Motor Skills*, *53*(1), 251–253. https://doi.org/10.2466/pms.1981.53.1.251

Wadey, R. (Ed.). (2020). *Sport injury psychology: Cultural, relational, methodological, and applied considerations*. Routledge.

Wiese-Bjornstal, D. M., Smith, A. M., Shaffer, S. M., & Morrey, M. A. (1998). An integrated model of response to sport injury: Psychological and sociological dynamics. *Journal of Applied Sport Psychology*, *10*(1), 46–69. https://doi.org/10.1080/10413209808406377

Williams, J. M., & Andersen, M. B. (1998). Psychosocial antecedents of sport injury: Review and critique of the stress and injury model. *Journal of Applied Sport Psychology*, *10*(1), 5–25. https://doi.org/10.1080/10413209808406375

Winkler, E. A., Yue, J. K., Burke, J. F., Chan, A. K., Dhall, S. S., Berger, M. S., . . . Tarapore, P. E. (2016). Adult sports-related traumatic brain injury in United States trauma centers. *Neurosurgical focus*, *40*(4), E4. https://doi.org/10.3171/2016.1.FOCUS15613

Zakrajsek, R. A., Fisher, L. A., & Martin, S. B. (2017). Certified athletic trainers' understanding and use of sport psychology in their practice. *Journal of Applied Sport Psychology*, *29*(2), 215–233. https://doi.org/10.1080/10413200.2016.1231722

Zakrajsek, R. A., Fisher, L. A., & Martin, S. B. (2018). Certified athletic trainers' experiences with and perceptions of sport psychology services for student-athletes. *The Sport Psychologist*, *32*(4), 300–310. https://doi.org/10.1123/tsp.2017-0119

Zakrajsek, R. A., Martin, S. B., & Wrisberg, C. A. (2016). National collegiate athletic association division I certified athletic trainers' perceptions of the benefits of sport psychology services. *Journal of Athletic Training*, *51*(5), 398–405. https://doi.org/10.4085/1062-6050-51.5.13

2 Biopsychosocial Risk Factors of Sport Injury

Andreas Ivarsson and Urban Johnson

Chapter Objectives

- To outline existing theoretical models explaining biopsychosocial injury risk factors.
- To summarize the most common biopsychosocial sport injury risk factors.
- To synthesize evidence in support of existing injury prevention programs.

Introduction

When participating in sport, an athlete can experience numerous stressors (e.g., Arnold & Fletcher, 2012). Without adequate strategies or resources to cope with stressors, the risk of acute and overuse injury is increased (e.g., Ivarsson et al., 2017; Tranaeus et al., 2022). Sport injuries are also associated with an increased risk for adverse consequences for the athlete, including increased risk of mental and physical illness and early career termination (e.g., Podlog et al., 2014). Such consequences can have long-lasting impact on the athlete many years after career termination. A study with 3,357 retired Olympians showed that of the sample, 32% continued to experience ongoing pain, and 36% reported functional limitations due to their previous sport injuries (Palmer et al., 2021).

Given high injury rates associated with sport participation (Åman et al., 2016), combined with several potential adverse long- and short-term consequences of sport injury, it is important to develop effective strategies to prevent sport injuries. An important first step in the development process is to identify risk factors that are likely to increase the possibility of sustaining a sport injury (Bahr, 2016). While several researchers have emphasized the importance of taking multiple factors into account when researching risk factors for injury (e.g., Bittencourt et al., 2016), much of previous research has focused on identifying and addressing physiological and/ or biomechanical injury risk factors. Over the past couple of years, however, an increased number of research studies has focused on psychosocial sport injury risk factors and their role in sport injury prevention. The purpose of this chapter is to provide an overview of the biopsychosocial risk factors associated with sport injury. More specifically, this chapter will (a) outline existing theoretical models that have been developed to explain biopsychosocial injury risk factors, (b) introduce the most common biopsychosocial sport injury risk factors, and (c) present an overview of existing injury prevention programs.

DOI: 10.4324/9781003295709-3

Theoretical Models for Psychosocial Risk Factors of Sport Injuries

Given the increased interest in psychological aspects related to sport injury prevention, several theoretical models have been developed. The focus within these models is to illustrate how the interaction between different psychological variables might be related to injury risk. In the next paragraphs, the models that have gained most attention within the literature will be presented.

The Revised Stress and Injury Model

One of the first theoretical models developed to explain the potential relationships between psychosocial variables and acute injury occurrence was the (revised) model of stress and athletic injury (Andersen & Williams, 1988; modified by Williams & Andersen, 1998). Within the model, the authors suggest that when placed in a potentially stressful situation, depending on the athlete's stress response, their injury risk may be amplified. The stress response is conceptualized as consisting of both cognitive appraisals and physiological and/or attentional changes, which are said to have a bidirectional relationship. According to the model, the stress response can be influenced by the interplay between various psychosocial factors, known as the injury antecedents. These are divided into three categories: personality factors, history of stressors, and coping resources. In the original model (Andersen & Williams, 1988), the authors suggested

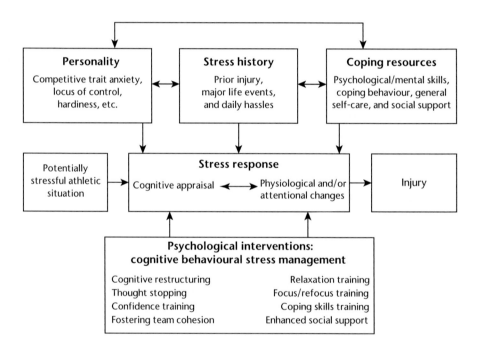

Figure 2.1 An amalgamated version of the revised stress and injury model.

that only history of stressors directly influenced the stress response, whereas both personality and coping variables have an indirect effect on stress responses through the history of stressors. Ten years later, however, the authors suggested that history of stressors could both influence and be influenced by an athlete's personality and coping resources, and therefore, they placed bidirectional arrows between the three psychosocial factors (Williams & Andersen, 1998). The revised model also posits that a range of psychological interventions influence/buffer the stress response and are therefore suggested to decrease acute sport injury risk.

The Overtraining Risks and Outcomes Model

The overtraining risks and outcomes model (Richardson et al., 2008) aims to illustrate how different psychosocial factors might influence the risk of overuse injuries. Within the model, the proposed factors are divided into four major categories of *risk factors*: intrapersonal variables (e.g., motivation, personality traits), interpersonal influences (e.g., past and present relationships with coaches, parents, friends), situational factors (e.g., poor performance, transitions in sport, major sport and non-sport events), and the sociocultural context (e.g., sport culture, societal influences). These risk factors are dynamic and intersecting in nature, ultimately affecting an athlete's beliefs and behaviors, particularly related to balancing stress load and recovery.

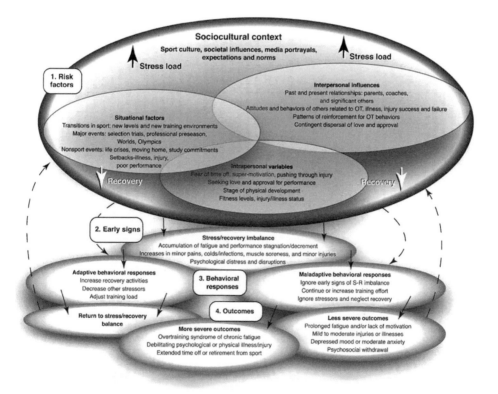

Figure 2.2 The overtraining risks and outcomes model.

Source: Used with permission of Human Kinetics, Inc., from *Overtraining Athletes: Personal Journey in Sport*, Sean O. Richardson, Mark B. Andersen, & Tony Morris, 2008; permission conveyed through Copyright Clearance Center, Inc.

If poorly managed, this can lead to *early signs* of stress/recovery imbalance, characterized by both physical and physiological (e.g., increased fatigue level, decrease in performance, muscle pain) and psychological (e.g., emotional distress, increased anxiety, emotional reactivity) signs and symptoms. The third step of the model outlines possible *behavioral responses* to the stress/recovery imbalance. If an athlete engages in adaptive behavioral responses (e.g., increase time in recovery activities, reduction of exposure to other stressors, or adjustment in training load), they are likely to return to a stress/recovery balance. Conversely, if an athlete engages in maladaptive behavioral responses (e.g., ignore the early signs of physical and/or psychological imbalance between stress/recovery, continue to increase training effort, or ignore stressors and neglect recovery), the resultant *outcome* of these behaviors is typically unfavorable. The *outcomes* are either less severe (e.g., prolonged fatigue, mild to moderate injuries or illnesses) or more severe (e.g., overtraining syndrome, debilitating psychological or physical injury, or retirement from sport).

The Biopsychosocial Sport Injury Risk Profile

The biopsychosocial sport injury risk profile (Wiese-Bjornstal, 2009, 2010) aims to illustrate how a combination of internal-intrinsic-personal and external-extrinsic-environmental factors contributes to an athlete's acute and chronic injury risk profile. The internal-intrinsic-personal

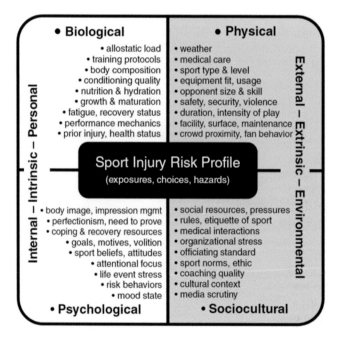

Figure 2.3 The biopsychosocial sport injury risk profile.

Source: Used with permission of John Wiley & Sons from Psychology and socioculture affect injury risk, response, and recovery in high-intensity athletes: A consensus statement, Diane M. Wiese-Bjornstal, *20*(Suppl. 2) 2010; Permission conveyed through Copyright Clearance Center, Inc.

factors include biological factors, such as allostatic load, body composition, nutrition and hydration, fatigue, recovery status, and health status. The psychological factors include perfectionism, coping, attitudes, attentional focus, life event stress, mood state, and risk behaviors. The external-extrinsic-environmental factors include physical factors, such as weather, medical care, sport type, opponent size and skill, and intensity of play, and sociocultural factors, such as social resources, rules, organizational stress, sport norms, and coaching quality. The model assumes a complex interaction between the biological and psychological characteristics and that this interplay influences the athlete's behavior when interacting with the physical and sociocultural environments. This will, in turn, increase injury risk vulnerability based on the resultant exposures, choices, and hazards.

The Biopsychosocial Model of Stress Athletic Injury and Health

The biopsychosocial model of stress athlete injury and health (Appaneal & Perna, 2014) aims to illustrate different pathways between stress demands and athlete health. The authors claim that this model is an independent extension of the revised model of stress and injury (Williams & Andersen, 1998). Alongside cognitive stress responses, the model also considers emotional, behavioral, and physiological stress responses as potential risk factors for acute and overuse injuries. The biopsychosocial model of stress athlete injury and health suggests that psychophysiological stressors, such as negative life event stress and intense physical training, have a direct relationship with increased injury and illness risk. The model also suggests that psychophysiological stressors also have an indirect effect on injury risk via behavioral (e.g., impaired self-care, poor sleep quality) or physiological (e.g., peripheral narrowing, stress hormone perturbation) mechanisms. These mechanisms are also proposed to have a bidirectional relationship with each other.

Psychosocial Risk Factors for Acute Sport Injuries

Much of the existing research on psychosocial risk factors has focused on acute injuries. Most of the research designs have utilized the revised model of stress and athletic injury (Williams & Andersen, 1998) as a framework for the selection of risk factors. In this section, while an apparent overlap between all the models outlined previously exists, we will first discuss the evidence on each of the psychosocial factors included in the revised model of stress and athletic injury (Williams & Andersen, 1998), followed by existing evidence on the role of several general well-being factors as a risk factor for acute sport injuries.

Stress Response

According to the revised model of stress and athletic injury (Williams & Andersen, 1998), an athlete's stress response to a potentially stressful event is hypothesized as having a direct effect on acute sport injury risk. This has been supported in the literature, as a meta-analysis by Ivarsson et al. (2017) found that stress response had the strongest relationship with acute sport injury risk. Over the past five years since the meta-analysis, several studies (e.g., McDonald et al., 2019) have mainly focused on different types of cognitive stress responses (e.g., attention, concentration, processing speed). The results from most studies have showed statistically significant relationships between varied cognitive functions and increased injury risk.

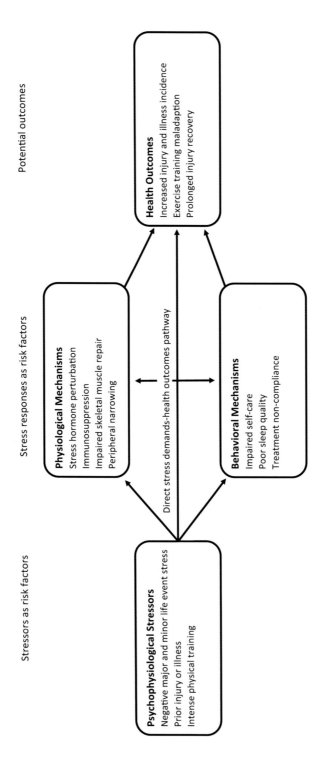

Figure 2.4 An adapted version of the biopsychosocial model of stress athletic injury and health.

Source: Adapted from Appaneal and Perna (2014).

Personality

Defined as "individual differences in characteristic patterns of thinking, feeling, and behaving" (American Psychological Association, 2022), certain personality variables have been hypothesized as having potential to either lower (e.g., hardiness) or increase (e.g., cognitive trait anxiety) individuals' stress response to a stressful situation, subsequently either decreasing or amplifying potential injury risk (Appaneal & Habif, 2013). Much of the research on personality traits as potential risk factors for injury to date has focused on trait anxiety and negative mood states (Ivarsson et al., 2017). While most existing research has found a significant relationship between a number of personality factors and injury occurrence, several studies have reported inconsistent findings (Ivarsson et al., 2017). Likewise, more adaptive traits, such as optimism (Wadey et al., 2013) and hardiness (Wadey et al., 2012), have also been found to influence stress response, subsequently decreasing acute sport injury risk.

History of Stressors

According to the revised model of stress and athletic injury (Williams & Andersen, 1998), the "history of stressors" factor includes major life events, daily events, and previous injures. Most of the existing published research has focused on the relationship between injury occurrence and history of stressors. To date, few studies (e.g., Smith et al., 1997) have reported contradictory results on the relationship between history of stressors and injury risk. However, for the most part, research has consistently provided support for a positive relationship between injury risk and high life stress (e.g., Hardy & Riehl, 1988), negative life event stress (e.g., Johnson & Ivarsson, 2011; Rogers & Landers, 2005), previous injury (e.g., Steffen et al., 2009), and daily hassles (e.g., Fawkner et al., 1999; Ivarsson et al., 2014). Indeed, a meta-analysis revealed that of the injury antecedents, history of stressors has the strongest association with injury risk (Ivarsson et al., 2017). One explanation for the preceding is that negative (or threatening) information is typically processed more thoroughly and has more severe and longer-lasting effects on behaviors than positive information.

Coping Resources

Coping, that is, "the cognitive and behavioral efforts to manage (master, reduce, or tolerate) a troubled person-environment relationship" (Folkman & Lazarus, 1985, p. 152), is proposed to influence the stress response by affecting both the cognitive appraisal of the stressors as well as the physiological and/or attentional changes to the stressful situation. Research focusing on coping strategies and injury occurrence is limited and lacks consistent results. For example, statistically significant negative relationships (i.e., lack of coping) were found between low levels of coping resources and injury occurrence (e.g., Hanson et al., 1992). In contrast, statistically significant positive relationships (i.e., ineffective coping) were found between injury occurrence and high levels of behavioral disengagement and self-blame (Ivarsson & Johnson, 2010) and injury occurrence and high prevalence of avoidance coping strategies (Maddison & Prapavessis, 2005).

Much of the coping resource research has focused on social support (for more on social support, see Chapter 18). Like coping strategies, social support research has also reported mixed results concerning the relationship between social support and injury risk. Specifically, a statistically significant negative relationship was found between low levels of social support and injury risk (e.g., Andersen & Williams, 1999). Several studies have found social support as a moderator in the stress–injury relationship (e.g., Maddison & Prapavessis, 2005; Patterson et al., 1998). A few studies have found non-statistically significant relationships between social support and injury occurrence (e.g., Hanson et al., 1992; Noh et al., 2005). Based on existing research evidence, one explanation for the rather weak direct relationship between coping and injury risk can be the stress-buffering hypothesis (Cassel, 1976; Cobb, 1976). The stress-buffering hypothesis assumes that coping resources such as social support will ameliorate or buffer the potential pathogenic effects of stressful events, stress, and stress responses, thus influencing injury risk (Maddison & Prapavessis, 2005; Rogers & Landers, 2005; Williams & Andersen, 1998).

General Well-Being Factors

Outside the injury risk factors outlined in the revised model of stress and athletic injury (Williams & Andersen, 1998), other general well-being factors have also been investigated as potential risk factors for sport injuries. For example, both sleep quantity (<7h/day; Johnston et al., 2020) and decreased sleep volume (Von Rosen et al., 2017) have been associated with increased injury risk. Johnston et al. (2020) also found that psychological/lifestyle distress reported in the seven days leading up to injury increased injury risk. In support, Van der Does et al. (2017) found that in the six weeks leading up to injury occurrence, athletes had experienced a decrease in social recovery and general well-being. Moreover, several other general well-being factors have been associated with injury risk, including symptoms of depression (Yang et al., 2014), emotional exhaustion, fatigue, and decreased fitness/injury (i.e., physical stress; Shrier & Hallé, 2011). These identified risk factors may also mediate the impact of stressors on injury risk.

Psychosocial Risk Factors for Overuse Injuries

In comparison to research focusing on psychosocial risk factors for acute injuries, even fewer studies have focused on psychosocial risk factors for overuse injuries. Existing research was recently summarized within a systematic review (Tranaeus et al., 2022), and thus far, only 14 research studies (9 quantitative and 5 qualitative) have investigated psychosocial risk factors for overuse injuries. The results of the systematic review identified 27 different psychosocial factors as potential injury risk factors. The results also revealed that several intrapersonal factors, such as personality traits, previous injuries, and neglecting warning signals and long-term consequences, had a potential effect on the risk of overuse injury. Several interpersonal and sociocultural factors were identified as potential injury risk factors. These included poor coach–athlete relationships, lack of social support, and pain normalization. The preceding findings are in support of the conceptualizations put forth in the overtraining risks and outcomes model (Richardson et al., 2008). More specifically, all the identified psychosocial sport injury risk factors can, often in combination with extensive training load, increase the odds for an athlete to engage in maladaptive behaviors. If an athlete repeatedly engages in these types of behaviors, the likelihood of sustaining an overuse injury is increased.

Psychological Interventions in Sport Injury Prevention

Consistent with the theoretical models presented in this chapter, many of the maladaptive psychosocial responses to stress can be managed or alleviated with a myriad of psychological strategies and interventions. Since the early 1990s, several research studies have developed and implemented psychological intervention programs with the goal to decrease sport injury risk.

The results from a review of literature (n = 5 intervention studies; Appaneal & Habif, 2013), a meta-analysis (n = 7 experimental studies; Ivarsson et al., 2017), and a systematic review of literature (n = 13 articles with 14 research studies; Gledhill et al., 2018) have concluded that athletes in intervention conditions have reported less injuries when compared to control conditions. Given the variability in methodologies and methods used in the intervention studies, it is important to acknowledge that these results have a moderate risk of bias. To date, research has investigated different psychological interventions, which can be generally divided into two main types based on philosophical underpinnings: cognitive behavioral interventions focused on psychological skills training (PST) and mindfulness/acceptance interventions.

Cognitive Behavioral Interventions

Cognitive behavioral interventions typically encompass a myriad of techniques, such as patient education, goal setting, and cognitive restructuring, to name a few. Psychological interventions aimed at decreasing sport injury risk have typically been focused on PST by educating the participants in different stress management techniques, such as imagery, relaxation, and goal setting (e.g., Johnson et al., 2005; Kerr & Goss, 1996; Olmedilla-Zafra et al., 2017). The interventions have varied in intervention length (range 1–36 weeks), frequency (range 1–16 sessions), and session duration (range 45–120 minutes). The interventions have also been conducted in different sports, such as gymnastics, soccer, rugby, and floorball.

Mindfulness/Acceptance Interventions

Mindfulness/acceptance interventions aim to help an individual stay focused on the present moment and accept thoughts and feelings without judgment. To date, at least two mindfulness/acceptance intervention research studies have also been published (Ivarsson et al., 2015; Zadeh et al., 2019). Both of these studies used soccer players and adopted the mindfulness acceptance commitment (MAC) approach (Gardner & Moore, 2007). The MAC approach consists of seven intervention sessions, where the focus is on the introduction and training of mindfulness/acceptance techniques.

Factors Affecting Psychological Intervention Success in Sport Injury Prevention

Despite limited research, the majority of what exists has demonstrated reduction in injury rates, irrespective of interventions used or design. Explanations of success can be broadly divided into two categories: specific and common factors (e.g., Mulder et al., 2017). *Specific factors* refer to aspects of treatment that are pertinent to a particular intervention strategy (e.g., adherence to the treatment protocol, treatment differences). *Common factors* refer to the aspects of treatment that are generic for all intervention strategies (e.g., empathy, working alliance). What follows is a discussion of pertinent specific and common factors and the reasons they may have influenced the intervention effectiveness.

Specific Factors

One potential explanation for psychological intervention success is likely to be attributable to the targeted nature of the intended outcomes. Most of the interventions have focused on stress management, and since both stress and subsequent stress responses are one of the key mechanisms for increased risk of injury, they likely result in successful outcomes. Many of the psychological interventions used in the research can down-regulate amygdala activation (Cozolino, 2010), a psychophysiological process that is associated with the ability to decrease the magnitude of stress response, and thus decrease the risk of injury.

Another explanation of success for some of the psychological interventions is the potential changes to attentional focus. It has been suggested that stress management and mindfulness practice are related to functional changes in the brain's attention systems (Hölzel et al., 2011), and that these changes can lead to increased attentional capacity to relevant cues in the environment (Cozolino, 2010). Since previous research has found peripheral vision narrowing to be a sport injury predictor (e.g., Rogers & Landers, 2005), increased attentional capacity might decrease injury risk by affording the athlete an opportunity to pay better attention toward important information (Clacy et al., 2013).

Common Factors

While research has used intervention strategies that have roots in different psychophysiological mechanisms (e.g., cognitive behavioral and mindfulness/acceptance-based approaches), the results have consistently demonstrated that psychosocial interventions are beneficial for reducing injury risk. In addition to the psychophysiological mechanism–based explanations earlier, it is likely that more common factors can explain the similarity in results across different intervention studies (Mulder et al., 2017; Wampold, 2015). One common factor that has gained attention in the literature is the quality of the professional relationship between the practitioner and the athlete. Research has found that having a high-quality, non-judgmental relationship in which the athlete feels comfortable is more likely to result in successful intervention outcomes when compared to professional relationship of lower quality (Andersen & Ivarsson, 2016).

Conclusion

Existing theoretical conceptualizations and empirical evidence suggest that biological, psychological, and social factors contribute to sport injury risk. Of the psychosocial factors, stress and stress response appear to have the strongest relationship with injury occurrence. Several mechanisms can provide a potential explanation for the stress–injury risk relationship. It is likely that physiological (e.g., stress hormone perturbation), cognitive (e.g., narrowed peripheral view, poorer decision-making), and behavioral (e.g., impaired self-care) stress responses predispose an athlete to stressful situations where they may not be able to successfully cope with stressors. Existing psychological intervention research has found a reduction in injury rates for the intervention group, suggesting benefits of integrating stress management strategies to sport injury prevention efforts.

Case Study

Katja is a talented 21-year-old basketball player playing for one of the best teams in Scandinavia. She aspires to play at an international level, hopefully professionally overseas. Over the past couple of weeks, Katja has experienced a generalized low mood, tiredness, and lack of motivation to train and compete. Some of it can be explained through increased physical training load over the past month, as the team prepares for a prestigious regional basketball tournament. Another reason for Katja's general lowness is stressors at home – her close relative has recently been hospitalized for a life-threatening illness. This has affected Katja – her thoughts are constantly spinning around and are filled with worries, such as "Will my close relative really get well again?" and "I want to be near the hospital if it gets really bad."

On the day of the tournament, Katja wakes up tired and finds herself unable to focus on the upcoming game. "I know this is unlike me, but I don't want to play today. I don't feel 'balanced' at the moment," Katja says to herself when driving to the tournament location. Since she is the star player on the team, she quickly brushes these thoughts out of her mind. "I cannot think about this. I know everyone, including my coaches, the spectators, and the media, is expecting me to play my 'A game' and lead the team to victory. I don't want to disappoint my teammates. I know they would understand if I told them what is going on, but I can't bear to let them down." As Katja walks to the locker room, she is aware of her inner voice talking to her: "You shouldn't play this game; you should first take care of yourself and your loved ones."

About 5 minutes into the game, in a moment of poor concentration, while dribbling, Katja trips and badly sprains her non-dominant ankle. The team sports medicine professional evaluates Katja's ankle and, after imaging, diagnoses her with a grade III lateral ankle sprain and ruptured ligaments.

Questions

1. Based on the case description, what psychosocial factors may have increased Katja's risk of sport injury?
2. What theory discussed in this chapter best explains Katja's case, and why?
3. If you had an opportunity to provide Katja some suggestions on how to reduce her risk of sport injury, what would you say? What evidence supports your suggestions?
4. To ensure successful recovery and return to participation, what critical success factors would you need to consider when treating Katja (within your future or current professional role)?

References

Åman, M., Forsblad, M., & Henriksson-Larsén, K. (2016). Incidence and severity of reported acute sports injuries in 35 sports using insurance registry data. *Scandinavian Journal of Medicine & Science in Sports*, *26*(4), 451–462. https://doi.org/10.1111/sms.12462

American Psychological Association. (2022). *APA dictionary of psychology*. https://dictionary.apa.org/

Andersen, M. B., & Ivarsson, A. (2016). A methodology of loving kindness: How interpersonal neurobiology, compassion, and transference can inform researcher-participant encounters and storytelling. *Qualitative Research in Sport, Exercise and Health*, *8*(1), 1–20. https://doi.org/10.1080/21596 76X.2015.1056827

Andersen, M. B., & Williams, J. M. (1988). A model of stress and athletic injury: Prediction and prevention. *Journal of Sport & Exercise Psychology*, *10*(3), 294–306. https://doi.org/10.1123/jsep.10.3.294

Andersen, M. B., & Williams, J. M. (1999). Athletic injury, psychosocial factors, and perceptual changes during stress. *Journal of Sports Sciences*, *17*(9), 735–741. https://doi.org/10.1080/026404199365597

Appaneal, R. N., & Habif, S. (2013). Psychological antecedents to sport injury. In M. Arvinen-Barrow & N. Walker (Eds.), *The psychology of sport injury and rehabilitation* (pp. 6–22). Routledge.

Appaneal, R. N., & Perna, F. M. (2014). Biopsychosocial model of injury. In R. C. Eklund & G. Tenen-baum (Eds.), *Encyclopedia of Sport and Exercise Psychology* (pp. 74–77). Sage Publishing. https://doi.org/10.4135/9781483332222.n30

Arnold, R., & Fletcher, D. (2012). A research synthesis and taxonomic classification of the organizational stressors encountered by sport performers. *Journal of Sport & Exercise Psychology, 34*(3), 397–429. https://doi.org/10.1123/jsep.34.3.397

Bahr, R. (2016). Why screening test to predict injury do not work – and probably never will. . .: A critical review. *British Journal of Sports Medicine, 50*(13), 776–780. https://doi.org/10.1136/bjsports-2016-096256

Bittencourt, N. F. N., Meeuwisse, W. H., Mendonca, L. D., Nettel-Aguirre, A., Ocarino, J. M., & Fonseca, S. T. (2016). Complex systems approach for sports injuries: Moving from risk factor identification to injury pattern recognition – narrative review and new concept. *British Journal of Sports Medicine, 50*(21), 1309–1314. https://doi.org/10.1136/bjsports-2015-095850

Cassel, J. C. (1976). The contribution of the social environment to host resistance. *American Journal of Epidemiology, 104*(2), 107–123. https://doi.org/10.1093/oxfordjournals.aje.a112281

Clacy, A. L., Sharman, R., & Lovell, G. P. (2013). Risk factors to sport-related concussion for junior athletes. *OA Sports Medicine, 1*(1), 4. https://doi.org/10.13172/2053-2040-1-1-566

Cobb, S. (1976). Social support as a moderator of life stress. *Psychosomatic Medicine, 38*(5), 300–314. https://doi.org/10.1097/00006842-197609000-00003

Cozolino, L. (2010). *The neuroscience of psychotherapy: Healing the social brain* (2nd ed.). Norton.

Fawkner, H. J., McMurray, N. E., & Summers, J. (1999). Athletic injury and minor life events: A prospective study. *Journal of Science and Medicine in Sport, 2*, 117–124. https://doi.org/10.1016/s1440-2440(99)80191-1

Folkman, S., & Lazarus, R. S. (1985). If it changes it must be a process: Study of emotion and coping during three stages of a college examination. *Journal of Personality and Social Psychology, 48*(1), 150–170. https://doi.org/10.1037/0022-3514.48.1.150

Gardner, F. L., & Moore, Z. E. (2007). *The psychology of enhancing human performance: The mindfulness-acceptance-commitment (MAC) approach*. Springer Publishing Co.

Gledhill, A., Forsdyke, D., & Murray, E. (2018). Psychological interventions used to reduce sports injuries: A systematic review of real-world effectiveness. *British Journal of Sports Medicine, 52*(15), 967–971. https://doi.org/10.1136/bjsports-2017-097694

Hanson, S. J., McCullagh, P., & Tonymon, P. (1992). The relationship of personality characteristics, life stress, and coping resources to athletic injury. *Journal of Sport & Exercise Psychology, 14*(3), 262–272. https://doi.org/10.1123/jsep.14.3.262

Hardy, C. J., & Riehl, R. E. (1988). An examination of the life stress-injury relationship among noncontact sport participants. *Behavioral Medicine, 14*(3), 113–118. https://doi.org/10.1080/08964289.1988.9935132

Hölzel, B. K., Lazar, S. W., Gard, T., Schumen-Oliver, Z., Vago, D. R., & Ott, U. (2011). How does mindfulness meditation work? Proposing mechanisms of action from a conceptual and neural perspective. *Perspectives on Psychological Science, 6*(6), 537–559. https://doi.org/10.1177/1745691611419671

Ivarsson, A., & Johnson, U. (2010). Psychological factors as predictors of injuries among senior soccer players: A prospective study. *Journal of Sports Science & Medicine, 9*(2), 347–352.

Ivarsson, A., Johnson, U., Andersen, M. B., Fallby, J., & Altem, M. (2015). It pays to pay attention: A mindfulness-based program for injury prevention with soccer players. *Journal of Applied Sport Psychology, 27*(3), 319–334. https://doi.org/10.1080/10413200.2015.1008072

Ivarsson, A., Johnson, U., Andersen, M. B., Tranaeus, U., Stenling, A., & Lindwall, M. (2017). Psychosocial factors and sport injuries: Meta-analyses for prediction and prevention *Sports Medicine, 47*(2), 353–365. https://doi.org/10.1007/s40279-016-0578-x

Ivarsson, A., Johnson, U., Lindwall, M., Gustafsson, H., & Altemyr, M. (2014). Psychosocial stress as a predictor of injury in elite junior soccer: A latent growth curve analysis *Journal of Science and Medicine in Sport, 17*(4), 366–370. https://doi.org/10.1016/j.jsams.2013.10.242

Johnson, U., Ekengren, J., & Andersen, M. B. (2005). Injury prevention in Sweden: Helping soccer players at risk. *Journal of Sport & Exercise Psychology, 27*(1), 32–38. https://doi.org/10.1123/jsep.27.1.32

Johnson, U., & Ivarsson, A. (2011). Psychological predictors of sport injuries among junior soccer players. *Scandanavian Journal of Medicine & Science in Sports, 21*(1), 129–136. https://doi.org/10.1111/j.1600-0838.2009.01057.x

Johnston, R., Cahalan, R., Bonnett, L., Maguire, M., Glasgow, P., Madigan, S., . . . Comyns, T. (2020). General health complaints and sleep associated with new injury within an endurance sporting population: A prospective study. *Journal of Science and Medicine in Sport, 23*(3), 252–257. https://doi.org/10.1016/j.jsams.2019.10.013

Kerr, G. A., & Goss, J. (1996). The effects of a stress management program on injuries and stress levels. *Journal of Applied Sport Psychology, 8*(1), 109–117. https://doi.org/10.1080/10413209608406312

Maddison, R., & Prapavessis, H. (2005). A psychological approach to the prediction and prevention of athletic injury. *Journal of Sport & Exercise Psychology, 27*(3), 289–310. https://doi.org/10.1123/jsep.27.3.289

McDonald, A. A., Wilkerson, G. B., McDermott, B. P., & Bonacci, J. A. (2019). Risk factors for initial and subsequent core or lower extremity sprain or strain among collegiate football players. *Journal of Athletic Training, 54*(5), 489–496. https://doi.org/10.4085/1062-6050-152-17

Mulder, R., Murray, G., & Rucklidge, J. (2017). Common versus specific factors in psychotherapy: Opening the black box. *Lancet Psychiatry, 4*(12), 953–962. https://doi.org/10.1016/S2215-0366(17)30100-1

Noh, Y.-E., Morris, T., & Andersen, M. B. (2005). Psychosocial factors and ballet injuries. *International Journal of Sport & Exercise Psychology, 3*(1), 79–90. https://doi.org/10.1080/1612197X.2005.9671759

Olmedilla-Zafra, A., Rubio, V. J., Ortega, E., & García-Mas, A. (2017). Effectiveness of a stress management pilot program aimed at reducing the incidence of sports injuries in young football (soccer) players. *Physical Therapy in Sport, 24*(2), 53–59. https://doi.org/10.1016/j.ptsp.2016.09.0031466-853X/

Palmer, D., Engebretsen, L., Carrard, J., Grek, N., Königstein, K., Maurer, D. J., . . . Soligard, T. (2021). Sports injuries and illnesses at the Lausanne 2020 Youth Olympic Winter games: A prospective study of 1783 athletes from 79 countries. *British Journal of Sports Medicine, 55*(17), 968–974. https://doi.org/10.1136/bjsports-2020-103514

Patterson, E., Smith, R., & Everett, J. (1998). Psychosocial factors as predictors of ballet injuries: Interactive effects of life stress and social support. *Journal of Sport Behavior, 21*, 101–112.

Podlog, L., Heil, J., & Schulte, S. (2014). Psychosocial factors in sports injury rehabilitation and return to play. *Physical Medicine and Rehabilitation Clinics, 25*(4), 915–930. https://doi.org/10.1016/j.pmr.2014.06.011

Richardson, S. O., Andersen, M. B., & Morris, T. (2008). *Overtraining athletes: Personal journeys in sport.* Human Kinetics.

Rogers, T. J., & Landers, D. M. (2005). Mediating effects of peripheral vision in the life event stress/athletic injury relationship. *Journal of Sport & Exercise Psychology, 27*(3), 271–288. https://doi.org/10.1123/jsep.27.3.271

Shrier, I., & Hallé, M. (2011). Psychological predictors of injuries in circus artists: An exploratory study. *British Journal of Sports Medicine, 45*(5), 433–436. https://doi.org/10.1136/bjsm.2009.067751

Smith, A. M., Stuart, M. J., & Wiese-Bjornstal, D. M. (1997). Predictors of injury in ice hockey players. *American Journal of Sports Medicine, 25*(4), 500–507. https://doi.org/10.1177/036354659702500413

Steffen, K., Pensgaard, A. M., & Bahr, R. (2009). Self-reported psychological characteristics as risk factors for injuries in female youth football. *Scandinavian Journal of Medicine & Science in Sports, 19*(3), 442–451. https://doi.org/10.1111/j.1600-0838.2008.00797.x

Tranaeus, U., Martin, S., & Ivarsson, A. (2022). Psychosocial risk factors for overuse injuries in competitive athletes: A mixed-studies systematic review. *Sports Medicine, 52*, 773–788. https://doi.org/10.1007/s40279-021-01597-5

Van der Does, H. T. D., Brink, M. S., Otter, R. T., Visscher, C., & Lemmink, K. A. P. M. (2017). Injury risk is increased by changes in perceived recovery of team sport players. *Clinical Journal of Sport Medicine, 27*(1), 46–51. https://doi.org/10.1097/JSM.0000000000000306

Von Rosen, P., Frohm, A., Kottorp, A., Fridén, C., & Heijne, A. (2017). Too little sleep and an unhealthy diet could increase the risk of sustaining a new injury in adolescent elite athletes. *Scandinavian Journal of Medicine & Science in Sports*, *27*(11), 1364–1371. https://doi.org/10.1111/sms.12735

Wadey, R., Evans, L., Hanton, S., & Neil, R. (2012). An examination of hardiness throughout the sport injury process. *British Journal of Health Psychology*, *17*(1), 103–128. https://doi.org/10.1111/j.2044-8287.2011.02025.x

Wadey, R., Evans, L., Hanton, S., & Neil, R. (2013). Effect of dispositional optimism before and after injury. *Medicine and Science in Sports and Exercise*, *45*(2), 387–394. https://doi.org/10.1249/mss.0b013e31826ea8e3

Wampold, B. E. (2015). How important are the common factors in psychotherapy? An update. *World Psychiatry*, *14*(3), 270–277. https://doi.org/10.1002/wps.20238

Wiese-Bjornstal, D. M. (2009). Sport injury and college athlete health across the lifespan. *Journal of Intercollegiate Sport*, *2*(1), 64–80. https://doi.org/10.1123/jis.2.1.64

Wiese-Bjornstal, D. M. (2010). Psychology and socioculture affect injury risk, response, and recovery in high-intensity athletes: A consensus statement. *Scandinavian Journal of Medicine & Science in Sports*, *20*, 103–111. https://doi.org/10.1111/j.1600-0838.2010.01195.x

Williams, J. M., & Andersen, M. B. (1998). Psychosocial antecedents of sport injury: Review and critique of the stress and injury model. *Journal of Applied Sport Psychology*, *10*(1), 5–25. https://doi.org/10.1080/10413209808406375

Yang, J., Cheng, G., Zhang, Y., Covassin, T., Heiden, E. O., & Peek-Asa, C. (2014). Influence of symptoms of depression and anxiety on injury hazard among collegiate American football players. *Research in Sports Medicine*, *22*(2), 147–160. https://doi.org/10.1080/15438627.2014.881818

Zadeh, M. M., Ajilchi, B., Salman, Z., & Kisely, S. (2019). Effect of a mindfulness programme training to prevent the sport injury and improve the performance of semi-professional soccer players. *Australasian Psychiatry*, *27*(6), 589–595. https://doi.org/10.1177/1039856219859288

3 Biopsychosocial Understanding of Sport Injury

Monna Arvinen-Barrow, Natalie C. Walker, and Caroline Heaney

Chapter Objectives

- To outline existing theoretical models explaining biopsychosocial responses to sport injury.
- To summarize the most common psychosocial responses to sport injury.
- To explain how psychological and social factors influence sport injury experience and recovery outcomes.

Introduction

Anyone who has ever experienced a sport injury – be it from the perspective of the athlete with injuries, parents, significant other, sport coach, sports medicine professional (SMP), or sport administrators – should be aware that the injury will have biological, psychological, and social consequences to the athlete and the various sociocultural systems in which they operate. Consideration of the biopsychosocial and sociocultural consequences of sport injury is imperative, as they can impact an athlete's reactions to the injury, rehabilitation, intermediate and overall rehabilitation outcomes, and the subsequent return to participation and/or transition out of sport (Brewer & Redmond, 2017; Kamphoff et al., 2013; Stambulova et al., 2007). The purpose of this chapter is to provide an overview of biopsychosocial responses to sport injury. More specifically, this chapter will (a) outline existing theoretical models that have been developed to explain the interaction between biological, psychological, and social responses to sport injury, and (b) introduce some of the most common biopsychosocial responses to injury. In doing so, the chapter makes a compelling case for the importance of understanding how psychological and social factors influence sport injury experience and recovery outcomes to support holistic recovery.

Theoretical Models for Psychosocial Responses to Sport Injury

Prompted by the research supporting the role of psychosocial factors in sport injury risk (see Andersen & Williams, 1999) and the development of the stress and injury model (Andersen & Williams, 1988), an increased curiosity to understand the role of psychological factors affecting post-injury responses has grown among sport psychology researchers (see Chapter 2 for more details). Herein, a brief summary of the historical development of theoretical models aiming to explain psychological responses to sport injury is presented. This is followed by a more detailed

DOI: 10.4324/9781003295709-4

outline of two of the most comprehensive models to date: the integrated model of psychological response to the sport injury and rehabilitation process (Wiese-Bjornstal et al., 1998) and the biopsychosocial model of sport injury rehabilitation (Brewer et al., 2002).

Historical Development of Psychological Response to Sport Injury

In the absence of scientific data, early theoretical conceptualizations of psychological responses to injury borrowed heavily from other psychology domains – namely, literature on responses to grief and stress (Brewer & Redmond, 2017). Models based on grief literature have typically adapted stage-based grief response models (e.g., Kübler-Ross, 1969) to sport injury and are founded on two main assumptions. First, when an athlete experiences a sport injury, they will perceive it as a loss of self (Brewer & Redmond, 2017). Second, to successfully navigate the perceived loss of self, the athlete with injury will move through sequential stages (Brewer & Redmond, 2017), which, in Kübler-Ross's (1969) model, are denial, bargaining, anger, depression, and acceptance (Brewer & Redmond, 2017).

While initially intuitively appealing, grief response models have since received criticism in sport injury psychology literature. First, strong evidence exists in support of injury responses being individual in nature, and not always is injury perceived as a loss (see Brewer, 2017), thus challenging the first assumption of the grief response models. Second, evidence also challenges the "stereotypic, invariant, sequence of reactions" (Brewer & Redmond, 2017, p. 61), therefore failing to account for inevitable oscillation between the different stages (Evans & Hardy, 1995). The word *denial* has also been questioned as potentially not being appropriate for all athletes with injuries. Walker et al. (2007) proposed that it should be reserved for athletes who are non-compliant during rehabilitation and who, despite education about their injury, refuse to accept its existence. In support, research has found athletes tend to downplay the severity of the injury and the limitations it can bring rather than outright denying its existence (Pearson & Jones, 1992).

To address the inherent assumed uniformity of athletes' psychological responses to injury in the grief response models, cognitive appraisal models were proposed as an alternative to account for individual differences (Brewer, 1994; Brewer & Redmond, 2017; Evans & Hardy, 1995; Walker et al., 2007). Grounded in the literature on stress and coping (Lazarus & Folkman,

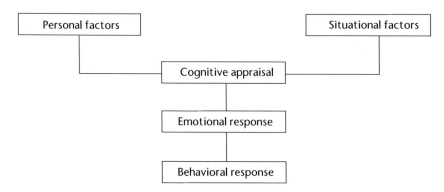

Figure 3.1 A typical cognitive appraisal model of psychological adjustment to athletic injury.

Source: Reprinted from Review and critique of models of psychological adjustment to athletic injury, Britton W. Brewer, *Journal of Applied Sport Psychology*. Copyright ©1994 Association for Applied Sport Psychology, reprinted by permission of Informa UK Limited, trading as Taylor & Francis Group, www. Tandfonline.com on behalf of Association for Applied Sport Psychology.

1984), the cognitive appraisal models posit that athletes' emotional and behavioral responses to their injury are a consequence of their cognitive appraisal or subjective interpretation of the injury. Influenced by a number of personal and situational factors, these cognitive appraisals are typically focused on the injury and its consequences and/or the athlete's ability to cope with it (Brewer, 1994; Evans & Hardy, 1995; Kolt, 2003).

The Integrated Model of Psychological Response to the Sport Injury and Rehabilitation Process

Given the increasing empirical evidence in support of both pre-injury (Andersen & Williams, 1988) and post-injury (Brewer, 1994; Evans & Hardy, 1995) models, Wiese-Bjornstal et al. (1998) proposed a model that is "marked by inherent flexibility and inclusiveness that allow the model to consider a multitude of possible predictors of psychological adjustment" (Brewer & Redmond, 2017, p. 62). The integrated model of psychological response to the sport injury and rehabilitation process (from now on referred to as the integrated model; Wiese-Bjornstal et al., 1998) proposes that grief response and cognitive appraisal models are not mutually exclusive. The model posits that the core assumption of the grief response (i.e., a sense of loss) does not happen in isolation but is an outcome of a primary cognitive appraisal. The integrated model also recognizes that a sense of loss can also lead to a myriad of emotional and behavioral responses commonly associated with grief (e.g., depression, anger, bargaining). In other words, the integrated model also provides support to the key constructs (but not the stage-like sequencing) of the stage models and the cognitive-affective-behavioral sequence of the cognitive appraisal models (Brewer, 1994).

At the core of the integrated model is a bidirectional cyclical relationship between cognitive appraisals and emotional and behavioral responses, representing the dynamic and changing nature of the psychological responses to the rehabilitation process and recovery outcomes. Known as the "dynamic core," this interaction between thoughts, emotions, and behaviors is also said to influence both physical (e.g., increased range of motion) and psychosocial (e.g., increased confidence) recovery outcomes. The clockwise arrows, representing the *more dominant* direction, indicate that cognitive appraisals (e.g., pain perceptions) affect emotional responses (e.g., fear of movement), which, in turn, affect behavior (e.g., reduced rehabilitation adherence) and subsequent recovery outcomes. The anti-clockwise arrows, which represent the *less dominant* direction, indicate that at times the reverse can occur and that multiple directional changes are also possible during rehabilitation (Brewer, 1994; Wiese-Bjornstal et al., 1998). To illustrate, cognitive appraisals (e.g., pain perceptions) affect behaviors (e.g., hesitancy in rehabilitation), which affect subsequent emotional responses (e.g., frustration) and new cognitive appraisals (e.g., slow rate of perceived recovery). The dynamic core should be viewed as a three-dimensional spiral that heads in an upward direction toward successful recovery or in a downward direction toward unsuccessful injury rehabilitation and recovery (Wiese-Bjornstal et al., 1998). It is also important to note that the physical and psychosocial recovery outcomes do not always happen simultaneously (Burland et al., 2019).

Consistent with the stress and athletic injury model (Andersen & Williams, 1988), the dynamic core is also influenced by a number of pre-injury factors (i.e., personality, history of stressors, coping resources, and interventions) that may have contributed to the sport injury occurrence. The model also assumes that once one is injured, the injury itself becomes a stressor, resulting in cognitive appraisals related to the demands and consequences of injury and resources available to cope with the said demands and consequences. The model also posits that many personal and situational factors will influence cognitive appraisals. Personal factors include injury-related

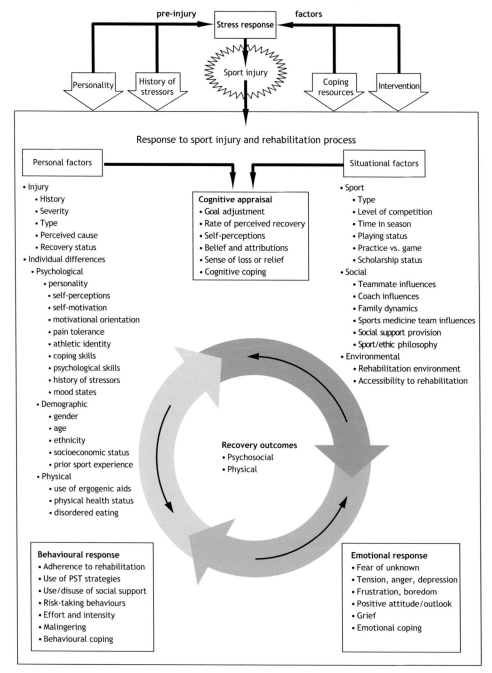

Figure 3.2 The integrated model of psychological response to the sport injury and rehabilitation process.

Source: Printed with permission from An integrated model of response to sport injury: Psychological and sociological dynamics, Diane M. Wiese-Bjornstal, Aynsley M. Smith, Shelly M. Shaffer, & Michael A, Morrey, *Journal of Applied Sport Psychology*. Copyright ©1998 Association for Applied Sport Psychology, reprinted by permission of Informa UK Limited, trading as Taylor & Francis Group, www.tandfonline.com on behalf of 1998 Association for Applied Sport Psychology.

factors and individual psychological, demographic, and physical differences. Situational factors include sport, social, and environmental factors (Wiese-Bjornstal et al., 1998).

Initially, the integrated model was developed to visually conceptualize existing research to help identify apparent knowledge gaps and guide future research designs. Since its original conceptualization, the integrated model has also been modified to explain psychology of concussion injury (Wiese-Bjornstal et al., 2015) and the role of religiosity in sport injury and the rehabilitation process (Wiese-Bjornstal, 2019a, 2019b). To date, the integrated model is regarded as the most comprehensive theoretical model explaining the psychosocial process of response to sport injury (Anderson et al., 2004; Brewer & Redmond, 2017; Kolt, 2003; Walker et al., 2007) and has been extensively used by researchers and practitioners (Wiese-Bjornstal, 2010).

The Biopsychosocial Model of Sport Injury Rehabilitation

One of the main critiques of the integrated model is its lack of explanation on *how* psychological factors influence, and are influenced by, the biological injury characteristics and the physical sport injury rehabilitation and recovery outcomes (Brewer, 2001; Brewer et al., 2002). To address this gap, Brewer et al. (2002) proposed the biopsychosocial model of sport injury rehabilitation (from now on referred to as the biopsychosocial model). The aim of the biopsychosocial model was to bridge the gap between the medical and psychological approaches to sport injury, to broaden the scope of research, and to augment, rather than replace, the existing models (Brewer et al.,

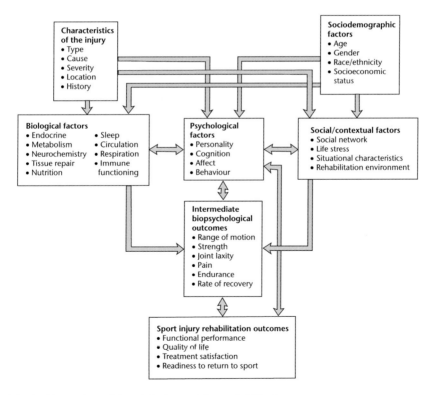

Figure 3.3 The biopsychosocial model of sport injury rehabilitation.

Source: Used with permission of Fitness Information Technology Inc., from *Medical and Psychological Aspects of Sport and Exercise*, D. L. Mostofsky and L. D. Zaichowsky (eds), by Britton W. Brewer (2002); permission conveyed through Copyright Clearance Center, Inc.

2002). The model acknowledges that sport injury recovery is a complex and dynamic matrix of biological, psychological, and social factors (Andersen, 2007) and, as such, offers a broad-based framework for understanding biopsychosocial responses to sport injury (Brewer, 2001).

Influenced by characteristics of the injury (e.g., type, cause, severity) and various sociodemographic factors (e.g., age, gender, race/ethnicity), at the core of the model is a bidirectional interaction between biological, psychological, and social/contextual factors. These factors are also conceptualized as having a direct effect on the intermediate biopsychological outcomes (e.g., perception of pain, range of motion, and rate of recovery), which in turn has a bidirectional relationship with sport injury rehabilitation outcomes (e.g., functional performance, readiness to return to participation). The model also highlights the bidirectional reciprocal relationship between psychological factors (i.e., personality, cognition, affect, and behavior), intermediate biopsychological outcomes, and sport injury rehabilitation outcomes (Brewer et al., 2002). Whilst the biopsychosocial model does not explicitly outline the cyclical relationship between cognitions, emotions, and behaviors as the integrated model, it does include a novel connection between the psychological and biological factors of injury by outlining the bidirectional relationship between the intermediate rehabilitation outcomes and psychological factors (Arvinen-Barrow & Granquist, 2020).

Biopsychosocial Responses to Injury

Research has identified numerous biological, psychological, and social factors as influencing sport injury risk and response to sport injury, rehabilitation, and return to participation. Given the overlap between the integrated model (Wiese-Bjornstal et al., 1998) and the biopsychosocial model (Brewer et al., 2002), this section will present a brief synthesis of current evidence of how pertinent biological, psychological, and social factors influence sport injury experience and recovery outcomes. This synthesis of research is not exhaustive but focuses on highlighting the importance of understanding the role of biopsychosocial factors in rehabilitation and return-to-participation process. By doing so, this section also emphasizes the usefulness of theoretical models when designing, implementing, and evaluating holistic injury rehabilitation protocols (Arvinen-Barrow & Granquist, 2020).

Psychological Factors

Both the integrated model (Wiese-Bjornstal et al., 1998) and the biopsychosocial model (Brewer et al., 2002) recognize the role of psychological factors as central to the sport injury, rehabilitation, and return to participation experience and outcomes. In the integrated model, a bidirectional cyclical process between cognitive appraisals and emotional and behavioral responses is proposed to influence recovery outcomes. This dynamic core is proposed to be influenced by personality (both pre-injury and post-injury person factor), among other factors. In the biopsychosocial model, these four psychological factors (cognition, affect, behavior, and personality) are proposed as a bidirectional conduit between biological and social-contextual factors.

Cognition/Cognitive Appraisal

Typically defined as a process by which potentially stressful events are evaluated for meaning and significance to individual well-being (Lazarus & Folkman, 1984), the central role of cognitive appraisal in sport injury has been well documented in the literature (Brewer & Redmond, 2017). In addition to cognitive appraisals, Brewer and Redmond (2017) stated that a number of other cognitive processes and factors are also relevant to an athlete's response to sport injury. These include self-related cognitions (e.g., Sparkes, 1998), attributions for injury (e.g., Osborne, 2017), cognitive content (e.g., Vergeer, 2006), cognitive coping strategies (e.g., Ruddock-Hudson et al., 2014), perceived benefits of injury (e.g., Wadey et al., 2016), injury-related perceptions (e.g., Clement et al., 2015), and cognitive performance (e.g., Taylor-Postma et al., 2022).

One of the dominant cognitive effects of injury are changes in athlete's self-perception (Brewer et al., 2002; Lattimore, 2017). Changes in athlete's self-esteem (Leddy et al., 1994), self-efficacy and/or self-confidence (Thomeé et al., 2007), and athletic identity (Brewer et al., 1993) have been reported by athletes with injuries. These findings are not surprising, as sport typically serves as a source of self-worth and self-definition for many athletes (Brewer & Redmond, 2017). Injury, by default, poses a threat to sport involvement, consequentially affecting thoughts about the self. Research has also found that in comparison to non-injured athletes, athletes with injuries tend to have lower global self-esteem that decreases following injury (e.g., Leddy et al., 1994). Athletes have also reported high levels of confidence at the start of rehabilitation that have declined during rehabilitation and then increased again as the injury recovery progressed (Brewer & Redmond, 2017). Self-identity can also change considerably during rehabilitation, with a decline in athletic identity typically occurring over the course of rehabilitation for those individuals requiring surgical procedures (Brewer et al., 2010).

Affect/Emotional Response

Defined as a "psychophysiological response to a particular intrapsychic feeling(s) that may or may not be outwardly manifested but that trigger an action or behavioral response" (Arvinen-Barrow & Granquist, 2020, p. 98), *emotional responses* to sport injuries have received the most research attention to date (Brewer & Redmond, 2017). There is a direct link between the psychological and biological aspects of injury, as existing research has "demonstrated that emotions can affect the injury process on a cellular level; unpleasant emotions are known to suppress our immune system, while pleasant emotions strengthen it" (e.g., Davidson et al., 2003; cited in Arvinen-Barrow & Clement, 2022, p. 201).

Depending on the initial cognitive appraisals of injury (Brewer & Redmond, 2017), most of the early emotional responses are unpleasant and have a negative valence. The most common affective response to injury is stress (Brewer & Petrie, 1995), and some of the typical emotional responses include anger, anxiety, apprehension, bitterness, confusion, depression, disappointment, dispiritedness, devastation, fear, frustration, helplessness, relief, resentment, and shock (Arvinen-Barrow & Granquist, 2020; Arvinen-Barrow et al., 2014; Brewer & Redmond, 2017; Madrigal & Gill, 2014). Emotional responses to injury are generally most salient immediately post-injury and tend to become less-intense over time (Brewer, 2017). During the reaction-to-rehabilitation phase (Kamphoff et al., 2013), fluctuation between emotions with positive valence (e.g., enthusiasm, excitement) and negative valence (e.g., depression, frustration, sadness) is common (Arvinen-Barrow & Clement, 2022; Arvinen-Barrow & Granquist, 2020; Clement & Arvinen-Barrow, 2020; Clement et al., 2015). Emotional responses are also likely to intensify as return to participation approaches (Brewer, 2017) and include a myriad of affective states, such as re-injury anxiety (Clement et al., 2015; Grindstaff et al., 2010; Walker & Thatcher, 2011; Walker et al., 2010), fear of re-injury (Rodriguez et al., 2019), frustration, nervousness, and excitement (Clement et al., 2015). While most emotional responses to injuries are likely to be sub-clinical in nature, it is important to recognize that instances of clinically meaningful levels of psychological distress have also been documented among athletes with injuries (Brewer et al., 1995) and thus warranting mental health referral (see Chapter 10). Equally, not all emotional responses to injury are negative. Some athletes with injuries perceive the time away from sport as a relief (Wadey et al., 2011). Being injured can also be an opportunity for (a) change and growth (Howells et al.,

2017; Lattimore, 2017), (b) learning more about the sport (Wadey et al., 2011), and (c) developing self-identity, resilience, and social relationships beyond sport (Wadey et al., 2019).

Behavior/Behavioral Response

According to Arvinen-Barrow and Granquist (2020), in the context of sport injury, *behavioral responses* can be defined as "actions an athletic patient displays during reactions to injury, rehabilitation, and return to participation phases that can either facilitate hinder successful healing and recovery" (p. 99). Such behaviors can be broadly divided into several categories: (a) treatment adherence; (b) use of ergonomic aides; (c) use of psychosocial strategies, including social support; (d) facilitative functional behaviors (e.g., sleep, nutrition, hydration); (e) risk-taking behaviors (e.g., substance abuse); and (f) behavioral coping (e.g., social support use; Arvinen-Barrow & Granquist, 2020; Lattimore, 2017; Wiese-Bjornstal et al., 1998).

Of the behavioral responses, adherence to rehabilitation has garnered the most research attention (Brewer & Redmond, 2017; Granquist & Brewer, 2013). Defined as the "extent to which an individual completes behaviors as part of a treatment regimen designed to facilitate recovery from injury" (Granquist & Brewer, 2013, p. 42), *adherence* has been associated with successful rehabilitation outcomes (Brewer & Redmond, 2017; Goddard et al., 2021). In support, under-adherence (i.e., not engaging in the rehabilitation protocol, completing too few exercise repetitions, poor attendance at rehabilitation sessions) has been associated with poorer overall rehabilitation outcomes (e.g., functional ability, strength, range of motion) and increased risk of re-injury (Granquist & Brewer, 2013). More recently, over-adherence (i.e., failing to comply with restrictions, doing too much too quickly, displaying excessive efforts to push through pain) has received attention in the literature and has been associated with a risk of returning to sport prematurely (Arvinen-Barrow & Granquist, 2020; Podlog et al., 2013).

Personality

Defined as "the enduring configuration of characteristics and behavior that comprises an individual's unique adjustment to life" (American Psychological Association, 2022), *personality* is typically considered to be "a complex, dynamic integration or totality shaped by many forces" (American Psychological Association, 2022). The American Psychological Association (2022) definition also defines personality characteristics to include person's major traits, interests, drives, values, self-concept, abilities, and emotional patterns. It also defines the forces that shape personality to include hereditary and constitutional tendencies, physical maturation, early training, identification with significant individuals and groups, culturally conditioned values and roles, and critical experiences and relationships.

Both the integrated model (Wiese-Bjornstal et al., 1998) and the biopsychosocial model (Brewer et al., 2002) recognize the role of personality as an integral psychological factor influencing sport injury and rehabilitation. Much like personality has been found to influence injury risk and occurrence (see Chapter 2), personality characteristics (e.g., trait beliefs about stress) have also been found to influence cognitive appraisals (Mansell, 2021). Personality traits of conscientiousness and agreeableness have been found to be predictive of adherence to rehabilitation (Hilliard et al., 2014), and neuroticism has been positively correlated with emotional disturbance (Brewer, 2017). Likewise, causal attributions of stable and personally controllable factors, cognitive appraisals of injury coping ability, rehabilitation self-efficacy, and self-esteem have been positively associated with rehabilitation adherence behavior (Brewer et al., 2002). Athletic identity is probably the most notable personality factor associated with sport injury and rehabilitation process. Athletic identity has been found to influence athlete engagement with rehabilitation

(Podlog et al., 2013), over-adherence, and premature return to sport (Podlog et al., 2013). It has also been found to influence pain-related maladaptive behaviors, such as pushing through pain and avoiding pain reporting (Tasiemski & Brewer, 2011), and to be a predictor of emotional disturbance (Brewer, 2017), anxiety, and depressive symptoms (Giannone et al., 2017).

Social/Contextual/Situational Factors

Both the integrated model (Wiese-Bjornstal et al., 1998) and the biopsychosocial model (Brewer et al., 2002) recognize the role of numerous social, contextual, and situational factors as influential in sport injury and rehabilitation. In the integrated model, these include selected pre-injury factors (history of stressors, coping resources) and situational factors (e.g., SMPs) that unidirectionally influence cognitive appraisals, emotional and behavioral responses, and recovery outcomes. In the biopsychosocial model, the same factors are proposed to have a bidirectional relationship with psychological and biological factors and unidirectional relationship with intermediate biopsychosocial outcomes.

Sport Factors

Sport-related factors, including type, competitive level, time of season, playing and scholarship status, have been found to influence post-injury responses. For example, Grindstaff et al. (2010) have found that playing status, team support, and state-of-the-art facilities can influence an athlete's responses to injury. Similarly, sport-related situational characteristics, such as competitive level and financial status, have been found to influence transition out of sport due to injury (Arvinen-Barrow, DeGrave et al., 2019; Arvinen-Barrow, Hurley et al., 2017; Park et al., 2013; Stoltenburg et al., 2011).

Social Factors

Social networks, including teammates, coaches, family, and sports medicine professionals (SMPs), have been found to influence post-injury responses. Evidence on the integral role of social support in injury is strong, and lack of social support has been found to negatively influence the rehabilitation process and recovery outcomes (see chapter 18; or Arvinen-Barrow & Pack, 2013). Sport injury has also been found to be a potential catalyst for change in social relationships (Lattimore, 2017), and increased risk of over-adherence has been related to coach and teammate approval of such behavior (Podlog et al., 2013). Support for the relationships between sport, sociodemographic, psychological, and social factors have also been found in the literature. Evidence in support of sport type, gender, nationality, and previous experiences with the SMP or sport psychology professional (SPP) has been found to influence athlete attitudes and expectations (cognitive appraisals) toward the SMP or SPP (social factor; Arvinen-Barrow et al., 2012; Arvinen-Barrow, Clement, Hamson-Utley et al., 2016; Clement et al., 2012; Ildefonso et al., 2020; Martin et al., 2001; Potter et al., 2003).

Environmental Factors

The rehabilitation environment that the sports medicine team creates has also been found to influence sport injury, rehabilitation, and the return to participation process. For example, in a single performance management team (Hess & Meyer, 2022), the sociocultural context of the team (multi- vs. interprofessional professional practice model), the individual struggles faced by the team members, and the functioning of the team were found to be important contributors for both team members' lived experience and rehabilitation outcomes (Hess & Meyer, 2022; for more on interprofessional practice, see Chapter 7).

Support for the importance of rehabilitation environment in post-operative success after anterior cruciate ligament reconstruction (ACL-R) has also been found in the literature. In a retrospective analysis of 676 patients, the only factor to significantly influence return to sport after ACL-R was participation in an additional return-to-sport program (i.e., change in rehabilitation environment; Franck et al., 2021). A clinical review of factors influencing post-operative success also concluded that consideration of psychosocial factors in ACL-R rehabilitation protocols is imperative in creating a positive and successful rehabilitation environment (Burland et al., 2019).

Biological Factors

The biopsychosocial model recognizes the role of biological factors (i.e., endocrine, metabolism, neurochemistry, tissue repair, nutrition, sleep, circulation, respiration, immune functioning) as central to the sport injury rehabilitation process and recovery outcomes. Influenced by injury characteristics and sociodemographic factors, the biological factors interact with psychological and social/contextual factors and directly influence intermediate biopsychosocial outcomes (e.g., range of motion, strength, pain) and, indirectly, overall sport injury rehabilitation outcomes (e.g., quality of life, readiness to return to participation, treatment satisfaction). Notwithstanding the importance of all biological factors in sport injury rehabilitation, from the psychosocial perspective, sleep and nutrition are likely to be the most important biological factors to consider. Both sleep and nutrition can influence cognitions, affect, behaviors, and other injury healing-related biological functions.

Sleep

Sleep is a particularly significant biological factor through the injury rehabilitation and recovery process. In general, adults are reported to require seven to nine hours of sleep (Watson, 2017). While the amount of sleep required to achieve optimal health and quality of life tends to decrease from birth to older adulthood, this might not be true for adult athletes. Research with 11 division I collegiate varsity basketball players found several positive physical, psychological, and performance effects of sleep (Mah et al., 2011). Extending sleep from baseline to minimum of ten hours a night resulted in better overall physical and mental well-being during practices and games, faster reaction time, decreased daytime sleepiness, increased vigor and decreased fatigue, faster timed sprint performance, and better free throw and three-point-shooting accuracy (Mah et al., 2011).

The importance of sleep during rehabilitation is particularly important as it can influence intermediate biopsychosocial outcomes, such as inflammation, pain, and rate of healing (Huang & Ihm, 2021; Lentz et al., 1999; Mullington et al., 2010; Wininger, 2007). Subsequently, sleep also has an influence on sport injury rehabilitation outcomes (e.g., functional performance, perceived quality of life). More specifically, lack of sleep/poor quality of sleep during the early stages of healing has been found to stimulate chronic inflammation, which promotes ongoing tissue damage and thus negatively effects rate of healing (Motivala, 2011; Mullington et al., 2010). Lack of sleep can also negatively affect (Huang & Ihm, 2021) and reduce (Lentz et al., 1999) pain threshold. Suboptimal sleep has also been reported to have a negative effect on mood and affect, known to negatively affect pain perceptions (Huang & Ihm, 2021). Impaired sleep is also both a risk factor and a symptom of depression (Steiger & Pawlowski, 2019), a common emotional response to sport injury (Appaneal et al., 2009; Mainwaring et al., 2004; Myers et al., 2004).

Likewise, suboptimal sleep can affect cognitive processing and thus increase the risk of injury (Huang & Ihm, 2021) and/or re-injury.

Nutrition

Much like sleep, nutrition can also be beneficial for injury rehabilitation and recovery. According to Knappenberger (2018, July), "optimal nutrition can play a key role in controlling inflammation, providing key nutrients for rebuilding injured tissue, minimizing muscle atrophy and supporting strength preservation and gain" (p. 14). Research has highlighted the importance of maintaining energy balance during injury, including high protein intake (Tipton, 2015). There is some preliminary evidence of using omega-3 fatty acids and creatine to counter injury-induced muscle loss (Tipton, 2015), and certain micronutrients (e.g., calcium, vitamin D, iron, electrolytes, and vitamin C) have been recommended as beneficial for injury recovery (Knappenberger, 2018, July). Given that nutrition can also affect mood (Martins et al., 2021), its role in biopsychosocial sport injury rehabilitation and recovery cannot be understated. According to Tipton (2015), "the overriding nutritional recommendation for injured exercisers should be to consume a well-balanced diet based on whole, minimally processed foods or ingredients made from whole foods" (p. 93). The diet should be assessed and tailored to each individual athlete's needs and adjusted based on the progress of healing, phases of recovery, and any changes in activity patterns (Tipton, 2015).

Pertinent Factors Affecting the Biopsychosocial Responses to Injury

Both the integrated model (Wiese-Bjornstal et al., 1998) and the biopsychosocial model (Brewer et al., 2002) recognize various factors as also influencing the biopsychosocial responses and outcomes of sport injury. What follows here is a brief introduction to the most pertinent ones, namely, pre-injury factors, characteristics of injury, sociodemographic factors, and selected physical factors.

Pre-Injury Factors

Evidence in support of pre-injury factors affecting post-injury psychological responses (see Wiese-Bjornstal et al., 1998) is limited when compared to their influence of injury risk. What is known is that personality *traits* (i.e., stable, consistent aspects of personality), as outlined earlier in the personality section, can influence post-injury psychological responses (Brewer, 2017; Hilliard et al., 2014; Mansell, 2021; Tasiemski & Brewer, 2011). Negative life event stress has also been found to predict post-injury mood disturbances, which was positively related to cognitive appraisals (Albinson & Petrie, 2003). Other pre-injury factors, such as coping skills, social support, and use of psychosocial strategies, have also been found to be beneficial post-injury (for more details, see Chapters 12–18), thus suggesting transferability from pre- to post-injury.

Characteristics of Injury

Various injury characteristics have also been found to be influential in port-injury responses. Injury *history* has been found to affect rehabilitation self-efficacy (Grindstaff et al., 2010), and injury *severity* has been found to influence athletes; need for social support (Ruddock-Hudson et al., 2012). Severe injuries that require long-term recovery have been associated with negative, inconsistent, and challenging emotional responses, whereas athletes with less-severe injuries that require a shorter recovery time tend to be more positive and optimistic (Ruddock-Hudson et al., 2012). Perceived cause of the injury (i.e., attributions) has also been found to influence post-injury responses (Brewer & Redmond, 2017).

Sociodemographic Factors

Existing research has also found that all athletes, regardless of sociodemographic and other marginalized factors, will experience biopsychosocial responses to their injury, rehabilitation, and return to participation process. For example, effects of age on wound (Gerstein et al., 1993) and bone fracture (Clark et al., 2017) healing are well reported in the literature. Research has also found gender differences in psychological responses to recovery after ACL-R before returning to sport (Lisee et al., 2020), cultural/country differences in athletes' expectations of SMPs (Arvinen-Barrow et al., 2016; Clement et al., 2012), racial differences in recovery and subjective experiences following a sport-related concussion (Yengo-Kahn et al., 2021), and sociocultural differences in access to medical care (Dawkins et al., 2021).

Physical Factors

Other physical health factors, such as the use of ergonomic aids, overall physical health status, and the presence of disordered eating, have also been proposed to influence biopsychosocial responses to injuries, recovery, and return to participation (Wiese-Bjornstal et al., 1998). For example, experiencing an injury while coping with a permanent disability that inhibits function can provide further biopsychosocial barriers and disturbances to the rehabilitation process. Athletes with maladaptive eating and weight control behaviors and attitudes are also more likely to experience post-injury psychosocial disturbances (Brewer & Redmond, 2017), partially due to nutritional deficits that have been found to negatively impact biological aspects of healing (Tipton, 2015). In such instances, it is imperative for SMPs and SPPs to assess any needs for referral to holistic care within professional competencies (for more on assessment and referral, see Chapter 10).

The Effects of Biopsychosocial Responses to Rehabilitation and Recovery Outcomes

Existing research has found significant empirical support for the bidirectional interaction between cognitive appraisals and emotional and behavioral responses (Wiese-Bjornstal, 2010, 2014; Wiese-Bjornstal et al., 2020), as well as the dynamic, cyclical nature across different phases of rehabilitation (Clement & Arvinen-Barrow, 2020; Clement et al., 2015; Ruddock-Hudson et al., 2014). Likewise, the effects of the aforementioned on intermediate and overall physical and psychosocial recovery outcomes have been well documented in the literature. For example, research with SMPs has highlighted the importance of maintaining a positive attitude (cognitive appraisal), low stress, anxiety, and depression (emotional responses), and rehabilitation adherence/compliance (behavioral response) in successfully coping with rehabilitation (Arvinen-Barrow et al., 2007; Clement et al., 2013; Francis et al., 2000; Heaney, 2006; Hemmings & Povey, 2002; Larson et al., 1996). Maladaptive cognitive appraisals and affective processes associated with catastrophizing have been proposed as "exerting effects on the neuromuscular, cardiovascular, immune, and neuroendocrine systems, and on the activity in the pain neuromatrix within the brain" (Campbell & Edwards, 2009, p. 97). In support, emotional responses associated with stress (i.e., depression and anger) have been found to affect wound healing (Christian et al., 2006) and non-compliance with rehabilitation (DiMatteo et al., 2000), to name a few.

Conclusion

The aim of this chapter was to provide an overview of biopsychosocial responses to sport injury. Both models presented in this chapter have one thing in common – they help emphasize the importance of biopsychosocial factors in sport injury rehabilitation. The most frequently researched psychosocial responses to sport injuries include social support and rehabilitation adherence (Evans & Brewer, 2022). Given the biopsychosocial nature of post-injury responses, it is imperative for SMPs, SPPs, and other sport professionals to ensure a holistic approach to injury rehabilitation and the return to participation process (Hess et al., 2019). While research evidence is ever growing, there appears to be gaps in "application-readiness of several subareas of sport injury psychology research" (Evans & Brewer, 2022, p. 1011), particularly as it relates to intervention efficacy and effectiveness.

Case Study

Hallie (they/them) is a 33-year-old Welsh field hockey player who recently sustained an Achilles tendon injury. Hallie is in the twilight of their international career but has one unfulfilled ambition – to compete at the Commonwealth Games. Hallie missed out on selection for the last Commonwealth Games due to similar injury and realizes that, given their age, qualifying for the next Games is likely to be the last chance to fulfil ambition.

Prior to the injury, Hallie's training had been going extremely well. Their past year can be characterized by "an excellent run of form," as Hallie has received numerous player of the match awards and their scoring statistics are best of their whole playing career.

Hallie is keen to return to full training as soon as possible. "I cannot wait to be back in play. The past six weeks have been incredibly frustrating, and I feel like I am angry ALL the time. I want to get selected to the team, and this useless wait time is not helping," Hallie vents to Kadi, the team physiotherapist. "I mean, I know I have been here before, and back then, I recovered quickly. But now the doctor and you keep telling me that due to my age and injury history" – Hallie rolls their eyes – "my recovery will take longer. What if I don't make it back on time and I miss my opportunity to play for Wales?"

Over the past three weeks, Kadi has also noticed Hallie yawning a lot. When Kadi asks Hallie about it, she responds abruptly, "It's no big deal. I mean, I am in constant pain, and that stops me from sleeping well. This has been going on for a while now, but it's fine. I know my thoughts are also wandering, and that keeps me awake. What if I don't make the team? I have to make the team. If I don't, why did I play this long?"

"How do you think the lack of sleep is affecting you?" Kadi asks Hallie.

"Well, I think it has made me irritable. I also don't eat much, and I feel like my head is spinning. But otherwise, I think I am fine. I just need to push through this pain, get these exercises done, and go back to the game," Hallie responds.

Kadi listens carefully to Hallie. After a short silence, Kadi responds, "I understand this all feels overwhelming. The first thing we need to do is to get your pain under control so you can sleep and eat better. I also think we should give our team psychologist a call. I think talking to them would be a great help so together we can create a plan to get you back to sport safely as soon as possible."

Questions

1. Based on the case description, what are Hallie's cognitive appraisals and emotional and behavioral responses to their situation?
2. What role does pain play in Hallie's biopsychosocial responses to their injury?
3. How might Hallie's cognitive appraisals and emotional and behavioral responses differ if the timing of the injury, their age, and their injury history had been different?
4. In your (future or current) professional role, what would be your next steps in providing care for Hallie? Consider the professional core competencies of your discipline or field and provide two (2) examples of psychological support that are within your (future or current) scope of practice and two (2) examples that would warrant referral.
5. Considering your (future or current) professional competencies, what advice would you give Hallie on their current sleep hygiene and its impact on their physical and psychosocial recovery?

References

Albinson, C. B., & Petrie, T. A. (2003). Cognitive appraisals, stress, and coping: Preinjury and postinjury factors influencing psychological adjustment to sport injury. *Journal of Sport Rehabilitation, 12*(4), 306–322. https://doi.org/10.1123/jsr.12.4.306

American Psychological Association. (2022). *APA dictionary of psychology*. https://dictionary.apa.org/

Andersen, M. B. (2007). Collaborative relationship in injury rehabilitation: Two case examples. In D. Pargman (Ed.), *Psychological bases of sport injuries* (3rd ed., pp. 219–236). Fitness Information Technology.

Andersen, M. B., & Williams, J. M. (1988). A model of stress and athletic injury: Prediction and prevention. *Journal of Sport & Exercise Psychology, 10*(3), 294–306. https://doi.org/10.1123/jsep.10.3.294

Andersen, M. B., & Williams, J. M. (1999). Athletic injury, psychosocial factors, and perceptual changes during stress. *Journal of Sports Sciences, 17*(9), 735–741. https://doi.org/10.1080/026404199365597

Anderson, A. G., White, A., & McKay, J. (2004). Athletes' emotional responses to injury. In D. Lavallee, J. Thatcher, & M. Jones (Eds.), *Coping and emotion in sport* (pp. 207–221). Nova Science.

Appaneal, R. N., Levine, B. R., Perna, F. M., & Roh, J. L. (2009). Measuring postinjury depression among male and female competitive athletes. *Journal of Sport & Exercise Psychology, 31*(1), 60–76. https://doi.org/10.1123/jsep.31.1.60

Arvinen-Barrow, M., & Clement, D. (2022). Role of emotions in sport injury. In M. C. Ruiz & C. Robazza (Eds.), *Feelings in sport: Theory, research, and practical implications for performance and well-being* (pp. 201–212). Routledge.

Arvinen-Barrow, M., Clement, D., & Bayes, N. (2012, July). Athletes attitudes towards physiotherapist. *International Journal of Multi-Disciplinary Studies and Sports Research, 2,* 324–334.

Arvinen-Barrow, M., Clement, D., Hamson-Utley, J. J., Zakrajsek, R. A., Kamphoff, C. S., Lee, S.-M., . . . Martin, S. B. (2016). Athletes' expectations about sport injury rehabilitation: A cross-cultural study. *Journal of Sport Rehabilitation, 25*(4), 338–347. https://doi.org/10.1123/jsr.2015-0018

Arvinen-Barrow, M., DeGrave, K., Pack, S. M., & Hemmings, B. (2019). Transitioning out of professional sport: The psychosocial impact of career-ending non-musculoskeletal injuries among male cricketers from England and Wales. *Journal of Clinical Sport Psychology, 13*(4), 629–644. https://doi.org/10.1123/jcsp.2017-0040

Arvinen-Barrow, M., & Granquist, M. D. (2020). Psychosocial considerations for rehabilitation of the injured athletic patient. In W. Prentice (Ed.), *Rehabilitation techniques for sports medicine and athletic training* (7th ed., pp. 93–116). SLACK Inc.

Arvinen-Barrow, M., Hemmings, B., Weigand, D. A., Becker, C. A., & Booth, L. (2007). Views of chartered physiotherapists on the psychological content of their practice: A national follow-up survey in the United Kingdom. *Journal of Sport Rehabilitation, 16*(2), 111–121. https://doi.org/10.1123/jsr.16.2.111

Arvinen-Barrow, M., Hurley, D., & Ruiz, M. C. (2017). Transitioning out of professional sport: The psychosocial impact of career-ending injuries among elite Irish rugby football union players. *Journal of Clinical Sport Psychology, 10*(1). https://doi.org/10.1123/jcsp.2016-0012

Arvinen-Barrow, M., Massey, W. V., & Hemmings, B. (2014). Role of sport medicine professionals in addressing psychosocial aspects of sport-injury rehabilitation: Professional athletes' views. *Journal of Athletic Training, 49*(6), 764–772. https://doi.org/10.4085/1062-6050-49.3.44

Arvinen-Barrow, M., & Pack, S. M. (2013). Social support in sport injury rehabilitation. In M. Arvinen-Barrow & N. Walker (Eds.), *The psychology of sport injury and rehabilitation* (pp. 117–131). Routledge.

Brewer, B. W. (1994). Review and critique of models of psychological adjustment to athletic injury. *Journal of Applied Sport Psychology, 6*, 87–100. https://doi.org/10.1080/10413209408406467

Brewer, B. W. (2001). Psychology of sport injury rehabilitation. In R. N. Singer, H. A. Hausenblas, & C. M. Janelle (Eds.), *Handbook of sport psychology* (pp. 787–809). John Wiley & Sons.

Brewer, B. W. (2017). Psychological responses to injury. In *Oxford research encyclopedia of psychology*. Oxford University Press.

Brewer, B. W., Andersen, M. B., & Van Raalte, J. L. (2002). Psychological aspects of sport injury rehabilitation: Toward a biopsychological approach. In D. L. Mostofsky & L. D. Zaichkowsky (Eds.), *Medical aspects of sport and exercise* (pp. 41–54). Fitness Information Technology.

Brewer, B. W., & Cornelius, A. E., Stephan, Y., & Van Raalte, J. (2010). Self-protective changes in athletic identity following anterior cruciate ligament reconstruction. *Psychology of Sport and Exercise, 11*(1), 1–5. https://doi.org/10.1016/j.psychsport.2009.09.005

Brewer, B. W., Petitpas, A. J., Van Raalte, J. L., Sklar, J. H., & Ditmar, T. D. (1995). Prevalence of psychological distress among patients at a physical therapy clinic specializing in sports medicine. *Sports Medicine, Training and Rehabilitation, 6*, 139–145.

Brewer, B. W., & Petrie, T. A. (1995). A comparison between injured and uninjured football players on selected psychological variables. *The Academic Athletic Journal, 10*, 11–18.

Brewer, B. W., & Redmond, C. J. (2017). *Psychology of sport injury*. Human Kinetics.

Brewer, B. W., Van Raalte, J. L., & Linder, D. E. (1993). Athletic identity: Hercules' muscles or Achilles' heel? *International Journal of Sport Psychology, 24*(2), 237–254.

Burland, J. P., Toonstra, J. L., & Howard, J. S. (2019). Psychosocial barriers after anterior cruciate ligament reconstruction: A clinical review of factors influencing postoperative success. *Sports Health: A Multidisciplinary Approach, 11*(6), 528–534. https://doi.org/10.1177/1941738119869333

Campbell, C. M., & Edwards, R. R. (2009). Mind-body interactions in pain: The neurophysiology of anxious and catastrophic pain-related thoughts. *Translational Research: The Journal of Laboratory and Clinical Medicine, 153*(3), 97–101. https://doi.org/10.1016/j.trsl.2008.12.002

Christian, L. M., Graham, J. E., Padgett, D. A., Glaser, R., & Kiecolt-Glaser, J. K. (2006). Stress and wound healing. *Neuroimmunomodulation, 13*(5–6), 337–346. https://doi.org/10.1159/000104862

Clark, D., Nakamura, M., Miclau, T., & Marcucio, R. (2017). Effects of aging on fracture healing. *Current Osteoporosis Reports, 15*(6), 601–608. https://doi.org/10.1007/s11914-017-0413-9

Clement, D., & Arvinen-Barrow, M. (2020). Psychosocial strategies for the different phases of sport injury rehabilitation. In A. Ivarsson & U. Johnson (Eds.), *Psychological bases of sport injuries* (4th ed., pp. 297–330). Fitness Information Technology.

Clement, D., Arvinen-Barrow, M., & Fetty, T. (2015). Psychosocial responses during different phases of sport injury rehabilitation: A qualitative study. *Journal of Athletic Training, 50*(1), 95–104. https://doi.org/10.4085/1062-6050-49.3.52

Clement, D., Granquist, M. D., & Arvinen-Barrow, M. (2013). Psychosocial aspects of athletic injuries as perceived by athletic trainers. *Journal of Athletic Training, 48*(4), 512–521. https://doi.org/10.4085/1062-6050-48.3.21

Clement, D., Hamson-Utley, J. J., Arvinen-Barrow, M., Kamphoff, C., Zakrajsek, R. A., & Martin, S. B. (2012). College athletes' expectations about injury rehabilitation with an athletic trainer. *International Journal of Athletic Therapy & Training, 17*(4), 18–27. https://doi.org/10.1123/ijatt.17.4.18

Dawkins, B., Renwick, C., Ensor, T., Shrinkins, B., Jayne, D., & Meads, D. (2021). What factors affect patients' ability to access healthcare? An overview of systematic reviews. *Tropical Medicine & International Health, 26*(10), 1177–1188. https://doi.org/10.1111/tmi.13651

DiMatteo, M. R., Lepper, H. S., & Croghan, T. W. (2000). Depression is a risk factor for noncompliance with medical treatment: Meta-analysis of the effects of anxiety and depression on patient adherence. *Archives of Internal Medicine*, *160*(14), 2101–2107.

Evans, L., & Brewer, B. W. (2022). Applied psychology of sport injury: Getting to – and moving across – The valley of death. *Journal of Applied Sport Psychology*, *34*(5), 1011–1028. https://doi.org/10.1080/10413200.2021.2015480

Evans, L., & Hardy, L. (1995). Sport injury and grief response: A review. *Journal of Sport & Exercise Psychology*, *17*, 227–245.

Francis, S. R., Andersen, M. B., & Maley, B. (2000). Physiotherapists' and male professional athletes' views on psychological skills for rehabilitation. *Journal of Science and Medicine in Sport*, *3*(1), 17–29. https://doi.org/10.1016/S1440-2440(00)80044-4

Franck, F., Saithna, A., Vieira, T. D., Pioger, C., Vigne, G., Le Guen, M., . . . Sonnery-Cottet, B. (2021). Return to sport composite test after anterior cruciate ligament reconstruction (K-STARTS): Factors affecting return to sport test score in a retrospective analysis of 676 patients. *Sports Health: A Multidisciplinary Approach*, *13*(4), 364–372. https://doi.org/10.1177/1941738120978240

Gerstein, A. D., Phillips, T. J., Rogers, G. S., & Gilchrest, B. A. (1993). Wound healing and aging. *Dermatologic Clinics*, *11*(4), 749–757.

Giannone, Z. A., Haney, C. J., Kealy, D., & Ogrodniczuk, J. S. (2017). Athletic identity and psychiatric symptoms following retirement from varsity sports. *International Journal of Social Psychiatry*, *63*(7), 598–601. https://doi.org/10.1177/0020764017724184

Goddard, K., Roberts, C. M., Byron-Daniel, J., & Woodford, L. (2021). Psychological factors involved in adherence to sport injury rehabilitation: A systematic review. *International Review of Sport and Exercise Psychology*, *14*(1), 51–73. https://doi.org/10.1080/1750984x.2020.1744179

Granquist, M. D., & Brewer, B. W. (2013). Psychological aspects of rehabilitation adherence. In M. Arvinen-Barrow & N. Walker (Eds.), *The psychology of sport injury and rehabilitation* (pp. 40–53). Routledge.

Grindstaff, J. S., Wrisberg, C. A., & Ross, J. R. (2010). Collegiate athletes' experience of the meaning of sport injury: A phenomenological investigation. *Perspectives in Public Health*, *130*(3), 127–135.

Heaney, C. (2006). Physiotherapists' perceptions of sport psychology intervention in professional soccer. *International Journal of Sport and Exercise Psychology*, *4*(1), 73–86. https://doi.org/10.1080/1612197X.2006.9671785

Hemmings, B., & Povey, L. (2002). Views of chartered physiotherapists on the psychological content of their practice: A preliminary study in the United Kingdom. *British Journal of Sports Medicine*, *36*(1), 61–64. https://doi.org/10.1136/bjsm.36.1.61

Hess, C. W., Grnacinski, S., & Meyer, B. B. (2019). A review of the sport-injury and -rehabilitation literature: From abstraction to application. *The Sport Psychologist*, *33*(3), 232–243. https://doi.org/10.1123/tsp.2018-0043

Hess, C. W., & Meyer, B. B. (2022). Lived experiences of an elite performance management team through injury rehabilitation: An interpretative phenomenological analysis. *Journal of Sport Rehabilitation*, *31*(2), 199–210. https://doi.org/10.1123/jsr.2021-0072

Hilliard, R. C., Brewer, B. W., Cornelius, A. E., & Van Raalte, J. L. (2014). Big five personality characteristics and adherence to clinic-based rehabilitation activities after ACL surgery: A prospective analysis. *The Open Rehabilitation Journal*, *7*, 1–5. https://doi.org/10.2174/1874943701407010001

Howells, K., Sarkar, M., & Fletcher, D. (2017). Can athletes benefit from difficulty? A systematic review of growth following adversity in competitive sport. *Progress in Brain Research*, *234*, 117–159. https://doi.org/10.1016/bs.pbr.2017.06.002

Huang, K., & Ihm, J. (2021). Sleep and injury risk. *Current Sports Medicine Reports*, *20*(6), 286–290. https://doi.org/10.1249/JSR.0000000000000849

Ildefonso, K., Blanton, J., Durwin, C., Arvinen-Barrow, M., & Kamphoff, C. (2020). A preliminary investigation into collegiate student-athletes' attitudes towards athletic trainers and sport psychology consultants. *The Journal of SPORT*, *8*(1), 56–75. https://oaks.kent.edu/sport/vol8/iss1/preliminary-investigation-collegiate-student-athletes-attitudes-towards-athletic

Kamphoff, C. S., Thomae, J., & Hamson-Utley, J. J. (2013). Integrating the psychological and physiological aspects of sport injury rehabilitation: Rehabilitation profiling and phases of rehabilitation. In M. Arvinen-Barrow & N. Walker (Eds.), *The psychology of sport injury and rehabilitation* (pp. 134–155). Routledge.

Knappenberger, K. (2018, July). Nutrition for injury recovery and rehabilitation: How to make sure your patients are receiving optimal fueling. *NATANews*, 14–17. www.nata.org/sites/default/files/nutrition-for-injury-recovery-and-rehabilitation.pdf

Kolt, G. S. (2003). Psychology of injury and rehabilitation. In G. S. Kolt & L. Snyder-Mackler (Eds.), *Physical therapies in sport and exercise* (pp. 165–183). Churchill Livingstone.

Kübler-Ross, E. (1969). *On death and dying*. MacMillan Ltd.

Larson, G. A., Starkey, C., & Zaichkowsky, L. D. (1996). Psychological aspects of athletic injuries as perceived by athletic trainers. *The Sport Psychologist*, *10*(1), 37–47. https://doi.org/10.1123/tsp.10.1.37

Lattimore, D. (2017). On the sidelines: An athlete's perspective of injury recovery. *Sport and Exercise Psychology Review*, *13*(2), 13–21. https://doi.org/10.53841/bpssepr.2017.13.2.13

Lazarus, R. S., & Folkman, S. (1984). *Stress, appraisal, and coping*. Springer Publishing Company.

Leddy, M. H., Lambert, M. J., & Ogles, B. M. (1994). Psychological consequences of athletic injury among high-level competitors. *Research Quarterly for Exercise and Sport*, *65*(4), 347–354. https://doi.org/10.1080/02701367.1994.10607639

Lentz, M. J., Landis, C. A., Rothermel, J., & Shaver, J. L. (1999). Effects of selective slow wave sleep disruption on musculoskeletal pain and fatigue in middle aged women. *The Journal of Rheumatology*, *26*(7), 1586–1592.

Lisee, C. M., DiSanti, J. S., Chan, M., Ling, J., Erickson, K., Shingles, M., & Kuenze, C. M. (2020). Gender differences in psychological responses to recovery after anterior cruciate ligament reconstruction before return to sport. *Journal of Athletic Training*, *55*(10), 1098–1105. https://doi.org/10.4085/1062-6050-558.19

Madrigal, L., & Gill, D. L. (2014). Psychological responses of division I female athletes through injury recovery: A case study approach. *Journal of Clinical Sport Psychology*, *8*(2), 276–298. https://doi.org/10.1123/wspaj.2014-0024

Mah, C. D., Mah, K. E., Kezirian, E. J., & Dement, W. C. (2011). The effects of sleep extension on the athletic performance of collegiate basketball players. *Sleep*, *34*(7), 943–950. https://doi.org/10.5665/SLEEP.1132

Mainwaring, L. M., Bisschop, S. M., Green, R. E. A., Antoniazzi, M., Comper, P., Kristman, V., . . . Richards, D. W. (2004). Emotional reaction of varsity athletes to sport-related concussion. *Journal of Sport & Exercise Psychology*, *26*(1). https://doi.org/10.1123/jsep.26.1.119

Mansell, P. C. (2021). Stress mindset in athletes: Investigating the relationships between beliefs, challenge and threat with psychological wellbeing. *Psychology of Sport and Exercise*, *57*, 102020. https://doi.org/10.1016/J.PSYCHSPORT.2021.102020

Martin, S. B., Akers, A., Jackson, A. W., Wrisberg, C. A., Nelson, L., Jason Leslie, P., & Laidig, L. (2001). Male and female athletes' and nonathletes expectations about sport psychology consulting. *Journal of Applied Sport Psychology*, *13*(1), 18–39.

Martins, L. B., Braga Tibães, J. R., Sanches, M., Jacka, F., Berk, M., & Teixeira, A. L. (2021). Nutrition-based interventions for mood disorders. *Expert Review of Neurotherapeutics*, *21*(3), 303–315. https://doi.org/10.1080/14737175.2021.1881482

Motivala, S. J. (2011). Sleep and inflammation: Psychoneuroimmunology in the context of cardiovascular disease. *Annals of Behavioral Medicine: A Publication of the Society of Behavioral Medicine*, *42*(2), 141–152. https://doi.org/10.1007/s12160-011-9280-2

Mullington, J. M., Simpson, N. S., Meier-Ewert, H. K., & Haack, M. (2010). Sleep loss and inflammation. *Best Practice & Research: Clinical Endocrinology & Metabolism*, *24*(5), 775–784. https://doi.org/10.1016/j.beem.2010.08.014

Myers, C. A., Peyton, D. D., & Jensen, B. J. (2004). Treatment acceptability in NCAA Division I football athletes: Rehabilitation intervention strategies. *Journal of Sport Behavior 27*(2), 165–169.

Osborne, R. E. (2017). Causal attribution of teammate injury: Intercultural sensitivity and "blame" for teammate injury. *International Journal of Sport & Society*, *8*(2), 1–14.

Park, S., Lavallee, D., & Tod, D. (2013). Athletes' career transition out of sport: A systematic review. *International Review of Sport and Exercise Psychology*, *6*(1), 22–53. https://doi.org/10.1080/17509 84X.2012.687053

Pearson, L., & Jones, G. (1992). Emotional effects of sports injuries: Implications for physiotherapists. *Physiotherapy*, *78*(10), 762–770.

Podlog, L., Gao, Z., Kenow, L., Kleinert, J., Granquist, M. D., Newton, M., & Hannon, J. (2013). Injury rehabilitation overadherence: Preliminary scale validation and relationships with athletic identity and self-presentation concerns. *Journal of Athletic Training*, *48*(3), 372–381. https://doi.org/10.4085/1062-6050-48.2.20

Potter, M., Gordon, S., & Hamer, P. (2003). Identifying physiotherapist and patient expectations in private practice physiotherapy. *Physiotherapy Canada*, *54*(4), 195–202.

Rodriguez, R. M., Marroquin, A., & Cosby, N. (2019). Reducing fear of reinjury and pain perception in athletes with first-time anterior cruciate ligament reconstructions by implementing imagery training. *Journal of Sport Rehabilitation*, *28*(4), 385–389. https://doi.org/10.1123/jsr.2017-0056

Ruddock-Hudson, M., O'Halloran, P., & Murphy, G. (2012). Exploring psychological reactions to injury in the Australian Football League (AFL). *Journal of Applied Sport Psychology*, *24*(4), 375–390. https://doi.org/10.1080/10413200.2011.654172

Ruddock-Hudson, M., O'Halloran, P., & Murphy, G. (2014). The psychological impact of long-term injury on Australian football league players. *Journal of Applied Sport Psychology*, *26*(4), 377–394. https://doi.org/10.1080/10413200.2014.897269

Sparkes, A. C. (1998). Athletic identity: An Achilles' heel to the survival of self. *Qualitative Health Research*, *8*(5), 644–664.

Stambulova, N., Stephan, Y., & Jäphag, U. (2007). Athletic retirement: A cross-national comparison of elite French and Swedish athletes. *Psychology of Sport and Exercise*, *8*(1), 101–118. https://doi.org/10.1016/j.psychsport.2006.05.002

Steiger, A., & Pawlowski, M. (2019). Depression and sleep. *International Journal of Molecular Sciences*, *20*(3), 607. https://doi.org/10.3390/ijms20030607

Stoltenburg, A. L., Kamphoff, C. S., & Lindstrom Bremer, K. (2011). Transitioning out of sport: The psychosocial effects of collegiate athletes' career-ending injuries. *Athletic Insight: Online Journal of Sport Psychology*, *11*(2), 1–11.

Tasiemski, T., & Brewer, B. W. (2011). Athletic identity, sport participation, and psychological adjustment in people with spinal cord injury. *Adapted Physical Activity Quarterly*, *28*, 233–250.

Taylor-Postma, R., Rider, J., & Otty, R. (2022). Functional cognition: An opportunity to highlight the role of occupational therapy in post-concussion care. *The Open Journal of Occupational Therapy*, *10*(2), 1–6. https://doi.org/10.15453/2168-6408.1909

Thomeé, P., Währberg, P., Börjesson, M., Thomeé, R., Eriksson, B. I., & Karlsson, J. (2007). Self-efficacy, symptoms and physical activity in patients with an anterior cruciate injury: A prospective study. *Scandinavian Journal of Medicine & Science in Sports*, *17*, 238–245.

Tipton, K. D. (2015). Nutritional support for exercise-induced injuries. *Sports Medicine*, *45*(1), 93–104. https://doi.org/10.1007/s40279-015-0398-4

Vergeer, I. (2006). Exploring the mental representation of athletic injury: A longitudinal case study. *Psychology of Sport and Exercise*, *7*(1), 99–114. https://doi.org/10.1016/j.psychsport.2005.07.003

Wadey, R., Evans, L., Evans, K., & Mitchell, I. D. (2011). Perceived benefits following sport injury: A qualitative examination of their antecedents and underlying mechanisms. *Journal of Applied Sport Psychology*, *23*(2), 142–158. https://doi.org/10.1080/10413200.2010.543119

Wadey, R., Podlog, L., Galli, N., & Mellalieu, S. D. (2016). Stress-related growth following sport injury: Examining the applicability of the organismic valuing theory. *Scandinavian Journal of Medicine & Science in Sports*, *26*(10), 1132–1139. https://doi.org/10.1111/sms.12579

Wadey, R., Roy-Davis, K., Evans, L., Howells, K., Salim, J., & Diss, C. (2019). Sport psychology consultants' perspectives on facilitating sport injury-related growth. *The Sport Psychologist, 33*(3), 244–255. https://doi.org/10.1123/tsp.2018-0110

Walker, N., & Thatcher, J. (2011). The emotional response to athletic injury: Re-injury anxiety. In J. Thatcher, M. V. Jones, & D. Lavallee (Eds.), *Coping and emotion in sport* (2nd ed., pp. 235–259). Routledge.

Walker, N., Thatcher, J., & Lavallee, D. (2007). Psychological responses to injury in competitive sport: A critical review. *The Journal of The Royal Society for the Promotion of Health, 127*(4), 174–180.

Walker, N., Thatcher, J., & Lavallee, D. (2010). A preliminary development of the re-injury anxiety inventory (RIAI). *Physical Therapy in Sport, 11*(1), 23–29. https://doi.org/10.1016/j.ptsp.2009.09.003

Watson, A. M. (2017). Sleep and athletic performance. *Current Sports Medicine Reports, 16*(6), 413–418. https://doi.org/10.1249/JSR.0000000000000418

Wiese-Bjornstal, D. M. (2010). Psychology and socioculture affect injury risk, response, and recovery in high-intensity athletes: A consensus statement. *Scandinavian Journal of Medicine & Science in Sports, 20*(s2), 103–111. https://doi.org/10.1111/j.1600-0838.2010.01195.x

Wiese-Bjornstal, D. M. (2014). Reflections on a quarter-century of research in sports medicine psychology. *Revista de Psicología del Deporte, 23*(2), 411–421.

Wiese-Bjornstal, D. M. (2019a). Christian beliefs and behaviours as health protective, resilience, and intervention factors in the context of sport injuries. In B. Hemmings, N. J. Watson, & A. Parker (Eds.), *Sport psychology and Christianity: Welfare, performance and consultancy* (pp. 54–70). Routledge.

Wiese-Bjornstal, D. M. (2019b). The integrated model of religiosity and psychological response to the sport injury and rehabilitation process: A Christian illustration. *Canadian Journal for Scholarship and the Christian Faith*. https://cjscf.org/wellness/356-2/

Wiese-Bjornstal, D. M., Smith, A. M., Shaffer, S. M., & Morrey, M. A. (1998). An integrated model of response to sport injury: Psychological and sociological dynamics. *Journal of Applied Sport Psychology, 10*(1), 46–69. https://doi.org/10.1080/10413209808406377

Wiese-Bjornstal, D. M., White, A. C., Russell, H. C., & Smith, A. M. (2015). Psychology of sport concussions. *Kinesiology Review, 5*, 169–189. https://doi.org/10.1123/kr.2015-0012

Wiese-Bjornstal, D. M., Wood, K. N., & Kronzer, J. R. (2020). Sport injuries and psychological sequelae. In G. Tenenbaum & R. C. Eklund (Eds.), *Handbook of sport psychology* (4th ed., pp. 751–772). John Wiley & Sons, Inc.

Wininger, S. R. (2007). Self-Determination theory and exercise behavior: An examination of the psychometric properties of the exercise motivation scale. *Journal of Applied Sport Psychology, 19*, 471–486.

Yengo-Kahn, A. M., Wallace, J., Jimenez, V., Totten, D. J., Bonfield, C. M., & Zuckerman, S. L. (2021). Exploring the outcomes and experiences of Black and White athletes following a sport-related concussion: A retrospective cohort study. *Journal of Neurosurgery Pediatrics, 28*(5), 516–525. https://doi.org/10.3171/2021.2.PEDS2130

4 Cultural, Institutional, and Relational Understanding of Sport Injury

*Samantha Glynn, Ross Wadey, Melissa Day,
and Ciara Everard*

Chapter Objectives

- To describe the multilevel model of sport injury.
- To outline the impact of relational, cultural, and institutional factors on sport injury.
- To illustrate how psychological experiences of athletes with injuries are produced by, within, and through social structures and associated environments and cultures.

Introduction

In the 21st century, the field of sport injury psychology continues to flourish and diversify, which can be evidenced from the numerous books (e.g., Arvinen-Barrow & Clement, 2019; Brewer & Redmond, 2017), review articles (e.g., Ivarsson et al., 2017; Putukian, 2016), and models that extend the way we conceptualize and theorize about sport injury (Brewer et al., 2002; Wadey et al., 2018). Yet aside from these significant advancements, a critical perusal of the sport injury psychology literature reveals a predominant lens on the injured athlete (Wadey & Day, 2022), with the spotlight of research remaining fixated on the "inner" world of athletes with injuries. Although the social context is acknowledged, primacy is given to the way athletes with injuries think and interpret the situations they find themselves in. This cognitive mono-perspective cannot be criticized for only being reductionist but also for locating the blame for injury and responses to injury squarely within the individual (e.g., "they" are not thinking correctly). By presenting injury in this way, the broader social context is left undertheorized and unchallenged. In this chapter, the authors aim to expand this view by encouraging the reader to broaden their analytical gaze to ensure that policies, practices, and resources are also put in place to support the welfare of all invested parties (Wadey & Day, 2022).

To help raise social consciousness, the purpose of this chapter is to describe the multilevel model of sport injury (MMSI; Wadey et al., 2018), which takes a systems perspective of sport injury. More specifically, this chapter will (a) review three levels of analysis within the MMSI (i.e., cultural, institutional, and relational) that can impact sport injury, (b) and contextualize each level with evidence-based examples. In doing so, the authors hope to illustrate how the psychological experiences of athletes with injuries are produced by, within, and through social structures and associated environments and cultures supporting them. To be clear from the outset and aligned with the MMSI, we do not see psychological experiences (e.g., mental illness) of athletes with injuries as located "in" an individual (i.e., determined, for example, by the person's biochemistry or genetics). Rather, this chapter views psychological experiences as a complex

DOI: 10.4324/9781003295709-5

and multifaceted phenomenon affected by biographical, experiential, physical, psychological, sociocultural, economic, and political factors (see Atkinson, 2018).

Multilevel Model of Sport Injury

The MMSI (Wadey et al., 2018) aims to take a systems perspective of sport injury. Not only does this model help broaden our analytical gaze, but it also provides a platform for systematic programs of research by illustrating how sport injury influences, and is influenced by, multiple levels. The model proposes five distinct yet relational levels of analysis: intrapersonal, inter-personal, institutional, cultural, and policy (see Figure 4.1). Within and across these levels of analysis, the MMSI can also accommodate additional models and theories to extend conceptual and theoretical understanding of sport injury as well as encourage theoretical integration and interdisciplinary research. Finally, the MMSI provides a useful framework for policymakers,

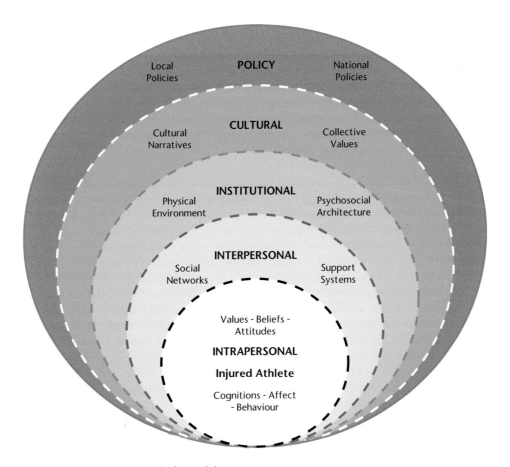

Figure 4.1 The multilevel model of sport injury.

Source: Copyright ©2018 from Multilevel model of sport injury (MMSI): Can coaches impact and be impacted by injury? by Ross Wadey, Melissa Day, Francesca Cavallerio, & Laura Martinelli. Reproduced by permission of Taylor and Francis Group, LLC, a division of Informa plc.

institutions, and various personnel (e.g., mental performance consultants, licensed mental health providers, licensed sport psychology professionals, sports medicine professionals, and sport professionals) to target their intervention strategies.

Intrapersonal Level

The first level, *intrapersonal*, reflects the characteristics of the individual (e.g., age, gender, ethnicity, social-economic status, values, beliefs); their embodied, subjective, and lived experiences; and the psychological skills they can learn and use to prevent injury and support their rehabilitation. Largely guided by Williams and Andersen's (1998) revised stress and injury model (see Chapter 2) and Wiese-Bjornstal et al.'s (1998) integrated model of psychological response to the sport injury and rehabilitation process (see Chapter 3), a significant body of research supports this level of analysis, which is concerned with injured athletes' thoughts (e.g., cognitive appraisals), feelings (e.g., distress), and behaviors (e.g., help seeking). For example, researchers have recently reviewed the differences between and within genders (Bunsell & Doidge, 2020), pain experienced (Atkinson, 2020), psychosocial strategies (Ledingham et al., 2020), and adherence to sport injury prevention programs (Brewer, 2020). These bodies of research have been critical toward enhancing our understanding of how athletes *experience* injury and can prevent or manage injury *themselves*. Yet while we can interpret this research from a broader cultural perspective, this body of research does not account for other levels of impact *beyond* the intrapersonal. The focus lies squarely with the individual; they are the problem (e.g., not thinking correctly) and the solution (e.g., they need to help themselves).

Interpersonal Level

The second level of analysis, *interpersonal*, focuses on formal and informal social networks and support systems and the relational impact of injury. Examples of interpersonal factors include social support, others' attitudes toward sporting injuries, and social processes (e.g., leadership, team dynamics, dyads, roles). The analytical gaze at this unit of analysis has tended to focus on the concept of social support and how support providers (e.g., coaches, physiotherapists, or interprofessional care teams) can be more athlete-centered (e.g., Arvinen-Barrow & Clement, 2019) and meet the needs of athletes with injuries (e.g., Rees et al., 2010). However, the research has largely been one-directional in nature (e.g., how can "we" help "them"). What researchers have not fully explored is how sport-related injuries can impact an athlete's support network (e.g., how can "they" impact "us") and how to better understand relationships between athletes with injuries and their support networks. Concepts such as vicarious trauma and vicarious growth are likely to be salient here when exploring the impact of injuries on others (see Martinelli & Day, 2020). Furthermore, the scope of the MMSI encourages the expansion of the conceptual remit beyond personal "needs" and more toward interpersonal units of analysis, such as care, compatibility, conflict, and power. Taking a more dyadic perspective will help identify new ways that athletes with injuries can work *with* others to strengthen relationships (Kerai, 2020).

Institutional Level

The third level, *institutional*, is concerned with the sport (e.g., type, level, norms, values), institutions and organizations (e.g., strategy, functioning, climate), physical environment (e.g., material provisions), psychosocial architecture (e.g., player welfare, key stakeholder relationships), and injury protocols (e.g., screening, surveillance, services). This unit of analysis has received less research attention in comparison to the previous two levels: intrapersonal and interpersonal. Examples include contextualized norms and values of the sport and how they influence overuse injuries (Cavallerio et al., 2016), how the rehabilitation environment can affect athletes' rehabilitation adherence (Niven, 2007; Wiese-Bjornstal, 2009), recommendations for screening and surveillance (Wiese-Bjornstal, 2009), and the psychological support mechanisms available for long-term injured athletes (Gervis et al., 2020). For example, Niven (2007) identified how rehabilitation environments can both support (e.g., encouraging climate) and undermine (e.g., poor access to resources) rehabilitation adherence. This level of analysis clearly foregrounds social responsibility. Rather than calling upon athletes with injuries to develop the resources to personally take care of themselves, it encourages that practices, resources, and pathways are put in places to support the athletes (Wadey et al., 2019).

Cultural Level

The fourth level, *cultural*, reflects the media, cultural narratives, and collective norms, traditions, and values (see McGannon & McMahon, 2020; Williams, 2020). Building upon the pioneering work of Sparkes and Smith (2005) and narrative inquiry (Frank, 2010b), this unit of analysis is perhaps best reflected by drawing on the work of Ciara Everard, who has explored how athletes story their injury experiences based on the narrative resources (e.g., resilience, merry-go-round, longevity) that their social and cultural worlds make available to them. These narrative resources were identified and illustrated to shape and frame how athletes made sense of their injury experiences. As Frank (2010b) described:

> People do not simply listen to stories. They become caught up, a phase that can be explained by another metaphor: stories get under people's skin. Once stories are under people's skin, they affect the terms in which people think, know and perceive.
>
> (p. 438)

Not only does this line of research raise social consciousness and how to theorize about sport injury, but it can also impact how to practice at a cultural (e.g., expanding the narrative environment), organizational (e.g., storytelling resources), and interpersonal (e.g., enable athletes to re-story their self and identity) level (Denison & Winslade, 2006; Sparkes & Partington, 2003).

Policy Level

Policy is the final level of analysis. That is, local and national policies. To illustrate, the minister for sport from the Department of Digital, Culture, Media, and Sport in the United Kingdom requested an independent report to the government by Baroness Grey-Thompson (2017) into the duty of care sport has toward its participants. One of the themes within the report of relevance was "safety, injury, and medical issues." Consequently, the report considers how the likelihood of injury could be lessened and whether improvements can be made to how sporting injuries are treated in the short and long term. Recommendations for this theme and others (e.g., "mental welfare") are put forward in the report that have implications that are directed at various levels. Intra/interindividual level, such as "staff, coaches, and athletes to receive mental health awareness training and support, which should be included as part of induction processes as well" (p. 32); institutional level, such as "NGB [National Governing Bodies] to strengthen links with

NHS [National Health Service], mental health teams, mental health charities, and community groups [with] [l]inks . . . considered through UK sport and Sport England" (p. 32); and policy level, such as "[g]overnments . . . consider[ing] the potential for an insurance scheme that all sports buy into that covers catastrophic injury" (p. 33). This duty of care report clearly provides a powerful illustration of the different units of analysis posed in the MMSI and how interventions can be targeted at each level.

Supporting Evidence for the MMSI: The Case of Mental Health Following Sport Injury

This section provides an evidence-based review of the MMSI by providing an example of the cultural, institutional, and relational factors and processes that impact and shape athletes' mental health following sport injury. Given that sport injuries have been identified to be one of the main triggers for athletes to experience a mental illness (Souter et al., 2018), which can include depression, generalized anxiety, eating disorders, substance use and abuse, and suicide ideation (e.g., Didymus & Backhouse, 2020; Foskett & Longstaff, 2018; Gervis et al., 2019; Gulliver et al., 2015; Putukian, 2016; Souter et al., 2018), we believe this is a timely example to illustrate the MMSI. Specifically, the following subsections focus on how relationships, institutions, and cultures impact mental health following sport injury.

Interpersonal Perspective

In the broader field of mental health in sport, the evidence suggests that athletes tend not to seek support for mental health concerns, with one of the main barriers being the *stigma* attached to mental illness in sport, which includes a perception that seeking help is a sign of "weakness" and so to be avoided (Gulliver et al., 2012). Historically, a stigma has and continues to exist around mental health, which can be defined as a sign of disgrace or discredit which arises when an individual lacks the attributes required to be an accepted member of a group and so disqualifies them from full social acceptance (Goffman, 1963). To understand how an athlete with injuries might become stigmatized with a cultural context at an interpersonal level, Goffman's (1959) dramaturgical model offers one perspective that can be embedded within the MMSI.

Here, Goffman's model uses the language of theater to characterize social interactions as performances (e.g., between coaches and athletes with injuries). People are suggested to select the appropriate role for any given situation, which they perform in public on what Goffman calls the *front stage*, while they prepare for their performances in the private *backstage* areas, away from the audience. In these social interactions, individuals are displaying their social identity, the one that is presented to and available for scrutiny by others. According to Goffman (1963), stigma arises when there is a discrepancy between a person's *virtual social identity* (i.e., what they ought to appear to be) and their *actual social identity* (i.e., what they privately experience themselves to be), with the gap between the two resulting in what Goffman calls a *spoiled identity*, which sets a person apart from others. Here, the concept of stigma helps us understand situations in which we do not grant athletes with injuries the deference they deserve because they deviate from the role expected in a given social context. Goffman (1963) calls this the *politics of identity*, which creates a divide between the "normals" (i.e., those who align with social expectations and perform normative roles) and the "stigmatized." The following example from an injured rhythmic gymnast (Cavallerio et al., 2016) provides an illustration of the politics of identity in action:

I smile wide, as a "good" gymnast would do at the end of a routine.

Soon, my smile turns to a frown. The music's over, the "mask" comes off. I don't want to look up. I don't want to hear Trudy's (coach's) comments. Tears well up in my eyes, but I try to fight them by looking upwards towards the lights, willing them back inside. "Don't cry. Please don't cry. Don't let Trudy see you cry. Just walk off the carpet." But hot tears start to stream down my face. I act quickly to try and wipe them away, but my efforts are futile. The gymnasts closest to me see my tears and I sense they feel my pain. I can see in their eyes the desire to help, sharing a look that also tells me they can't, and they continue to practice their routines. Slowly, I manage to get to my feet. I turn to Trudy.

"Oh, come on Sally! Not tears again. What's your excuse now? Are you in pain again? You look fine to me," shouts Trudy.

I say nothing.

What's wrong with **you***? shouts Trudy. I really don't have time for this.*

She turns her back to me. I walk off the carpet. Tears continue to stream down my face. My body is shaking from all the pain. I want to scream. I want to shout. I want Trudy to understand the pain. I just don't know how.

(Cavallerio et al., 2016, p. 105)

This social exchange in the preceding example provides an illustration of how pain and injury are produced by, within, and through social structures. It shows how Sally has internalized and now holds the same beliefs about the ideal social identity as other gymnasts (i.e., being "tough" and pushing *through* pain) but who is unable to maintain this outward or *front-stage* performance to others (i.e., "But hot tears start to stream down my face. I act quickly to try and wipe them away, but my efforts are futile") and reveals an inappropriate behavior in her culture (i.e., outwardly crying). In doing so, Sally is aware of her perceived "failing" through the enacted stigma from her coach ("She turns her back to me"). Furthermore, and extending Goffman's theorizing, this example also illustrates how dominant power hierarchies with a sporting context (i.e., coach) serve to reinforce behaviors that are normalized. After all, "it takes power to stigmatize" (Link & Phelan, 2001, p. 375). Lastly, this lived example of stigmatization also illustrates another pressing concern, which is Sally's difficulty in expressing *how* she's feeling ("I want to scream. I want to shout. I want Trudy to understand the pain. I just don't know how."), which is a salient barrier to help seeking for mental health concerns (Gulliver et al., 2012).

An Institutional Perspective

Given recent research that has stressed the critical importance of considering the organizational features of sport environments that contribute to mental health concerns in professional athletes (e.g., Poucher et al., 2021), this subsection is concerned with organizational systems. It also highlights how the physical environment and the individuals and groups of people who comprise the organization can help and hinder mental health following sport injury. To expand, Poucher et al. (2021) recently explored stakeholders' perceptions of how high-performance sport organizations impact athletes' mental health. Semi-structured interviews were conducted with 18 stakeholders from United Kingdom's high-performance sport system (e.g., heads of performance support, physiotherapists, sport psychology practitioners, mental health managers, and cultural leads). Three primary mechanisms of support for high-performance athletes were identified: (a) performance lifestyle advisors (e.g., to help athletes develop interests beyond their sport), (b) financial assistance (e.g., to afford additional support staff), and (c) mental health and sport psychology staff. Regarding the latter mechanism, this included the importance of mental health training for staff. For example:

> If support staff are able to learn, through a mental health first aid course, the warning signs that may indicate an athlete is not mentally well they may be able to spot mental ill health sooner, and thereby help athletes earlier and avoiding reactive referrals at times of crisis.
>
> (p. 5)

Yet in a recent review paper of the psychological support mechanisms available to athletes with injuries, Gervis et al. (2020) identify that these primary mechanisms of support were not available.

To identify the current rehabilitation practices available for long-term injured football players in the United Kingdom, Gervis et al. (2020) invited 75 heads of medical departments to complete a survey. Whilst recognizing that long-term injured players experience clinical mental health concerns (e.g., anxiety, depression; see also Gervis et al., 2019), findings revealed that most clubs had limited access to sport psychology professionals, and sports medicine professionals were almost entirely responsible for providing psychological support throughout rehabilitation. To expand, in response to the question "Do you have staff trained in the psychology of injury?", more than half (55%) of clubs did not have staff with expertise. Where training was indicated, limited formal education was identified (e.g., part of a physiotherapy or sport science undergraduate degree). These findings highlight the limited context- and population-specific appropriate training for support staff in professional football clubs and raise questions about their ability to support mental health, especially given that staff were not trained to identify, refer, or treat mental health concerns. For example, 62% of clubs reported "never" or only "occasionally" screening for psychological issues. Clubs who "never" screened for psychological concerns also had no psychologically trained professionals in their treatment staff. The implication here is that where clubs do not screen and have no qualified staff, there is a heightened risk that players living with mental health concerns go unsupported. The authors concluded that "the duty of care shown towards their injured players is deficient, neglectful and possibly negligent" (p. 23), which highlights the importance of the institution unit of analysis within the MMSI. It also demonstrates the need to provide environments that support mental health of athletes and provides pathways for those who are living with mental illness.

A Cultural Perspective

Given that "most aspects of sport, and therefore, sport injuries, are fundamentally as much social and cultural in nature as they are personal" (Wiese-Bjornstal, 2019, p. 18), this subsection aims to illustrate the importance of understanding how our cultures can impact mental health following sport injury. One form of inquiry that has been recommended to enhance our understanding of how the broader cultural landscape might shape injured athletes' experiences is narrative inquiry (Williams, 2020). It is proposed that humans live *storied lives*, and to make sense of and give meaning to our own experiences (e.g., sport injury), we formulate and share stories (Douglas & Carless, 2006). Through a narrative lens, it is understood that although individuals might tell unique stories or tales of our experiences, we draw upon the narrative scripts available within our cultures to shape our storytelling (Frank, 2013). Furthermore, narratives are not only resources for telling stories; they are also actors, in that they do things *on, in, for*, and *with* us (Frank, 2010a). In other words, narratives are crucial actors in helping create and shape experiences through the ordering of events (Williams, 2020). For example, narratives work *for* people by providing a map or destination to follow, and act *on* people by teaching what to pay attention to and how to respond to certain actions.

Given that narratives resources are theorized to enable athletes to make sense of their experiences (e.g., injury), to imbue our experiences with meaning, and that they can do things on, in, for, and with us (Frank, 2012), this inspired Everard et al. (2021) to explore the narratives that shape injured athletes' experiences. A total of 42 interviews were collected with elite track athletes, and the dataset was analyzed using dialogical narrative analysis. Six narrative typologies were identified (i.e., resilience, merry-go-round, longevity, pendulum, snowball, and more-to-me). For example, the merry-go-round narrative reflects a cyclical plot of highs and lows where chronic and recurring sports injuries continually affected athletes' mental health and sporting careers. This narrative encompassed a dynamic and temporal plotline as athletes' stories started with "what could be," shifted to "what should be," and ended reflecting on "what could have been." Trapped in a "revolving door" of injury and rehabilitation, the merry-go-round narrative reflects the relegation of athletes to the confinement of ongoing rehabilitation and the tumultuous journey it incurs (Everard et al., 2021). One athlete reported, "It was just that constant cycle, get injured, do your rehab, work back to the track and it could be a few weeks, or a few months and you would be right back at the beginning again" (p. 5). The latter stages of this merry-go-round were characterized by a lack of empathy and understanding from peers, institutions, and coaches, which increased feelings of low self-worth and isolation. One athlete reported, "I just avoided being around the track and that question, are you still injured then? People only care when you are relevant but when you're no longer relevant you're just cast aside" (p. 5). As a result, athletes were left questioning their sense of purpose within the sport. The following example (Everard et al., 2021) illustrates how athletes' internalization of the merry-go-round narrative had a devastating impact on their mental health:

> I remember being on a training session and I was like what am I doing with my life? What is the point of this? I'm losing money, I've had my funding cut, I've had my contract cut, two years in a row. All these negative thoughts and I just stopped and burst into tears in the middle of the session. It was a mental breakdown; I'm telling you because I couldn't control it. I knew my mind had gone. I was exhausted physically, I was malnourished, mentally I was ill. I was just done.
>
> (p. 5)

Conclusion

Although the field of sport injury psychology has continued to evolve and expand in its advancement of theory, research, and practice, it has remained individualistic over time by focusing on the "inner" world of athletes' thoughts and feelings and use of self-care strategies to help them help themselves. This chapter aimed to challenge the reader to broaden their analytical gaze to consider relationships, institutions, and cultures. Rather than continuing to encourage athletes just to "toughen up" and think more "positively," through the MMSI lens, the vision for the field of sport injury psychology is to work toward providing an evidence base that informs polices, practices, and resources to support the welfare of all invested parties.

Case Study

Cian's been sat in the car for the last 45 minutes. He stares at the training pitch, watching his friends and reflecting on his career. The words of his physiotherapist continue to reverberate around his mind: "I'm sorry, Cian, I'm so sorry. It's over. You must stop playing. You must think about your long-term health. Your future." He takes another two painkillers and washes them down with a swig of vodka from his "water" bottle to numb the pain. The vodka mixes with the feelings of despair and sense of loss that swell within. *What future? There is no future,* he thinks to himself. He desperately wants to cry. He wants to talk. Open up. Just talk.

He opens the car door, grabs a pack of mints to cover up the smell of vodka, and makes his way to the training pitch to relay the information from his physiotherapist to the club. His teammate Conor sees him and runs up to him. "Cian, great to see you back! How are you?" An opening. Cian takes a long deep breath. He imagines himself telling Conor the news from his physiotherapist and exposing how he feels overwhelmed, alone, lost, suicidal. *Say something, Cian, just say something!* He thinks to himself. As he looks up, Enda, his coach, brushes past. "Nice of you to join us, Cian, I was starting to forget what you looked like" and then keeps walking to start training. Cian looks down and takes a long deep breath. As he inhales, he feels a multitude of insecurities and vulnerabilities being pushed down. He looks up and smiles at Conor. Before he has the chance to speak, Conor says, "You look ready to me, Cian. Just keep up with your rehab and stay strong, mate. You'll be back before you know it. We need you." As Conor runs off to join the others in training, Cian returns to the safety of his car and takes another swig from his water bottle. *Why won't you open up?* He thinks to himself.

Questions

1. How would you describe and interpret Cian's psychological experience?
2. Using the multilevel model of sport injury as a theoretical lens, how might this framework help us further understand and locate Cian's experience?
3. If you could re-story Cian's experience, how would you like it to go, and why?
4. To help promote and encourage help-seeking behaviors by injured athletes, what would you advise, and why? Make sure to consider your (future or current) professional core competencies and scope of practice.

References

Arvinen-Barrow, M., & Clement, D. (Eds.). (2019). *The psychology of sport and performance injury: An interprofessional case-based approach.* Routledge.

Atkinson, M. (2018). *Sport, mental illness and sociology.* Emerald Publishing.

Atkinson, M. (2020). Pain and injury. In R. Wadey (Ed.), *Sport injury psychology: Cultural, relational, methodological, and applied considerations* (pp. 58–66). Routledge.

Brewer, B. W. (2020). Three decades later. In R. Wadey (Ed.), *Sport injury psychology: Cultural, relational, methodological, and applied considerations* (pp. 180–188). Routledge.

Brewer, B. W., Andersen, M. B., & Van Raalte, J. L. (2002). Psychological aspects of sport injury rehabilitation: Toward a biopsychological approach. In D. L. Mostofsky & L. D. Zaichkowsky (Eds.), *Medical aspects of sport and exercise* (pp. 41–54). Fitness Information Technology.

Brewer, B. W., & Redmond, C. J. (2017). *Psychology of sport injury*. Human Kinetics.

Bunsell, T., & Doidge, M. (2020). Gender matters! In R. Wadey (Ed.), *Sport injury psychology: Cultural, relational, methodological, and applied considerations* (pp. 41–49). Routledge.

Cavallerio, F., Wadey, R., & Wagstaff, C. R. D. (2016). Understanding overuse injuries in rhythmic gymnastics: A 12-month ethnographic study. *Psychology of Sport and Exercise*, *25*, 100–109. https://doi.org/10.1016/j.psychsport.2016.05.002

Denison, J., & Winslade, J. (2006). Understanding problematic sporting stories : Narrative therapy and applied sport psychology. *Junctures: The Journal for Thematic Dialogue*, *6*, 99–105. https://hdl.handle.net/10289/4061

Didymus, F., & Backhouse, S. H. (2020). Coping by doping? A qualitative inquiry into permitted and prohibited substance use in competitive rugby. *Psychology of Sport and Exercise*, *49*, 101680. https://doi.org/10.1016/j.psychsport.2020.101680

Douglas, K., & Carless, D. (2006). Performance, discovery, and relational narratives among women professional tournament golfers. *Women in Sport and Physical Activity Journal*, *15*(2), 14–27. https://doi.org/10.1123/wspaj.15.2.14

Everard, C., Wadey, R., & Howells, K. (2021). Storying sports injury experiences of elite track athletes: A narrative analysis. *Psychology of Sport and Exercise*, *56*, 102007. https://doi.org/10.1016/j.psychsport.2021.102007

Foskett, R. L., & Longstaff, F. (2018). The mental health of elite athletes in the United Kingdom. *Journal of Science and Medicine in Sport*, *21*(8), 765–770. https://doi.org/10.1016/j.jsams.2017.11.016

Frank, A. W. (2010a). In defence of narrative exceptionalism. *Sociology of Health & Illness*, *32*(4), 511–675. https://doi.org/10.1111/j.1467-9566.2010.01240_3.x

Frank, A. W. (2010b). *Letting stories breathe: A socio-narratology*. University of Chicago Press.

Frank, A. W. (2012). Narrative psychiatry: How stories can shape clinical practice (review). *Literature and Medicine*, *30*(1), 193–197. https://doi.org/10.1353/lm.2012.0009

Frank, A. W. (2013). *The wounded storyteller: Body, illness, and ethics*. University of Chicago Press.

Gervis, M., Pickford, H., & Hau, T. (2019). Professional Footballers' Association counselors' perceptions of the role long-term injury plays in mental health issues presented by current and former players. *Journal of Clinical Sport Psychology*, *13*(3), 451–468. https://doi.org/10.1123/jcsp.2018-0049

Gervis, M., Pickford, H., Hau, T., & Fruth, M. (2020). A review of the psychological support mechanisms available for long-term injured footballers in the UK throughout their rehabilitation. *Science & Medicine in Football*, *4*(1), 22–29. https://doi.org/10.1080/24733938.2019.1634832

Goffman, E. (1959). *The presentation of self in everyday life*. Doubleday.

Goffman, E. (1963). *Stigma: Notes on the management of spoiled identity*. Prentice-Hall, Inc.

Grey-Thompson, T. (2017). *Duty of care in sport: Independent report to the government*. www.gov.uk/government/publications/duty-of-care-in-sport-review

Gulliver, A., Griffiths, K. M., & Christensen, H. (2012). Barriers and facilitators to mental health help-seeking for young elite athletes: A qualitative study. *BMC Psychiatry*, *12*(1), 157. https://doi.org/10.1186/1471-244X-12-157

Gulliver, A., Griffiths, K. M., Mackinnon, A., Batterham, P. J., & Stanimirovic, R. (2015). The mental health of Australian elite athletes. *Journal of Science and Medicine in Sport*, *18*(3), 255–261. https://doi.org/10.1016/j.jsams.2014.04.006

Ivarsson, A., Johnson, U., Andersen, M. B., Tranaeus, U., Stenling, A., & Lindwall, M. (2017). Psychosocial factors and sport injuries: Meta-analyses for prediction and prevention *Sports Medicine*, *47*(2), 353–365. https://doi.org/10.1007/s40279-016-0578-x

Kerai, S. (2020). Physiotherapist – injured-athlete relationship: Toward a cultural and relational understanding. In R. Wadey (Ed.), *Sport injury psychology: Cultural, relational, methodological, and applied considerations* (pp. 92–100). Routledge.

Ledingham, K., Williams, T., & Evans, L. (2020). Experimental psychological response to injury studies: Why so few? In R. Wadey (Ed.), *Sport injury psychology: Cultural, relational, methodological, and applied considerations* (pp. 125–134). Routledge.

Link, B. G., & Phelan, J. C. (2001). Conceptualizing stigma. *Annual Review of Sociology, 27*(1), 363–385. www.jstor.org/stable/2678626

Martinelli, L., & Day, M. (2020). It's impacted me too" Where does vicarious growth fit in? In R. Wadey, M. Day, & K. Howells (Eds.), *Growth following adversity in sport* (pp. 47–58). Routledge.

McGannon, K. R., & McMahon, J. (2020). Sport media research: Examining the benefits for sport injury psychology and beyond. In R. Wadey (Ed.), *Sport injury psychology: Cultural, relational, methodological, and applied considerations* (pp. 33–40). Routledge.

Niven, A. (2007). Rehabilitation adherence in sport injury: Sport physiotherapists' perceptions. *Journal of Sport Rehabilitation, 16*(2), 93–110. https://doi.org/10.1123/jsr.16.2.93

Poucher, Z., Tamminen, K. A., & Wagstaff, C. R. (2021). Organizational systems in British sport and their impact on athlete development and mental health. *The Sport Psychologist, 35*(4), 270–280. https://doi.org/10.1123/tsp.2020-0146

Putukian, M. (2016). The psychological response to injury in student athletes: A narrative review with a focus on mental health. *British Journal of Sports Medicine, 50*(3), 145–149.

Rees, T., Mitchell, I., Evans, L., & Hardy, L. (2010). Stressors, social support and psychological responses to sport injury in high- and low-performance standard participants. *Psychology of Sport and Exercise, 11*(6), 505–512. https://doi.org/10.1016/j.psychsport.2010.07.002

Souter, G., Lewis, R., & Serrant, L. (2018). Men, mental health and elite sport: A narrative review. *Sports Medicine Open, 4*(1), 57. https://doi.org/10.1186/s40798-018-0175-7

Sparkes, A. C., & Partington, S. (2003). Narrative practice and its potential contribution to sport psychology: The example of flow. *The Sport Psychologist, 17*(3), 292–317. https://doi.org/10.1123/tsp.17.3.292

Sparkes, A. C., & Smith, B. (2005). When narratives matter: Men, sport, and spinal cord injury. *Journal of Medical Ethics: Medical Humanities, 31*(2), 81–88. https://doi.org/10.1136/jmh.2005.000203

Wadey, R., & Day, M. (2022). Challenging the status quo of sport injury psychology to advance theory, research, and applied practice: An epilogue to a special issue. *Journal of Applied Sport Psychology, 34*(4), 1029–1036. https://doi.org/10.1080/10413200.2022.2100006

Wadey, R., Day, M., Cavallerio, F., & Martinelli, L. (2018). Multilevel model of sport injury (MMSI): Can coaches impact and be impacted by injury? In R. Thelwell & M. Dicks (Eds.), *Professional advances in sports coaching: Research and practice* (pp. 336–357). Routledge. https://doi.org/10.4324/9781351210980

Wadey, R., Roy-Davis, K., Evans, L., Howells, K., Salim, J., & Diss, C. (2019). Sport psychology consultants' perspectives on facilitating sport injury-related growth. *The Sport Psychologist, 33*(3), 244–255. https://doi.org/10.1123/tsp.2018-0110

Wiese-Bjornstal, D. M. (2009). Sport injury and college athlete health across the lifespan. *Journal of Intercollegiate Sport, 2*(1), 64–80. https://doi.org/10.1123/jis.2.1.64

Wiese-Bjornstal, D. M. (2019). Sociocultural aspects of sport injury and recovery. In E. O. Acevedo (Ed.), *The Oxford encyclopedia of sport, exercise, and performance psychology* (pp. 841–863). Oxford University Press.

Wiese-Bjornstal, D. M., Smith, A. M., Shaffer, S. M., & Morrey, M. A. (1998). An integrated model of response to sport injury: Psychological and sociological dynamics. *Journal of Applied Sport Psychology, 10*(1), 46–69. https://doi.org/10.1080/10413209808406377

Williams, J. M., & Andersen, M. B. (1998). Psychosocial antecedents of sport injury: Review and critique of the stress and injury model. *Journal of Applied Sport Psychology, 10*(1), 5–25. https://doi.org/10.1080/10413209808406375

Williams, T. J. (2020). Narratives matter! Storying sport injury experiences. In R. Wadey (Ed.), *Sport injury psychology: Cultural, relational, methodological, and applied considerations* (pp. 13–24). Routledge.

5 Psychosocial Understanding of Sport-Related Concussion

J. Jordan Utley, Judi Schack-Dugré, and Karen Menard

Chapter Objectives

- To explain sport-related concussion and the development of post-concussion symptoms.
- To outline the integrated model of psychological response to the sport concussion injury and rehabilitation process.
- To outline the roles of sport psychology and sports medicine professionals as members of an interprofessional SRC care team.

Introduction

Defined as "a traumatic brain injury induced by biomechanical forces" (McCrory et al., 2017, p. 839), *sport-related concussion* (SRC) is a common injury for participants at all levels of play and across different sports worldwide. SRC is classified as a mild traumatic brain injury (mTBI), thus considered to be on the less-severe end of the brain injury continuum (Harmon et al., 2013). Nevertheless, concussion injury has been declared a public health problem (Register-Mihalik et al., 2020), and this designation is due to many factors, such as improved awareness and research around the short-term and long-term effects of concussion.

While the short-term effects of SRC injury usually resolve within ten days, subsequently allowing return to sport participation (McCrory et al., 2017), long-term effects of SRC have been reported in 10–30% of cases (Cnossen et al., 2018). As many as 40% (Voormolen et al., 2019) to 64% (Bannon et al., 2020) of those diagnosed with mTBI experience post-concussion symptoms (formerly known as post-concussion syndrome) six months after injury onset. Defined as a collection of symptoms that fail to resolve in a usual time frame, affecting quality of life for 10–15% of SRC patients (Skjeldal et al., 2022), *post-concussion symptoms* can have significant long-term consequences. Voormolen et al. (2019) conveyed that mTBI patients ($n = 599$) with computed tomography (CT) scan abnormalities reported a significantly lower health-related quality of life, and nearly half were dissatisfied with post-injury functioning.

Contemporary research has focused on understanding the application of a biopsychosocial approach to SRC recovery, specifically as it relates to prolonged concussion symptoms influencing symptom presentation and persistence. Research also posits that biological, psychological, and sociological factors exist on a continuum and interact to shape the concussion recovery process. As a consequence, SRC care should address biological, psychological, and sociological factors (Register-Mihalik et al., 2020). Care should also include professionals trained to address the psychological and sociological impact of SRC as they are uniquely prepared to contribute to SRC rehabilitation in meaningful ways. Effective SRC care requires interprofessional

DOI: 10.4324/9781003295709-6

collaboration and continued communication between different professionals, with a goal to promote successful recovery. In the case of lingering post-concussion symptoms, care often includes referrals to specific experts who are not members of the primary interprofessional care team (Register-Mihalik et al., 2020). However, while interprofessional SRC care is recommended, this is rarely achieved in practice. The purpose of this chapter is to provide an overview of current understanding of biopsychosocial aspects of sport-related concussion. Specifically, this chapter will (a) introduce SRC and post-concussion symptoms, (b) outline the integrated model of psychological response to the SRC injury and rehabilitation process (Wiese-Bjornstal et al., 2015), (c) introduce most common biopsychosocial responses to SRC, and (d) highlight the roles of sport psychology (SPP) and sports medicine professionals (SMP) as members of an interprofessional SRC care team.

Overview of Sport-Related Concussion

Concussion injury is unlike other sport injuries – as there may be no physical indicator of dysfunction. The existing SRC consensus statement (McCrory et al., 2017) recognizes the central role of psychological and social factors in concussion diagnosis, symptom management, and recovery. Furthermore, if psychological and social factors are left unmanaged, they can contribute to post-concussion symptoms (Register-Mihalik et al., 2020).

Concussion Symptoms

While the symptomatic experience following a concussion will vary by individual, SRC is commonly diagnosed using the following clinical domains: (a) patient symptoms (somatic, cognitive, and emotional), (b) physical signs, (c) balance impairment, (d) behavioral changes, (e) cognitive impairment, and (f) sleep disturbances (McCrory et al., 2017). Common *somatic symptoms* can include headache and nausea. *Cognitive symptoms* can include confusion and inability to concentrate. *Emotional symptoms* include emotional lability (i.e., expression of excessive emotions and mood swings), usually resolving within ten days. *Physical signs* include, but are not limited to, (a) loss of consciousness, (b) retrograde or anterograde amnesia, (c) neurological deficits, and (d) *balance impairment. Behavioral signs* (e.g., irritability, isolation) are also considered a part of the diagnosis of SRC. Of central importance to sport and competition, *cognitive impairment* (e.g., slowed reaction time) and *sleep/wake disturbances* are commonly utilized to make the diagnosis (McCrory et al., 2017).

Psychological symptoms (e.g., cognitive and emotional symptoms, behavioral changes) are more common than once assumed (Rose et al., 2015). However, not all SRC patients experience them, and the reason some SRC patients do not develop psychological symptoms remains unclear (Skjeldal et al., 2022). The literature on SRC suggests that immediate circumstances following SRC may contribute to the development of post-concussion symptoms, including difficulty sleeping, depressed mood, increased negative stressors, and a perception of lacking social support (Iverson et al., 2021).

Post-Concussion Symptoms

Symptoms that fail to resolve within the usual time frame that results in a decrease in quality of life are commonly called post-concussion *symptoms* (Skjeldal et al., 2022). Post-concussion symptoms were formerly referred to as post-concussion *syndrome* (i.e., "a set of symptoms or conditions that occur together and suggest the presence of a certain disease or an increased chance of developing the disease" (National Cancer Institute, 2022, para 1). This terminology change was prompted for two main reasons: (a) the definition of *syndrome* is diagnostically inaccurate to describe symptoms experienced post-concussion, and (b) the term *syndrome* might have a negative connotation (Polinder et al., 2018; Skjeldal et al., 2022). Existing research has found that negative symptom perception is linked to less-favorable prognosis (Leddy et al., 2016). Even more salient, negative perceptions may also act as symptom-sustaining agents and even reinforce symptoms leading to extended recovery times (Næss-Schmidt et al., 2022).

Post-concussion symptoms can best be described as a constellation of somatic, cognitive, and emotional patient signs experienced on a continuum, with some hypothesized to be influenced by the individuals' family, medical, and psychosocial history (Register-Mihalik et al., 2020). Common *somatic* post-concussion symptoms include headache, fatigue, sleep disturbance, dizziness, photophobia, and phonophobia, visual disturbance, nausea, and tinnitus, of which post-concussive headache is the most prevalent symptom (Ashina et al., 2021). Common *cognitive* and *emotional* post-concussion symptoms include impaired concentration and memory, word-finding difficulty, and slowed cognition, as well as anxiety and depressed/altered mood (Dwyer & Katz, 2018; Fure et al., 2021; Hove et al., 2021; Voormolen et al., 2019).

The Integrated Model of Psychological Response to the Sport Concussion Injury and Rehabilitation Process

The integrated model of psychological response to the sport concussion injury and rehabilitation process (from now on referred to as the sport-concussion model; Wiese-Bjornstal et al., 2015) aims to provide an evidence-based conceptual framework for understanding the dynamic nature of biopsychosocial responses to SRC. In doing so, the model provides a useful tool to understand the interrelationships between various critical elements of the rehabilitation and recovery process. According to the sport-concussion model, and consistent with the stress and athletic injury model (Williams & Andersen, 1998), psychological risk factors that exist prior to SRC will influence both the individual's stress response to a stressful situation, which can amplify the risk of experiencing SRC, impacting the post-injury psychological response and rehabilitation process. These pre-injury psychological risk factors include *personality* (including attention-deficit/hyperactivity disorder or other brain-related disabilities), *history of stressors* (including post-traumatic stress disorder, life event stress), *coping resources* (e.g., coping style, social support), and any previous *interventions*, such as prior SRC education.

After experiencing SRC, along with pre-injury risk factors, several *personal factors* (e.g., injury characteristics and individual psychological, demographic, physical/behavioral differences) and *situational factors* (e.g., sport, social, and the environment) are proposed to influence the *neurobiological*, *psychogenic*, and *pathophysiological causes* of post-concussion symptoms. These will subsequently influence an individual's *cognitive symptoms and appraisals*, *affective symptoms and responses*, and *behavioral symptoms and responses* to SRC in a cyclical and bidirectional manner. This dynamic cognitive-affective-behavioral cycle will, in turn, influence the overall psychological outcomes of SRC. The model also proposes that both the dynamic cognitive-affective-behavioral cycle and the *psychological outcomes* are influenced by post-injury psychological care, including *assessments*, *providers*, and *interventions*.

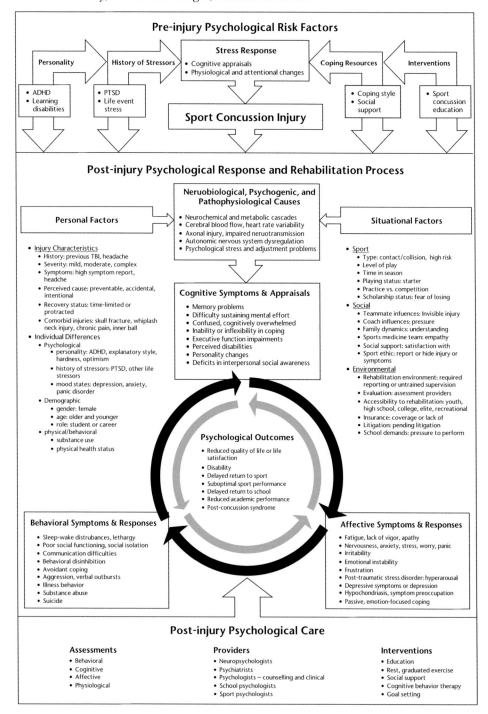

Figure 5.1 The integrated model of psychological response to the sport concussion injury and rehabilitation process.

Source: Reprinted with permission, from Diane M. Wiese-Bjornstal, Andrew C. White, Hayley C. Russell, & Aynsley M. Smith, 2005, Psychology of sport concussions, *4*(2), 169–189, https://doi.org/10.1123/kr.2015-0012.

Biopsychosocial Responses to Sport-Related Concussion

Research has yielded support for various factors contributing to the individual's SRC rehabilitation and recovery. What follows here is a brief summary of existing evidence to date as outlined by the sport-concussion model (Wiese-Bjornstal et al., 2015). Personality, sex, participation in organized sport, and concussion history have been studied in relation to their susceptibility to SRC and/or post-concussion symptoms. Existing literature has also highlighted the relation of various personal and situational factors to the responses to SRC and post-concussion recovery outcomes. According to the sport-concussion model, situational factors include the social, environmental, and economic implications, related to the neurobiological, psychogenic, and pathophysiological causes of symptoms and appraisals. Research indicates that existing neurobiological attributes, the physical burden of these symptoms, social support deficits, and perceived delayed recovery times may affect the incidence and severity of post-concussion symptoms (Register-Mihalik et al., 2020).

Pre-Injury Psychological Factors

The psychological pre-injury factors that have been supported in the literature as affecting post-concussion symptom risk include resilience, biological sex, SRC history, and involvement in organized sport. Additional pre-injury factors also associated with post-concussion symptoms include personality dispositions, life stress, mental health status, and premorbid pain (Skandsen et al., 2021). What follows here is a brief discussion of selected research evidence to date for each of the pre-injury factors outlined in the Wiese-Bjornstal et al. (2015) model.

Personality

Athletes ($n = 332$; aged 13 to 25) with lower levels of resilience have reported feeling less "back to normal" and increased symptom aggravation with physical and mental activity at three months post-SRC, compared to their more resilient counterparts (Bunt et al., 2021). In addition, high resilience levels in SRC patients have been found to correlate positively with personality traits of extroversion, agreeableness, and conscientiousness and negatively with pessimism, ADHD symptoms, and neuroticism (Skandsen et al, 2021). While this data suggests personality variable of resilience as being a key factor affecting SRC recovery, additional research to determine the strength of the relationship between resilience levels post-SRC with pre-SRC is warranted.

Sex Differences

A recent meta-analysis on SRC found that females reported a higher incidence and number of symptoms in comparison to males (Merritt et al., 2019). In comparison to males, females also appear to perform inferiorly on visual memory assessments post-concussion (Merritt et al., 2019) and are consistently associated with increased reporting of lingering post-concussion symptoms (Silverberg et al., 2015). Additional research has identified that hormones present in females during childbearing years may also affect SRC symptom experience (Bazarian et al., 2010). While existing research has identified biological sex differences in concussion symptom incidence, number, and duration of post-concussion symptoms, additional research is needed.

Sport-Related Concussion (SRC) History

Sport-related concussion history is also suggested to play a role in symptoms and recovery. Research assessing the influence of age at first SRC on post-concussion symptoms in collegiate athletes revealed sociodemographic equity, premorbidities, and sport type (contact, limited-contact, and non-contact sports) as impactful to clinical and cognitive outcomes, more so than age (Moody et al., 2022).

Participation in Organized Sports

Involvement in organized sport (leading to an SRC event) appears to provide a buffer to experiencing post-concussion symptoms and/or reducing the chronic nature of symptoms as compared to non-SRC mTBIs (Beauchamp et al., 2021). In related research with non-sport population, lower levels of education on mTBI in adults has been linked to higher incidence of post-concussion symptoms (Silverberg et al., 2015). The sport-concussion model hypothesizes that SRC education impacts resulting symptoms and appraisals of SRC injury; an athlete's knowledge of SRC and the potential for post-concussion symptoms may influence their experience of symptoms and the cognitive appraisals they form that shape their recovery.

Post-Injury Psychological Responses

Post-concussion symptoms are hypothesized to be the consequence of a continued cascade of the initial neurobiological changes, resulting in autonomic nervous system dysfunction (Purkayastha et al., 2019). Existing neurobiological attributes (i.e., individual differences in how the brain functions, including concentration and word-finding), the physical burden of these symptoms (i.e., post-concussion headache), psychosocial factors (e.g., being isolated from typical social support), and receiving less than expected evaluation of recovery progress from the SRC care team have also been found to affect the incidence and severity of post-concussion symptoms (Register-Mihalik et al., 2020). Case studies focused on post-concussion symptom resolution (including headache) have made the connection between neurobiological SRC causes and proposed psychosocial interventions (Hamson-Utley et al., 2019), supporting the theoretical conceptualizations proposed by Wiese-Bjornstal et al. (2015).

Social Support

Social support can influence post-SRC thoughts, feelings, and behaviors through relationships with teammates, coaches, SMPs, and family and significant others (Roderbourg et al., 2022). Research has connected both the social support provision and satisfaction with the support to post-concussion recovery. For example, disparities between desired and received social support negatively affect recovery (Roderbourg et al., 2022). Social support, community engagement, family dynamics, and lifestyle may also influence the development and persistence of post-concussion symptoms in adults (Silverberg & Iverson, 2011; Stålnacke, 2007) and children (Lumba-Brown et al., 2018). Lumba-Brown et al. (2018) also found that perceived pressure to perform (socially and behaviorally) during SRC recovery was common and considered to be a detractor to post-concussion recovery (Roderbourg et al., 2022).

Neurobiological, Psychogenic, and Pathophysiological Causes

The basic physiology of SRC is best described as a neurometabolic cascade of decreased cerebral blood flow (Purkayastha et al., 2019). The reduction in cerebral blood flow is proposed to be the cause for many of the acute concussion symptoms (Register-Mihalik et al., 2020). Even mild SRC may result in a temporary reduction in cerebral blood flow and cause cellular metabolic changes, such as receptor sensitivity and membrane regulation (Giza & Hovda, 2001; Howell & Southard, 2021). Research has also proposed an altered dynamic functional network connectivity in the brain (Biagianti et al., 2020) which could be linked to post-concussion symptoms, such as photophobia, phonophobia, and dizziness (Skjeldal et al., 2022).

Post-Concussion Symptom Persistence

Numerous demographics, pre-injury psychological factors, and post-injury psychological responses have been found to influence post-concussion symptom persistence. Age, level of education, and pre-injury mental health issues that co-exist with post-injury psychological responses of maladaptive coping and emotional distress have been found to be important recovery predictors at six months post-concussion (van der Naalt et al., 2017). Persistence of post-concussion symptoms has also been associated with high anxiety sensitivity (Wood et al., 2014), low resilience (Sullivan et al., 2016), and limited or maladaptive coping (Scheenen et al., 2017). Persistent post-concussion symptoms have also been found to leave patients feeling alone and unsure of how to manage their symptoms (Skjeldal et al., 2022).

Pressure to Return Participation

Athletes may feel the pressure of returning to participation from parents, coaches, teammates, and themselves. Such pressure is often linked to negative emotions related to loss of health and fitness, difficulties with absence of normal daily routines, and missing support of teammates as a consequence of being away from the sport setting (Kegelaers et al., 2022; McKay & Mellalieu, 2021). A qualitative case series of athletes' (*n* = 3) reintegration into sport participation post-concussion revealed a mismatch between self-pressure and perceived pressure from teammates and the desired and received social support (Caron et al., 2021). Athletes may also feel financial pressures to return to participation, particularly with elite athletes who depend on sport as a livelihood (Hamson-Utley et al., 2019).

Post-Injury Psychological Outcomes

The psychological post-injury outcomes include "experiences of somatic, cognitive, and emotional symptoms over months or even years . . . leading to functional limitations and quality of life" (Skandsen et al., 2021, p. 1102). Persistent psychological burden influences the biopsychosocial aspects of athlete recovery, which in turn may lead to self-injurious behaviors (Cassidy et al., 2014). A systematic review by Cassidy et al. (2014) concluded that poor pre-concussion mental health is associated with overall SRC recovery and can contribute to increased injury-related stress. Most SRC patients recover over one year, but persistent symptoms are more likely to be present in patients with more acute symptoms and higher emotional stress (Cassidy et al., 2014).

Recovery Status

Recent research has examined a constellation of personal factors associated with speed of recovery following mTBI. Skandsen et al. (2021) found that females (non-athletes) who scored lower on resilience and higher on pessimism, were employed less than full-time, and reported pre-concussion injury pain, headache, mental health problems, poor sleep quality, and significant negative life events recovered significantly slower than those in the control group at three months post-mTBI. A systematic review of the mTBI prognosis in adults concluded that slower recovery rate is associated with an increased number of initial cognitive deficits, premorbid physical health status, higher injury-related stress, persistent acute concussion symptoms (i.e., nausea, vomiting, headache), and high emotional distress (Cassidy et al., 2014).

Health-Related Quality of Life

Research has found SRC to be associated with short-term disablement and lower health-related quality of life (McGuine et al., 2019). Health-related quality of life may also be highly relevant to SRC as an insight into the recovery trajectory, including type and extent of the practical outcomes (von Steinbuechel et al., 2016). Research in the general population suggests that post-concussion symptoms correlate with lower levels of health-related quality of life and life satisfaction (van der Vlegel et al., 2021). Same is true with the athletic population, as deficits in health-related quality of life have been associated with time away from sport (Houston et al., 2016). In a longitudinal research with high school recreational and competitive athletes ($n = 125$), initial reports of disablement (high symptom score) and low health-related quality of life post-SRC stayed consistent until athletes reintegrated into sport, when the scores returned to baseline (McGuine et al., 2019). These findings were supported by Williamson and Wallace (2022), who proposed that adolescent athletes appear to rebound to baselines once back in sport regardless of recovery duration.

Health-related quality of life post-SRC also has financial implications. Parallels can be drawn between elite athletes returning to participation and the general population returning to work. The societal costs of mTBI include direct and indirect expenses related to seeking care and the value of missed time from work and/or reduced work efficiency (Burke et al., 2015; van der Vlegel et al., 2021). Financial pressures may contribute to the urgency to return to participation and create maladaptive thoughts and feelings associated with the inability to do so. The identification of mTBI as a public health problem coupled with a moderate number of patients (beyond athletes) with post-concussion symptoms creates the potential for substantial economic burden (Maas et al., 2017).

Interprofessional Approach to Sport-Related Concussion Care

Effective sport-related concussion management requires an interprofessional team of medical and health professionals working collaboratively to improve clinical outcomes (Institute of Medicine (IOM), 2015; World Health Organization, 2010). Building a team that includes essential knowledge, skills, and resources to facilitate a successful SRC recovery is a challenge, particularly as each athlete experiences clinical symptoms along a continuum. Some symptoms may be absent altogether, while some are a driving agent of daily dysfunction, thus dictating the need for various professionals to collaborate to advance recovery. Given the biopsychosocial nature of SRC (Wiese-Bjornstal et al., 2015), treatment should consider (a) physical factors that impact their patient's function and (b) psychosocial deficits that may stem from impairments impacting the patient's ability to engage and function in their roles, tasks, and activities (Gentry et al., 2018). Such approach lends to a holistic and balanced (Gentry et al., 2018; Gentry et al., 2021) athlete-centered approach to care. A biopsychosocial approach has been deemed most appropriate for concussion diagnosis and the treatment of post-concussion symptoms (Register-Mihalik et al., 2020).

Interprofessional SRC Care Team

The interprofessional SRC care team, by definition, should integrate perspectives from no less than two different professional backgrounds, with a goal to provide comprehensive, highest-quality care to the patient by working together with patients, families, and communities (Interprofessional Education Collaborative Expert Panel, 2011; World Health Organization, 2010). An interprofessional care plan should include "values and ethics for professional practice, identification of roles and responsibilities, interprofessional communication, and teamwork" (Interprofessional Education Collaborative Expert Panel, 2011). In SRC rehabilitation, potential professionals include, but are not limited to, physicians, athletic trainers, occupational therapists, physical therapists, and sport psychologists.

Each of the professionals listed can provide professional expertise that is necessary for successful SRC rehabilitation. For example, an athletic trainer (or other SMPs) is "typically the first providers to identify and evaluate injured persons and are integral in the post injury management and return to play decision-making process" (Broglio et al., 2014, p. 245). An occupational therapist has the competency to address physical and psychosocial limitations that influence functional independence and to provide a graded return to activity and school (DeMateo et al., 2017; Finn, 2019). A physical therapist (or physiotherapist) has the competency to address visual, oculomotor, cervical, balance, and vestibular impairments and make return to participation decisions (American Physical Therapy Association (APTA), 2019, 2020; Schneider & Gagnon, 2017). Sport psychology professionals, depending on their educational background and training (for more on role delineation and continuum of care, see Association for Applied Sport Psychology, 2021; Jones et al., 2022), can assist in psychological assessment and mental health screening and implement cognitive and behavioral interventions. In addition, clinically trained SPPs can also provide counseling for grief, depression, loss, and suicidal ideation. They can also address anger and aggression, sport participation and performance-related social issues, career transitions, and identity crisis, to name a few (American Psychological Association, 2023). Combining best practices in SRC management with effective interprofessional collaboration between different professionals will improve a safe return to participation (Kenrick-Rochon et al., 2020).

Building a Post-Concussion Care Plan

Upon establishing the interprofessional SRC care team (for more on interprofessional practice in sport injury, see Chapter 7), members of the team should collaboratively establish rehabilitation and recovery goals and interventions to meet the needs of the patient. Rest until asymptomatic is no longer the recommended care plan (Rytter et al., 2021; Silverberg et al., 2020). Instead, using a theoretical model (Wiese-Bjornstal et al., 2015) as a guide, a three-pronged care plan that addresses biological, psychological, and sociological factors is proposed as a model for best practice in post-concussion recovery (Register-Mihalik et al., 2020). Since post-concussion symptom recovery is highly individualized, existing research is yet to determine a standardized, evidence-based SRC care plan (Skjeldal et al., 2022). Thus, presenting interventions aimed at the biological, psychological, and sociological aspects of post-concussion recovery will provide an outline of potential elements of an individualized care plan.

Biological Post-Concussion Interventions

Biological post-concussion interventions should be designed and implemented based on the unique circumstances of the individual athlete and guided by the extent of the present SRC symptoms. For example, it is important to establish prior SRC history if previous SRC was diagnosed by a sports medicine professional, and history of any prior sub-concussive impacts (Polinder et al., 2018). It is important to note that symptom severity and physical brain injury have a weak correlation and that post-concussion symptoms can also be seen in athletes with non-mTBI injuries (Polinder et al., 2018). Many biological symptoms of SRC can be treated with interventions addressing autonomic, vestibulo-ocular, or cervical spine dysfunction. Notice that these areas and interventions will overlap as biological symptoms are intimately interwoven with one another.

Table 5.1 Predominant Autonomic Dysfunction Symptoms, Targeted Treatments, and Consulting Practitioners

Predominant Symptom(s)	Targeted Treatment(s)	Consulting Practitioner(s)
Abnormalities with sweating (too much or too little)	Behavior modification	Athletic trainer
	Coping strategies	Exercise physiologist
Blurry vision or reduced pupillary light reflex	Goal-setting strategies	Occupational therapist
Chest pain/discomfort with exertion	Neuroinflammation reduction	Physician
	Pacing activities	Physiotherapist
Depression	Relaxation strategies	Physical therapist
Fatigue	Supervised and prescribed/graded exercise testing/sessions that may require oxygen supplementation	Sport therapist
Headache		Sport psychologist
Light and sound sensitivity		
Orthostatic hypotension (fainting when standing up)	Visual integration	
	Work/play/environment analysis	
Unusual shortness of breath		
Vertigo		

Autonomic Dysfunction

Disruption to the autonomic system following mTBI can be broad and have significant consequences for the individual (Esterov & Greenwald, 2017). Autonomic dysfunction has also been correlated with depression (Esterov & Greenwald, 2017), highlighting the psychophysiological impact of SRC. The autonomic nervous system consists of two systems – sympathetic and parasympathetic – and functions as an unconscious regulator of critical functions within the body (Cleveland Clinic, 2023a). The sympathetic system prepares the body to respond when the "fight-or-flight" response has been activated to a perceived threat. The parasympathetic nervous system generally works to maintain homeostasis in the body and regulates the cardiovascular system, multiple endocrine and exocrine glands, while also innervating smooth muscle.

Vestibulo-Ocular Symptoms

Disruption to the vestibulo-ocular system can result in symptoms such as movement-related dizziness, blurry vision, difficulty maintaining balance with head movements, and nausea. Vestibulo-ocular symptoms are frequently present following an SRC, and dizziness is considered a risk factor for a prolonged recovery (Wallace & Lifshitz, 2016). Vestibulo-ocular symptoms can be intimately linked with cervical spine region injury, and treatment can occur concurrently due to the anatomical redundancies of these two regions (Wallace & Lifshitz, 2016). Normal function of the vestibulo-ocular reflex coordinates eye movement with head movement to provide clear vision during motion and maintenance of balance (Andreas et al., 2021; Sinnott et al., 2019; Wallace & Lifshitz, 2016). Normal function is necessary in carrying out activities of daily living (e.g., walking and driving), and it is important in higher-demand activities (e.g., sports).

Cervical Spine Dysfunction

Disruption to the cervical spine can cause multiple symptoms, such as whiplash, neck pain, and headaches, following SRC (Morin et al., 2016). Soft tissue or spinal injury including neurological structures subjected to trauma in the cervical region can be challenging to treat without

Table 5.2 Predominant Vestibulo-Ocular Dysfunction Symptoms, Targeted Treatments, and Consulting Practitioners

Predominant Symptom(s)	Targeted Treatment(s)	Consulting Practitioner(s)
Disrupted balance (during ambulation)	Balance/vestibular rehabilitation	Athletic trainer
Dizziness	Cervical spine rehabilitation (soft tissue condition, segmental mobility, functional strength, and active range of motion)	Exercise physiologist
Vestibular symptoms (vertigo)		Occupational therapist
Visual dysfunction		Physician
	Coping strategies	Physiotherapist
	Gait training	Physical therapist
	Neuroinflammation reduction	Sport therapist
	Postural re-education	Sport psychologist
	Relaxation strategies	Vision therapist
	Visual integration	
	Work/play/environment analysis	

Table 5.3 Predominant Cervical Spine Dysfunction Symptoms, Targeted Treatments, and Consulting Practitioners

Predominant Symptom(s)	Targeted Treatment(s)	Consulting Practitioner(s)
Fatigue	Behavior modification	Athletic trainer
Headache	Cervical spine rehabilitation (soft tissue condition, segmental mobility, functional strength, and active range of motion)	Exercise physiologist
Whiplash symptoms (soft tissue injury – guarding/ spasm, shortening, tenderness to palpation, reduced range of motion and blood flow)		Occupational therapist
		Physician
	Postural re-education	Physiotherapist
	Relaxation strategies	Physical therapist
	Sleep/wake cycles	Sport therapist
	Work/play/environment analysis	Sport psychologist

triggering a symptom. Post-traumatic headaches are reported as one of the most incapacitating symptoms following SRC. Physical, behavioral, and pharmacological interventions are frequently incorporated into treatment. Normal function of the cervical spine protects the spinal cord, supports the head to allow for movement, and provides a protective passageway for vertebral arteries (Cleveland Clinic, 2023b).

Psychological Post-Concussion Interventions

Psychological post-concussion interventions should be designed and implemented based on the unique circumstances of the individual athlete and guided by the extent of the present SRC symptoms. For example, it is important to establish prior SRC psychological history, as these symptoms may be exacerbated following SRC (McCrory et al., 2017). Interventions related to the psychological well-being of the post-concussed athlete are paramount. SPPs and SMPs can contribute to SRC recovery and quality of life by addressing psychosocial factors within their scope of practice. Psychological pre-concussion risk factors are considered important in influencing how an athlete may respond to an SRC (Wiese-Bjornstal et al., 2015). For example, psychological factors (e.g., lack of concentration, attentional focus shifts due to an attention-deficit disorder) that may have predisposed an athlete to SRC are likely to carry over to post-concussion. Post-injury, numerous psychosocial responses (e.g., irritability, anxiety, depression, cognitive changes, and mood swings) are likely to influence biological symptoms and physical and psychosocial SRC rehabilitation and recovery (Wiese-Bjornstal et al., 2015).

Sleep

Given the significant amount of biological disruption and neurometabolic requirements for healing following an SRC (Giza & Hovda, 2001; Wallace & Lifshitz, 2016), the athlete's ability to rest is essential for restorative processes to occur (Doherty et al., 2021). Sleep disturbances are common symptoms of SRC, and lack of sleep may cause or contribute to comorbidities, such as mood swings, anxiety, fatigue, cognitive deficits, and increased perceptions of pain. Sleep disturbances can also slow recovery and may perpetuate non-recovery (Considine et al., 2021). As such, not just sleep, but *effective* sleep, is a necessary component of recovery. Screening for sleep efficacy and understanding an athlete's sleep cycle may require adaptations to the athlete's plan of care and/or referral for a sleep assessment, both of which may contribute to the recovery outcomes. Cognitive behavioral therapy has also been found to be effective in regulating sleep disorders post-concussion (Vaduvathiriyan et al., 2020).

Nutrition

As the body's metabolic needs are enhanced following SRC, it is logical to assume that as the healing progresses, intentional nutrition consumption would be important. The consumption of appropriate amounts of calories and macronutrients, especially proteins, has been found beneficial for reducing length of hospital stay during the acute phase of SRC (Finnegan et al., 2022). In the later stages of recovery, the use of supplements such as omega-3 fatty acids and vitamin has been found to have a positive effect on some athletes with mTBI (Finnegan et al., 2022).

Cognitive-Emotional Disturbances

Mood changes, such as sadness, irritability, anxiety, hypervigilance, and sleep disturbance (Kontos et al., 2012; Sandel et al., 2017), have a significant effect on the athlete's recovery and return to play. If not treated properly, mood changes can become chronic post-concussive symptoms and cause functional impairment, especially in patients with pre-existing clinical conditions. The need to understand and address SRC emotional disturbances (e.g., coping, depression, anxiety, and post-traumatic stress) is important to manage any possible negative behavioral consequences (Clement & Arvinen-Barrow, 2013; Kontos et al., 2017; Scheenen et al., 2017). These cognitive-emotional disturbances can hinder the athlete's ability to feel connected to the team and ultimately return to participation.

Functional Cognitive Disturbances

Functional cognition is "the cognitive ability to perform daily life tasks" (Giles et al., 2020, p. 2); therefore, impaired cognition may significantly impact an individual's ability to return to daily activities that require higher-level cognition (Taylor-Postma et al., 2022). Cognitive fatigue and impairments are identified as clinical symptoms following SRC (Covassin & Elbin, 2010; Sandel et al., 2017). Symptoms may include low energy, fatigue, and significant disturbances

Table 5.4 Predominant Cognitive-Affective Symptoms, Targeted Treatments, and Consulting Practitioners

Predominant Symptom(s)	Targeted Treatment(s)	Consulting Practitioner(s)
Anxiety	Behavioral management	Athletic trainer
Apathy	Coping strategies	Cognitive psychologist
Depression	Journaling	Certified Mental Performance Consultant
Fatigue	Patient education on post-concussion symptoms	
Hypervigilance		Exercise psychologist
Irritability	Positive self-talk	Licensed clinical mental health professional
Mood swings	Relaxation strategies	
Ruminative thinking	Self-regulation strategies	Occupational therapist
Self-esteem concerns (tied to sport)	Sleep regulation	Physician
	Stress management	Physical therapist
Sleep disruption	Short-term goal setting	Physiotherapist
Stress	Work/play/environment analysis	Sports therapist
		Sport psychologist

Table 5.5 Predominant Functional Cognitive Disturbance Symptoms, Targeted Treatments, and Consulting Practitioners

Predominant Symptom(s)	Targeted Treatment(s)	Consulting Practitioner(s)
Catastrophizing	Cognitive rehabilitation	Athletic trainer
Cognitive fatigue	Establish routines	Cognitive psychologist
Confusion	Goal setting	Licensed clinical mental health professionals
Delayed executive functioning	Journaling	
Difficulty concentrating	Pacing to minimize cognitive load	Occupational therapist
Difficulty sequencing	Sleep regulation	Physical therapist
Disorientation	Stress management	Physiotherapist
Fatigue, low energy	Work/play/environment analysis	Sport professionals
Short-term memory; difficulties with recall		Sport psychologist
Sleep disruption		
Stress		

to concentration, attention, and memory. Athletes tend to minimize these functional cognitive symptoms for fear of being withheld from sport or due to lack of awareness of the signs of SRC (Covassin & Elbin, 2010). Interventions that focus on stress management and/or coping can be used (Hove et al., 2021; Voormolen et al., 2019) to facilitate return to daily activities, including sport. Normal functional cognition shows as an ability to problem-solve and complete daily tasks while considering shifting in contextual and environmental factors (Giles et al., 2020). To achieve normal functional cognition, the interprofessional team can guide the athletes in gaining competence with activities of daily living, essential functions, and return to participation.

Table 5.6 Predominant Social Disturbance Symptoms, Targeted Treatments, and Consulting Practitioners

Predominant Symptom(s)	Targeted Treatment(s)	Consulting Practitioner(s)
Anxiety	Coping skills	Athletic trainer
Depression	Establish routines	Cognitive psychologist
Self-esteem concerns (related to sports)	Goal setting	Licensed clinical mental health occupational therapist
	Journaling	
Social isolation	Social support, including peer, family, team, and coach	Physical therapist
		Physiotherapist
	Work/play/environment analysis	Sports professionals
		Sport psychologist

Social

The athlete's status and connection with their team members are an important part of the sport experience (Caron et al., 2021), highlighting the importance of reintegration into the team structure following an SRC. Addressing the connection between an athlete's personal and social identities, identifying underlying feelings of the pressure to return, and recognizing possible challenges of providing (and receiving) social support are paramount for SRC recovery (Caron et al., 2021). Athletes with mTBI symptoms may also have trouble with social relationships (Bannon et al., 2020), thus recognizing that each athlete's social needs may vary. To facilitate successful social integration, members of the sport community should be educated about SRCs, how to effectively communicate with and provide support to athletes with SRC (Roderbourg et al., 2022).

Conclusion

The role of implementing a biopsychosocial approach to SRC rehabilitation was explored in this chapter. The chapter defined SRC, post-concussion symptoms, and addressed the terminology change from sports-related concussion *syndrome* to sports-related concussion *symptoms*. The integrated model of psychological response to the sport concussion injury and rehabilitation process (Wiese-Bjornstal et al., 2015) was introduced to the reader, followed by evidence in support of various biological, psychological, and social factors influencing SRC risk, rehabilitation, and return to participation. The necessity of adopting an interprofessional approach to SRC rehabilitation was outlined, and suggestions for areas of targeted treatment interventions were identified.

Case Study

Grace started participating in triathlons when she was 28. Over the past five years, since turning 40, she has been winning the top three finishing times in just about every race. The week after Grace turned 45, she was hit by a car on a training bike ride and sustained multiple orthopedic injuries. Following surgery to stabilize her left acetabulum, femur, tibia, and fibula, and left ulna and radius, the nurses noticed that Grace was increasingly agitated and was having a hard time following commands. Initially, the surgeon told Grace's husband, Eric, that the anesthesia caused agitation and confusion; however, the symptoms worsened as the anesthesia wore off.

Grace complained to her nurse, "I have a splitting headache, and I can't pay attention to what my husband is saying to me!" The nurse reached out to the doctor, and following a brief exam, the doctor ordered an MRI. The MRI revealed that Grace had sustained a mild concussion from the accident. Two days later, Grace was discharged from the hospital with discharge instructions that included orthopedic precautions and follow-up care. Grace was also instructed to eliminate screen time and to "rest her eyes and take it easy" for the next two weeks.

Six months later, Grace's range of motion and strength returned, but she struggled to run short distances. After one of the training runs, Grace called her mom, Savannah, in distress and began to cry. "I feel like everything is falling apart around me. I can't even run down the block without getting a headache! Besides that, everything is blurry. I'm having a hard time reading notes on the refrigerator, and I get super anxious when trying to read my phone, even though I made it large print. I can't sleep through the night, and I am always mad at Eric!"

Later that same day, Savannah dropped by to bring Eric and Grace dinner. When Grace went to the bathroom, Savannah mentioned the phone call she had earlier with Grace to Eric, who responded, "I am not surprised. Grace seems to have a hard time driving from one place to another, and she hardly makes dinner anymore. She used to love to cook, and now the kitchen seems to make her agitated and anxious."

The next day, Savannah called Grace and asked her if she could bring meals over. Grace became defensive and yelled, "Stop treating me like a baby! I do not need your help." In the evening, Grace shares her outburst with Eric. "I know I should not have yelled at my mom. It's like something just came over me, and I cannot help it. I don't know what is wrong with me."

Eric hugged Grace and said, "You have been complaining about visual disturbances, insomnia, cognitive dysfunction, bad runs and bike rides for a long time now. I feel you are constantly stressed and that is limiting your daily function. Ever since the accident . . . I feel like the '*new Grace*' is not the same as the '*old Grace*,' and it has impacted your quality of life and . . . our relationship." Grace was quiet. Eric continued, "I know this is not what you want to hear, but . . . I think you need to see your primary care physician to get this figured out."

Grace's primary care physician issued an interprofessional care. Her post-concussion symptom rehabilitation plan included exercise therapy, vestibular therapy, sleep therapy, stress/emotion management, functional cognition management, and sport/life re-entry.

Questions

1. Consistent with the integrated model of psychological response to the sport concussion injury and rehabilitation process, what pre- and post-injury factors are important to consider when designing Grace's post-concussion care plan?
2. What personal and situational factors are influencing Grace's neurobiological, psychogenic, and pathophysiological causes of SRC?
3. In Grace's case, who should make up her interprofessional SRC care team, and why?
4. What biological and psychological interventions that are within your professional competencies would you implement in Grace's care, and why?

References

American Physical Therapy Association (APTA). (2019). *The physical therapist's role in management of individuals with concussion: HOD P06-19-40-14*. www.apta.org/siteassets/pdfs/policies/pt-management-concussion.pdf

American Physical Therapy Association (APTA). (2020). *Protecting student athletes from concussions act* (H.R.5611/S.2600). www.apta.org/advocacy/issues/position-paper-protecting-student-athletes-from-concussions-act#

American Psychological Association. (2023). *Sports psychology*. www.apa.org/ed/graduate/specialize/sports

Andreas, N., Molitor, W., & Dubisar, L. (2021). Managing concussion: Occupational therapy's role in evaluating and treating athletes. *OT Practice*. www.aota.org/publications/ot-practice/ot-practice-issues/2021/managing-concussion

Ashina, H., Eigenbrodt, A. K., Seifert, T., Sinclair, A. J., Scher, A. I., Schytz., H. W., . . . Ashina, M. (2021). Post-traumatic headache attributed to traumatic brain injury: Classification, clinical characteristics, and treatment. *The Lancet Neurology*, *20*(6), 460–469. https://doi.org/10.1016/S1474-4422(21)00094-6

Association for Applied Sport Psychology. (2021). *AASP statement on the continuum of mental health & relationship to performance. A response to the conversation supporting Naomi Osaka and Simon Biles*. Retrieved November 13, from https://appliedsportpsych.org/media/news-releases-and-association-updates/aasp-statement-on-the-continuum-of-mental-health-and-relationship-to-performance-a-response-to-the-conversation-supporting/

Bannon, S., Greenberg, J., Golden, J., O'Leary, D., & Vranceanu, A. M. (2020). A social blow: The role of interpersonal relationships in mild traumatic brain injury. *Psychosomatics*, *61*(5), 518–526. https://doi.org/10.1016/j.psym.2020.04.003

Bazarian, J. J., Blyth, B., Mookerjee, S., He, H., & McDermott, M. (2010). Sex differences in outcome after mild traumatic brain injury. *Journal of Neurotrauma*, *27*(3), 527–539. https://doi.org/10.1089/neu.2009.1068

Beauchamp, F., Boucher, V., Neveu, X., Ouellet, V., Archambault, P., Berthelot, S., . . . Le Sage, N. (2021). Post-concussion symptoms in sports-related mild traumatic brain injury compared to non-sports-related mild traumatic brain injury. *Canadian Journal of Emergency Medicine*, *23*(2), 223–231. https://doi.org/10.1007/s43678-020-00060-0

Biagianti, B., Stocchetti, N., Brambilla, P., & Van Vleet, T. (2020). Brain dysfunction underlying prolonged post-concussive syndrome: A systematic review. *Journal of Affective Disorders*, *1*(262), 71–76. https://doi.org/10.1016/j.jad.2019.10.058

Broglio, S., Cantu, R., Guskiewicz, K., Kutcher, J., Palm, M., & Valovich McLeod, T. (2014). National Athletic Trainers' Association position statement: Management of sport concussion. *Journal of Athletic Training*, *49*(2), 245–265. https://doi.org/10.4085/1062-6050-49.1.07

Bunt, S., Meredith-Duliba, T., Didehhani, N., Hynan, L., LoBue, C., Stokes, M., . . . Cullum, C. M. (2021). Resilience and recovery from sports related concussion in adolescents and young adults. *Journal of Clinical and Experimental Neuropsychology*, *43*(7), 677–688. https://doi.org/10.1080/13803395.2021.1990214

Burke, M., Fralick, M., Nejatbakhsh, N., Tartaglia, M., & Tator, C. (2015). In search of evidence-based treatment for concussion: Characteristics of current clinical trials. *Brain Injury*, *29*(300), 300–305. https://doi.org/10.3109/02699052.2014.974673

Caron, J. G., Benson, A. J., Steins, R., McKenzie, L., & Bruner, M. W. (2021). The social dynamics involved in recovery and return to sport following a sport-related concussion: A study of three athlete-teammate-coach triads. *Psychology of Sport and Exercise*, *52*, 101824. https://doi.org/10.1016/j.psychsport.2020.101824

Cassidy, J. D., Cancelliere, C., Carroll, L. J., Côté, P., Hincapié, C. A., Holm, L. W., . . . Borg, J. (2014). Systematic review of self-reported prognosis in adults after mild traumatic brain injury: Results of the international collaboration on mild traumatic brain injury prognosis. *Archives of Physical Medicine and Rehabilitation*, *95*(3), S132–S151. https://doi.org/10.1016/j.apmr.2013.08.299

Clement, D., & Arvinen-Barrow, M. (2013). Sport medicine team influences in psychological rehabilitation: A multidisciplinary approach. In M. Arvinen-Barrow & N. Walker (Eds.), *The psychology of sport injury and rehabilitation* (pp. 156–170). Routledge.

Cleveland Clinic. (2023a). *Autonomic nervous system.* https://my.clevelandclinic.org/health/body/23273-autonomic-nervous-system

Cleveland Clinic. (2023b). *Cervical spine.* https://my.clevelandclinic.org/health/articles/22278-cervical-spine

Cnossen, M., van der Naalt, J., Spikman, J., Nieboer, D., Yue, J., Windler, E., . . . Lingsma, H. (2018). Prediction of persistent post-concussion symptoms after mild traumatic brain injury. *Neurotrauma, 35*(22), 2691–2698. https://doi.org/10.1089/neu.2017.5486

Considine, C., Huber, D., Niemuth, A., Thomas, D., McCrea, M., & Nelson, L. (2021). Relationship between sport-related concussion and sleep based on self-report and commercial actigraph measurement. *Neurotrauma Reports, 2*(1), 214–223. https://doi.org/10.1089/neur.2021.0008

Covassin, T., & Elbin, R. (2010). The cognitive effects and decrements following concussion. *Open Access Journal of Sports Medicine, 12*(1), 55–61. https://doi.org/10.2147/oajsm.s6919

DeMateo, C., Reed, N., & Stazyk, K. (2017). The role of the occupational therapist in concussion management: What can the occupational therapist do? In I. Gagnon & A. Ptito (Eds.), *Sport concussions: A complete guide to recovery and management.* CRC Press. https://doi.org/10.1201/9781315119328

Doherty, R., Madigan, S., Nevill, A., Warrington, G., & Ellis, J. (2021). The sleep and recovery practices of athletes. *Nutrients, 13*(4), 1330. https://doi.org/10.3390/nu13041330

Dwyer, B., & Katz, D. (2018). Postconcussion syndrome. *Handbook of Clinical Neurology, 158*(3), 163–178. https://doi.org/10.1016/B978-0-444-63954-7.00017-3

Esterov, D., & Greenwald, B. (2017). Autonomic dysfunction after mild traumatic brain injury. *Brain Science, 7*(8), 100. https://doi.org/10.3390/brainsci7080100

Finn, C. (2019). Occupational therapists' perceived confidence in the management of concussion: Implications for occupational therapy education. *Occupational Therapy International, 9245153.* https://doi.org/10/1155/2019/9245153

Finnegan, E., Daly, E., Pearce, A., & Ryan, L. (2022). Nutritional interventions to support acute mTBI recovery. *Frontiers in Nutrition, 9,* 977728. https://doi.org/10.3389/fnut.2022.977728

Fure, S., Howe, E., Spjelkavik, Ø., Roe, C., Rike, P., Olsen, A., . . . Lovstad, M. (2021). Post-concussion symptoms three months after mild-to-moderate TBI: Characteristics of sick-listed athletes referred to specialized treatment and consequences of intracranial injury. *Brain Injury, 35*(9), 1054–1064. https://doi.org/10.1080/02699052.2021.1953593

Gentry, K., Snyder, K., Barstow, B., & Hamson-Utley, J. J. (2018). The biopsychosocial model: Application to occupational therapy practice. *The Open Journal of Occupational Therapy, 6*(4). https://doi.org/10.15453/2168-6408.1412

Gentry, K., Snyder, K., & Hamson-Utley, J. J. (2021). Clinical utility of the adapted biopsychosocial model: An initial validation through peer review. *The Open Journal of Occupational Therapy, 9*(2). https://doi.org/10.15453/2168-6408.1750

Giles, G. M., Edwards, D. F., Baum, C., Furniss, J., Skidmore, E., Wolf, T., & Leland, N. E. (2020). Making functional cognition a professional priority. *American Journal of Occupational Therapy, 74*(1), 090010. https://doi.org/10.5014/ajot.2020.741002

Giza, C., & Hovda, D. (2001). The neurometabolic cascade of concussion. *Journal of Athletic Training, 36*(3), 228–235. www.ncbi.nlm.nih.gov/pmc/articles/PMC155411/

Hamson-Utley, J. J., Kamphoff, C., & Oshikoya, C. (2019). Reactions to a circus injury: Jan Smith, an aerial performer, Cirque du Soleil. In M. Arvinen-Barrow & D. Clement (Eds.), *The psychology of sport and performance injury: An interprofessional, case-based approach* (pp. 27–41). Routledge.

Harmon, K. G., Drezner, J., Gammons, M., Guskiewicz, K., Halstead, M., Herring, S., . . . Roberts, W. (2013). American medical society for sports medicine position statement: Concussion in sport. *Clinical Journal of Sport Medicine, 23*(1), 1–18. https://doi.org/10.1136/bjsports-2012-091941

Houston, M., Bay, R., & Valovich McLeod, T. (2016). The relationship between post-injury measures of cognition, balance, symptom reports and health-related quality-of-life in adolescent athletes with concussion. *Brain Injury, 30*(7), 891–898. https://doi.org/10.3109/02699052.2016.1146960

Hove, K., Lodden, C., Mock, E., Roe, M., Schultz, L., & Jones, J. (2021). Implementation of biofeedback interventions for the treatment of adults with postconcussion syndrome. *American Journal of Occupational Therapy*, *75*(S2), 7512520388p7512520381. https://doi.org/10.5014/ajot.2021.75S2-RP388

Howell, D., & Southard, J. (2021). The molecular pathophysiology of concussion. *Clinical Sports Medicine*, *40*(1), 39–51. https://doi.org/10.1016/j.csm.2020.08.001

Institute of Medicine (IOM). (2015). *Institute of medicine report*. https://me-pedia.org/wiki/Institute_of_Medicine_report

Interprofessional Education Collaborative Expert Panel. (2011). *Core competencies for interprofessional collaborative practice: Report of an expert panel*. www.aacnnursing.org/Portals/42/Population%20Health/IPECReport.pdf

Iverson, G., Silverberg, N., & Zasler, N. (2021). Mild traumatic brain injury. In N. Zasler, D. Katz, & Z. R (Eds.), *Brain injury medicine* (3rd ed.). Springer Publishing Company. https://doi.org/10.1891/9780826143051.0028

Jones, M., Zakrajsek, R., & Eckenrod, M. (2022). Mental performance and mental health services in NCAA D1 athletic departments. *Journal for Advancing Sport Psychology in Research*, *2*(1), 4–18. https://doi.org/10.55743/0000010

Kegelaers, J., Wylleman, P., Defruyt, S., Praet, L., Stambulova, N., Torregrossa, M., . . . De Brandt, K. (2022). The mental health of student-athletes: A systematic scoping review. *International Review of Sport and Exercise Psychology*, *14*(1), 1–34. https://doi.org/10.1080/1750984X.2022.2095657

Kenrick-Rochon, S., Quesnele, J., Aldisera, T., Laurence, M., & Grenier, S. (2020). Does interprofessional concussion management improve recovery in varsity athletes? A year to year effectiveness-implementation hybrid study. *Physical Therapy in Sport*, *47*, 32–39. https://doi.org/10.1016/j.ptsp.2020.10.008

Kontos, A. P., Deitrick, J. M., Collins, M. W., & Mucha, A. (2017). Review of vestibular and oculomotor screening and concussion rehabilitation. *Journal of Athletic Training*, *52*(3), 256–261. https://doi.org/10.4085/1062-6050-51.11.05

Kontos, A. P., Elbin, R., Schatz, P., Covassin, T., Henry, L., Pardini, J., & Collins, M. (2012). A revised factor structure for the post-concussion symptom scale: Baseline and postconcussion factors. *The American Journal of Sports Medicine*, *40*(10), 2375–2384. https://doi.org/10.1177/0363546512455400

Leddy, J., Baker, J., & Willer, B. (2016). Active rehabilitation of concussion and post-concussion syndrome. *Physical Medicine and Rehabilitation Clinics*, *27*(2), 437–454. https://doi.org/10.1016/j.pmr.2015.12.003

Lumba-Brown, A., Yeates, K. O., Sarmiento, K., Breiding, M. J., Haegerich, T. M., Gioia, G. A., . . . Timmons, S. D. (2018). Centers for disease control and prevention guideline on the diagnosis and management of mild traumatic brain injury among children. *JAMA Pediatrics*, *172*(11), e182853. https://doi.org/10.1001/jamapediatrics.2018.2853

Maas, M., Adelson, P., & Andelic, N. (2017). Traumatic brain injury – integrated approaches to improving clinical care and research. *The Lancet Neurology*, *16*(12), 987–1048. https://doi.org/10.1016/S1474-4422(17)30371-X

McCrory, P., Meeuwisse, W., Dvorak, J., Aubry, M., Bailes, J., Broglio, S., . . . Vos, P. E. (2017). Consensus statement on concussion in sport – the 5th international conference on concussion in sport held in Berlin, October 2016. *British Journal of Sports Medicine*, *51*(11), 838–847. https://doi.org/10.1136/bjsports-2017-097699

McGuine, T., Pfaller, A., Kliethermes, S., Schwarz, A., Hetzel, S., Hammer, E., & Broglio, S. (2019). The effect of sport-related concussion injuries on concussion symptoms and health-related quality of life in male and female adolescent athletes: A prospective study. *The American Journal of Sports Medicine*, *47*(14), 3514–3520. https://doi.org/10.1177/0363546519880175

McKay, C. D., & Mellalieu, S. D. (2021). When injuries lead to retirement: Calling it a day. In C. D. McKay (Ed.), *The mental impact of sports injury* (pp. 153–166). Routledge.

Merritt, V. C., Padgett, C. R., & Jak, A. J. (2019). A systematic review of sex differences in concussion outcome: What do we know? *The Clinical Neuropsychologist*, *33*(6), 1016–1043. https://doi.org/10.1080/13854046.2018.1508616

Moody, J., Hayes, J., Buckley, T., Schmidt, J., Broglio, S., McAllister, T., . . . CARE Consortium Investigators. (2022). Age of first concussion and cognitive, psychological, and physical outcomes in

NCAA collegiate student athletes. *Sports Medicine*, *52*(11), 2759–2773. https://doi.org/10.1007/s40279-022-01719-7

Morin, M., Langevin, P., & Fait, P. (2016). Cervical spine involvement in mild traumatic brain injury: A review. *Journal of Sports Medicine*, 1590161. https://doi.org/10.1155/2016/1590161

Næss-Schmidt, E. T., Thastum, M. M., Stabel, H. H., Odgaard, L., Pedersen, A. R., Rask, C. U., . . . Nielsen, J. F. (2022). Interdisciplinary intervention (GAIN) for adults with post-concussion symptoms: A study protocol for a stepped-wedge cluster randomised trial. *Trials*, *23*(1), 613 https://doi.org/10.1186/s13063-022-06572-7

National Cancer Institute. (2022). *Dictionary of cancer terms*. www.cancer.gov/publications/dictionaries/cancer-terms/def/syndrome

Polinder, S., Cnossen, M. C., Real, R. G., Covic, A., Gorbunova, A., Voormolen, D. C., . . . Von Steinbuchel, N. (2018). A multidimensional approach to post-concussion symptoms in mild traumatic brain injury. *Frontiers in Neurology*, *9*, 1113. https://doi.org/10.3389/fneur.2018.01113

Purkayastha, S., Williams, B., Murphy, M., Lyng, S., Sabo, T., & Bell, K. (2019). Reduced heart rate variability and lower cerebral blood flow associated with poor cognition during recovery following concussion. *Autonomic Neuroscience*, *220*, 102548. https://doi.org/10.1016/j.autneu.2019.04.004

Register-Mihalik, J., DeFreese, J. D., Callahan, C., & Carneiro, K. (2020). Utilizing the biopsychosocial model in concussion treatment: Post-traumatic headache and beyond. *Current Pain and Headache Reports*, *24*(8), 44. https://doi.org/10.1007/s11916-020-00870-y

Roderbourg, L., Bianco, T., Sweet, S., & Caron, J. (2022). Desired and received social support following a sport-related concussion: Discrepancies between student-athletes and their social network. *Journal of Exercise, Movement, and Sport (SCAPPS Refereed Abstracts Repository)*, *53*(1). www.scapps.org/jems/index.php/1/article/view/2841.

Rose, S., Fischer, A., & Heyer, G. (2015). How long is too long? The lack of consensus regarding the post concussion syndrome diagnosis. *Brain Injury*, *29*(7–8), 798–803. https://doi.org/10.3109/02699052.2015.1004756

Rytter, H., Graff, H., Henriksen, H., Aaen, N., Hartvigsen, J., Hoegh, M., . . . Callesen, H. (2021). Non-pharmacological treatment of persistent post concussion symptoms in adults: A systematic review and meta-analysis and guideline recommendation. *JAMA Network Open*, *4*(11). https://doi.org/10.1001/jamanetworkopen.2021.32221

Sandel, N., Reynolds, E., Cohen, P., Gillie, B., & Kontos, A. (2017). Anxiety and mood clinical profile following sport-related concussion: From risk factors to treatment. *Sport, Exercise, and Performance Psychology*, *6*(3), 304–323. https://doi.org/10.1037/spy0000098

Scheenen, M., Spikman, J., De Koning, M., Van Der Horn, H., Roks, G., Hageman, G., & van der Naalt, J. (2017). Patients "at risk" of suffering from persistent complaints after mild traumatic brain injury: The role of coping, mood disorders, and post-traumatic stress. *Journal of Neurotrauma*, *34*(1), 31–37. https://doi.org/10.1089/neu.2015.4381

Schneider, K., & Gagnon, I. (2017). Physiotherapy and concussion: What can the physiotherapist do? In I. Gagnon & A. Ptito (Eds.), *Sport concussions: A complete guide to recovery and management*. CRC Press. https://doi.org/10.1201/9781315119328

Silverberg, N., Gardner, A., Brubacher, J., Panenka, W., Li, J., & Iverson, G. (2015). Systematic review of multivariable prognostic models for mild traumatic brain injury. *Journal of Neurotrauma*, *32*(8), 517–526. https://doi.org/10.1089/neu.2014.3600

Silverberg, N., Iaccarino, M., Panenka, W., Iverson, G., McCulloch, K., Dams-O'Connor, K., . . . McCrea, M. (2020). Management of concussion and mild traumatic brain injury: A synthesis of practice guidelines. *Archives of Physical Medicine and Rehabilitation*, *101*(2), 382–393. https://doi.org/10.1016/j.apmr.2019.10.179

Silverberg, N., & Iverson, G. (2011). Etiology of the post-concussion syndrome: Physiogenesis and psychogenesis revisited. *NeuroRehabilitation*, *29*(4), 317–329. https://doi.org/10.3233/NRE-2011-0708

Sinnott, A., Elbin, R., Collins, M., Reeves, V., Holland, C., & Kontos, A. (2019). Persistent vestibular-ocular impairment following concussion in adolescents. *Journal of Science and Medicine in Sport*, *22*(12), 1292–1297. https://doi.org/10.1016/j.jsams.2019.08.004

Skandsen, T., Stenberg, J., Follestad, T., Karaliute, M., Saksvik, S., Einarsen, C., . . . Iverson, G. (2021). Personal factors associated with postconcussion symptoms 3 months after mild traumatic brain injury. *Archives of Physical Medicine and Rehabilitation, 102*(6), 1102–1112. https://doi.org/10.1016/j.apmr.2020.10.106

Skjeldal, O. H., Skandsen, T., Kinge, E., Glott, T., & Solbakk, A. K. (2022). Long-term post-concussion symptoms. *Tidsskrift for Den norske legeforening, 142*(12). https://doi.org/10.4045/tidsskr.21.0713

Stålnacke, B. M. (2007). Community integration, social support and life satisfaction in relation to symptoms 3 years after mild traumatic brain injury. *Brain Injury, 21*(9), 933–942. https://doi.org/10.1080/02699050701553189

Sullivan, K., Kempe, C., Edmed, S., & Bonanno, G. (2016). Resilience and other possible outcomes after mild traumatic brain injury: A systematic review. *Neuropsychology Review, 26*(2), 173–185. https://doi.org/10.1007/s11065-016-9317-1

Taylor-Postma, R., Rider, J., & Otty, R. (2022). Functional cognition: An opportunity to highlight the role of occupational therapy in post-concussion care. *The Open Journal of Occupational Therapy, 10*(2), 1–6. https://doi.org/10.15453/2168-6408.1909

Vaduvathiriyan, P., Ludwig, R., & Siengsukon, C. (2020). Does cognitive – behavioral therapy (CBT) for insomnia improve sleep outcomes in individuals with traumatic brain injury (TBI)? A scoping review. *American Journal of Occupational Therapy, 74*(4), 7411515427p7411515421. https://doi.org/10.5014/ajot.2020.74S1-PO6728

van der Naalt, J., Timmerman, M., de Koning, M., van der Horn, H., Scheenen, M., Jacobs, B., & Spikman, J. (2017). Early predictors of outcome after mild traumatic brain injury (UPFRONT): An observational cohort study. *The Lancet Neurology, 16*(7), 532–540. https://doi.org/10.1016/S1474-4422(17)30117-5

van der Vlegel, M., Polinder, S., Mikolic, A., Kaplan, R., von Steinbuechel, N., Plass, A., . . . The Center-Tbi Participants and Investigators. (2021). The association of post-concussion and post-traumatic stress disorder symptoms with health-related quality of life, health care use and return-to-work after mild traumatic brain injury. *Journal of Clinical Medicine, 10*(11), 2473. https://doi.org/10.3390/jcm10112473

von Steinbuechel, N., Covic, A., Polinder, S., Kohlmann, T., Cepulyte, U., Poinstingl, H., . . . Truelle, J.-L. (2016). Assessment of health-related quality of life after TBI: Comparison of a disease-specific (QOLIBRI) with a generic (SF-36) instrument. *Behavioral Neurology*, 7928014. https://doi.org/10.1155/2016/7928014

Voormolen, D., Ponder, S., von Steinbuechel, N., Vos, P., Cnossen, M., & Haagsma, J. (2019). The association between post-concussion symptoms and health-related quality of life in patients with mild traumatic brain injury. *Injury, 50*(5), 1068–1074. https://doi.org/10.1016/j.injury.2018.12.002

Wallace, B., & Lifshitz, J. (2016). Traumatic brain injury and vestibulo-ocular function: Current challenges and future prospects. *Eye Brain, 8*, 153–164. https://doi.org/10.2147/EB.S82670

Wiese-Bjornstal, D., White, A., Russell, H., & A, S. (2015). Psychology of sport concussions. *Kinesiology Review, 4*(2), 169–189. https://doi.org/10.1123/kr.2015-0012

Williams, J. M., & Andersen, M. B. (1998). Psychosocial antecedents of sport injury: Review and critique of the stress and injury model. *Journal of Applied Sport Psychology, 10*(1), 5–25. https://doi.org/10.1080/10413209808406375

Williamson, M. M., & Wallace, J. (2022). Consequences of sport-related concussion on health-related quality of life in adolescents: A critically appraised topic. *Journal of Sport Rehabilitation, 32*(1), 107–114. https://doi.org/10.1123/jsr.2022-0232

Wood, R., O'Hagan, G., Williams, C., McCabe, M., & Chadwick, N. (2014). Anxiety sensitivity and alexithymia as mediators of postconcussion syndrome following mild traumatic brain injury. *Journal of Head Trauma Rehabilitation, 29*(1), E9–E17. https://doi.org/10.1097/HTR.0b013e31827eabba

World Health Organization. (2010). *The world health organization report 2010*. www.who.int/publications/i/item/9789241564021

6 Psychosocial Understanding of Patellofemoral Pain

Ken Ildefonso and Monna Arvinen-Barrow

Chapter Objectives

- To define patellofemoral pain, its prevalence, and prognosis.
- To synthesize existing research on psychosocial factors in patellofemoral pain.
- To outline a conceptual framework for understanding psychosocial experiences of recreational running with patellofemoral pain.

Introduction

Patellofemoral pain (PFP) is a chronic knee injury characterized by pain around or behind the patella (Crossley et al., 2016). The injury typically progresses from an insidious onset to constant or recurring discomfort and often presents itself with mild effusion or antalgic gait. The incidence of PFP is estimated as 1 in 14 adolescents and 1 in 5 adults (Smith, Selfe et al., 2018). PFP is also common among runners, accounting for approximately 17% ($n = 1{,}776$) of all running-related musculoskeletal injuries among non-ultramarathon runners (Kakouris et al., 2021) and 17% ($n = 606$) of all lower-extremity injuries among recreational, collegiate, and professional runners (Francis et al., 2019).

The majority of PFP risk factor and prognosis research has adopted a pathomechanical perspective (Francis et al., 2019; Martinelli et al., 2022; Neal et al., 2019; Smith, Selfe et al., 2018). The results appear to be inconsistent at best, possibly due to a lack of understanding of the role of psychosocial factors in PFP (Crossley et al., 2016; Hott et al., 2020; Neal et al., 2019; Vicenzino et al., 2022). Indeed, existing systematic reviews, meta-analyses, and consensus statements on PFP have concluded that psychosocial constructs influence the PFP experience in ways that are not yet understood (Crossley et al., 2016; Neal et al., 2019; Powers et al., 2017; Vicenzino et al., 2022). To address this gap, the purpose of this chapter is to provide an overview of current understanding of psychosocial aspects of PFP. The chapter will (a) synthesize existing research on psychosocial factors in patellofemoral pain, (b) outline a new conceptual framework for understanding psychosocial experiences of recreational running with patellofemoral pain, and (c) propose logical next steps in advancing understanding of psychosocial experiences of patellofemoral pain.

Synthesis of Existing Psychosocial Patellofemoral Pain Literature

Thus far, existing psychosocial PFP literature (for a thorough review, see Ildefonso, 2023) has focused on understanding the role of selected psychosocial constructs in PFP risk, prognosis,

DOI: 10.4324/9781003295709-7

and overall experience. These include fear-avoidance beliefs, pain catastrophizing, kinesiophobia, anxiety and depression, pain self-efficacy, coping strategies, and patient education.

Fear-Avoidance Beliefs

Fear-avoidance beliefs have been defined as exaggerated perceptions of pain that motivate an individual to avoid experiencing pain or taking part in painful activities as opposed to confronting them, often resulting in negative psychological (e.g., anxiety, depression) and physical (e.g., loss of mobility) consequences over time (Lethem et al., 1983). The original fear-avoidance model by Lethem et al. (1983) suggests that exaggerated perceptions of pain produces substantial fear toward an acute or chronic pain problem. Those fears are presumed to facilitate the execution of psychological and behavioral strategies to dissociate pain experiences and behaviors from potentially painful sensations (Lethem et al., 1983).

Existing research has found high fear-avoidance beliefs negatively influence PFP patients' pain, perceived function, and physical activity participation (Mansfield & Selhorst, 2018; Piva, Fitzgerald, Irrgang et al., 2009; Piva, Fitzgerald, Wisniewski et al., 2009; Selhorst, Fernandez-Fernandez et al., 2020; Selhorst et al., 2021). Fear-avoidance beliefs have also been found to influence deficits in objective function and levels of physical activity intensity (Glaviano et al., 2017, 2019; Glaviano & Saliba, 2018). PFP patients' fear-avoidance beliefs may also decrease after watching a psychologically informed educational video (Selhorst et al., 2021; Selhorst, Hoehn et al., 2020).

Pain Catastrophizing

Catastrophizing is a common cognitive distortion that is characterized by an inclination toward overestimation or magnification of serious potential consequences (Ellis, 1962). *Pain catastrophizing* has been defined as "an exaggerated negative mental set brought to bear during actual or anticipated painful experiences" (Sullivan et al., 2001, p. 52). Pain catastrophizing as a construct has long been accepted in chronic pain research, but its inaugural development is unknown and without theory (Sullivan et al., 2001). Early chronic pain literature has, however, suggested that pain catastrophizing is an emotional state (Pincus et al., 2010; Sullivan et al., 2001; Vlaeyen & Linton, 2000), a characterization that is somewhat inconsistent yet complementary with the general definition of catastrophizing, as stated earlier. The role of pain catastrophizing in PFP can be explained using the fear-avoidance model of chronic pain (FAMC; Leeuw et al., 2007). The FAMC assumes pain catastrophizing reflects the cognitive aspects (i.e., catastrophic thinking) of the misinterpretation of chronic pain. The FAMC presumes individuals appraise their chronic pain as either catastrophic or as non-threatening. A non-threatening appraisal results in confronting one's pain and, in turn, facilitates recovery. A catastrophic appraisal results in fear, and the anticipation of pain causes anxiety to develop. Fear/anxiety, in turn, facilitates avoidance behaviors, disuse of the injured extremity, disability, and depression (Leeuw et al., 2007).

Pain catastrophizing research has explored its relationships with pain, perceived function, objective function, physical activity level, and kinesiophobia. Pain catastrophizing has been observed to be high during the initial phases of rehabilitation, decrease over time, and have an influence on the PFP experience that is minimal at best. The latter is supported by qualitative research – as only one study has supported the presence of pain catastrophizing among PFP patients (Glaviano et al., 2022).

Kinesiophobia

By definition, *kinesiophobia* refers to "an excessive, irrational, and debilitating fear of physical movement and activity resulting from a feeling of vulnerability to painful injury or (re)injury" ("Kinesiophobia," 2007, p. 1036). Much like other fears, kinesiophobia is a negative emotional state that develops in response to stressful situations (for the tripartite model, see Clark & Watson, 1991). Originally, kinesiophobia was presumed to be a phobic process that directly caused pain-related behaviors in chronic pain patients (Miller et al., 1991). Founded on Miller et al.'s (1991) definition, Vlaeyen et al. (1995) developed the cognitive behavioral model of fear of movement/(re)injury (CBM) to explain how kinesiophobia moderates the relationship between chronic low back pain and physical activity avoidance behaviors. The CBM presumes that patients who exhibit pain catastrophizing can develop kinesiophobia, which will lead to persistent avoidance of activities that would increase pain, resulting in disuse of the injured extremity, disability, and depression (Vlaeyen et al., 1995).

Research has focused on the relationship between kinesiophobia and perceived pain, perceived function, perceived disability, fear-avoidance beliefs, pain catastrophizing, physical activity participation, objective functions, and biomechanical factors, such as lower-extremity muscular strength. These relationships have reportedly been inconsistent (Barton et al., 2019; de Oliveira Silva et al., 2018; Doménech et al., 2014; Doménech et al., 2013; Holden et al., 2021; Hott et al., 2022; Maclachlan et al., 2020; Maclachlan et al., 2018). Evidence also suggests that kinesiophobia is task/activity-specific and subpopulation-dependent (Bagheri et al., 2021; de Oliveira Silva et al., 2018; Greaves et al., 2021; Hott, Brox, Pripp, Juel, & Liavaag, 2019; Priore et al., 2019; Smith, Moffatt et al., 2018). Much like pain catastrophizing (de Oliveira Silva et al., 2018), kinesiophobia appears to not have an effect on the physical PFP rehabilitation outcomes (Greaves et al., 2021; Holden et al., 2021; Hott, Brox, Pripp, Juel, & Liavaag, 2019). It is also possible that kinesiophobia is related to and/or influenced by other psychosocial variables, such as PFP patients' desire and uncertainty related to participation in physical activity and further injury (Smith, Moffatt et al., 2018).

Anxiety and Depression

From a cognitive psychology perspective, anxiety and depression are considered comorbid negative emotional states (Eysenck & Fajkowska, 2018). *Anxiety* refers to physiological hyperarousal or fear, often associated with hypervigilance and/or expectations of future events (Eysenck & Fajkowska, 2018). *Depression* refers to an absence of positive affect, or sadness, often associated with anhedonia (i.e., inability to feel pleasure) and/or thoughts of past experiences (Eysenck & Fajkowska, 2018). According to the tripartite model of anxiety and depression (Clark & Watson, 1991), the symptoms of anxiety and depression are categorized into three factors: negative affect, positive affect, and physiological hyperarousal. Both anxiety and depression are characterized by negative affect and negative mood states, including irritability, fear, and disgust. What differentiates anxiety and depression are *positive affect* and *physiological hyperarousal*. Along with negative affect, anxiety is characterized by physiological hyperarousal, such as increased heart rate, sweaty palms, shortness of breath, and lightheadedness. Depression is characterized by the absence of positive affect and heightened presence of negative mood states, such as loneliness and sadness. Theoretically, the roles of anxiety and depression in PFP are explained through the FAMC (Leeuw et al., 2007). Fear of pain and pain anxiety are consequences of pain catastrophizing, the former in the presence of pain and the latter in anticipation of it. In turn, avoidance behaviors become a means of eluding pain, facilitating injured extremity disuse, disability, and depression (Leeuw et al., 2007).

Research on anxiety and depression among the PFP population has focused on potential relationships with pain, perceived and objective function, disability, fear-avoidance beliefs, pain catastrophizing, and kinesiophobia. Depression and anxiety have also been used as efficacy measurements in rehabilitation intervention research. Neither anxiety nor depression has been found to be a predictor of pain (Doménech et al., 2014; Doménech et al., 2013; Holden et al., 2021), but both anxiety and depression have been inversely associated with perceived function – higher anxiety and/or depression is associated with decreased perceived function (Piva, Fitzgerald, Irrgang et al., 2009; Wride & Bannigan, 2019). Depression, but not anxiety, has been found to predict perceived disability (Doménech et al., 2013; Maclachlan et al., 2018). Rehabilitation interventions (i.e., patient education, patellar taping, and stretching/strengthening exercises) have been found to reduce short- and long-term anxiety (Clark et al., 2000; Holden et al., 2021) and short- but not long-term depression (Clark et al., 2000; Maclachlan et al., 2019). Qualitative research has also found that physiotherapy interventions focused on physical rehabilitation may facilitate PFP patients' confidence in overcoming setbacks (Smith et al., 2019), and that anxiety could be a response to emotional uncomfortability, uncertainty, and worry (Robertson et al., 2017; Smith et al., 2019).

Pain Self-Efficacy

Self-efficacy refers to individuals' beliefs in their ability to perform a specific task or behavior (Bandura, 1977). Self-efficacy of people in chronic pain (i.e., pain self-efficacy) "incorporates not just the expectation that a person could perform a particular behavior or task, but also their confidence in being able to do it despite their pain" (Nicholas, 2007, p. 153). No explicit theoretical framework exists to explain the mechanisms through which pain self-efficacy influences individuals' experiences with PFP. The self-efficacy and knee pain mediation model, developed for osteoarthritic pain (SEKPM-Model; Rejeski et al., 1998), can explain how self-efficacy and pain influence health outcomes of patients with knee pain. The model suggests a linear relationship between exercise therapy and health outcomes that is mediated by the relationship between self-efficacy and pain. Patients who experience pain and have high self-efficacy are likely to perform exercise therapy tasks well, leading to better functional outcomes. Patients who experience knee pain and have low self-efficacy are presumed to avoid painful tasks (Rejeski et al., 1998).

Pain self-efficacy has been researched as an outcome among those with PFP, using pre- and post-intervention designs to explore its relationships with pain, perceived function, kinesiophobia, anxiety and depression, and health-related quality of life. Results suggest the prevalence of pain self-efficacy among PFP patients is less common than other psychosocial constructs, such as anxiety (de Oliveira Silva et al., 2018; Hott, Brox, Pripp, Juel, & Liavaag, 2019; Hott, Brox, Pripp, Juel, Paulsen et al., 2019; Maclachlan et al., 2019). Recent quantitative (Hott et al., 2022) and qualitative (Barber et al., 2022; Manojlović et al., 2022) research has provided support for pain self-efficacy in mediating the relationship exercise therapy and patient education have with pain and return to run. No pain self-efficacy research among the PFP population has explored the known sources of self-efficacy (Bandura, 1977), including include past accomplishments, vicarious experiences, physiological/affective states, and verbal feedback (Bandura, 1977). It is also not known if the patient education interventions that examined changes in pain self-efficacy were designed considering the theoretical assumptions of how self-efficacy is facilitated.

Coping Strategies

Coping refers to "cognitive and behavioral efforts to master, reduce, or tolerate the internal and/or external demands that are created by a stressful transaction" (Folkman, 1984, p. 843) and is typically an emotion-focused or problem-focused strategy a person uses in response to threatening or challenging situations (Folkman, 1984). *Emotion-focused coping* refers to strategies where an individual attempts to regulate their emotions, whereas *problem-focused coping* refers to strategies aimed at managing a cause of distress (Folkman, 1984). The transactional theory of stress and coping (Lazarus & Folkman, 1984) suggests coping strategies influence how individuals address stressful situations by mediating the relationship between one's controllability beliefs and the effectiveness of their cognitive and/or behavioral efforts (for more on coping, see Chapter 12).

Research investigating PFP coping strategies has explored their associations with pain catastrophizing, kinesiophobia, perceived function, and disability. Findings suggest adult patients use cognitive and behavioral coping strategies, such as resting, ignoring pain sensations, and distraction, to cope with PFP (Ak & No, 2018; Bagheri et al., 2021; Thomeé et al., 2002; Witvrouw et al., 2000). Participation in mindfulness intervention has the potential to help overlook pain sensations and distract from the pain (Bagheri et al., 2021). In addition, cognitive coping strategies, including prayer and hope, have also been associated with perceptions of pain and disability (Doménech et al., 2013), but not perceptions of function (Van Middlekoop et al., 2017).

Patient Education

Patient education is a cognitive behavioral strategy defined as a structured learning experience aimed to influence knowledge and health-related behaviors (Sluijs, 1991). In PFP research, patient education has been defined as a clinician providing patient-specific advice on suspected etiologies, proposed options for treatment, and expectation management (Bosshardt et al., 2021). A recent systematic review and meta-analysis by Winters et al. (2021) concluded that patient education intervention, when coupled with exercise, orthoses, or patellar taping/mobilization, is most effective at three months following diagnosis. As a standalone intervention, patient education has been found to be as effective as when combined with any physical intervention at 12 months following diagnosis (Winters et al., 2021; for more on patient education, see Chapter 13).

Pertinent Gaps in Psychosocial Patellofemoral Pain Research

Based on a thorough review of existing psychosocial PFP literature (Ildefonso, 2023), it is apparent that existing psychosocial PFP research is limited with inconsistent findings. Much of it has adopted quantitative research designs, with one of two research foci. First, research has aimed to identify and report on the existence of specific psychosocial constructs with PFP patients, namely, fear-avoidance beliefs, pain catastrophizing, kinesiophobia, anxiety, depression, pain self-efficacy, and coping strategies (e.g., Hott et al., 2022; James et al., 2021; Maclachlan et al., 2018; Pazzinatto et al., 2022). Second, the research has aimed to compare and/or investigate potential changes, differences, and relationships between specific psychosocial constructs and physical PFP outcomes, such as perceived pain and/or function (e.g., Bagheri et al., 2021; Doménech et al., 2014; Glaviano et al., 2019; Maclachlan et al., 2019). A few intervention studies have investigated the effects of patient education on PFP prognosis, and a handful of research studies (e.g., Robertson et al., 2017; Smith, Moffatt et al., 2018; Smith et al., 2019) have also adopted a qualitative design, with results suggesting that there are more psychosocial constructs that influence the PFP experience than those explored quantitatively.

The review (Ildefonso, 2023) also revealed inconsistencies in how the different psychosocial constructs (i.e., fear-avoidance beliefs, pain catastrophizing, kinesiophobia, anxiety, depression, pain self-efficacy, and coping strategies) are defined and operationalized in the literature. For example, *pain catastrophizing*, a psychosocial construct frequently studied in PFP research, has been defined as a cognitive coping strategy, a cognitive appraisal related to pain, an emotional response, and even a behavior (de Oliveira Silva et al., 2018; Doménech et al., 2014; Piva, Fitzgerald, Irrgang et al., 2009; Priore et al., 2019; Selhorst et al., 2021). In a similar manner, *kinesiophobia* has been defined and theorized in PFP research as a cognitive appraisal (de Oliveira Silva et al., 2018; Hott et al., 2022; Miller et al., 1991; Selhorst, Hoehn et al., 2020; Vlaeyen et al., 1995), which is inconsistent with its core definition that classifies it as a negative emotional state that develops in response to stressful situations (for the tripartite model, see Clark & Watson, 1991). Without clear definitions and construct clarity, it is not surprising that existing psychosocial PFP research has also lacked theoretically based research designs, grounded in psychological theory. An absence of conceptual framework has prohibited researchers from understanding *how* psychosocial constructs influence the PFP experience, prognosis, and intervention outcomes.

Psychosocial Experiences of Recreational Running with Patellofemoral Pain

To address the apparent theoretical gap in existing PFP research, Ildefonso et al. (in preparation) used a Straussian grounded theory (Corbin & Strauss, 2015) research design with a sample ($n = 10$) of recreational runners. The purpose of this research was to (a) document recreational runners' perceived psychosocial experiences with PFP and (b) develop a conceptual framework for recreational runners' perceived psychosocial experiences with PFP. What follows here is the resultant conceptual framework, consisting of five theoretical categories that explain the perceived psychosocial experiences of recreational running with PFP: *who*, *what*, *how*, *why*, and *psychosocial outcomes*.

The Conceptual Framework for Psychosocial Experiences of Recreational Runners with Patellofemoral Pain

The conceptual framework (Ildefonso et al., in preparation) suggests recreational runners are individuals *who* have prominent personal characteristics that influence their perceived psychosocial experiences of recreational running with PFP. The conceptualization also suggests that dominant psychosocial responses are *what* recreational runners experience when running with PFP. Those experiences influence and are influenced by *how* they address the perceived cause of their psychosocial responses and the reasons *why* they respond in the ways they do. All of which influence and are influenced by *psychosocial outcomes*. Theoretically, *who* recreational runners are, *what* they experience when recreational running with PFP, *how* they respond, *why* they respond in the ways they do, and their *psychosocial outcomes* combine to create a set of interrelated overarching psychosocial constructs for which a vast amount of subconstructs influence the perceived psychosocial experiences of recreational runners with PFP.

Who

The theoretical category *who* refers to the prominent personal characteristics of the participants who provided their psychosocial experiences of recreational running with PFP. In the sample of ten recreational runners with PFP, Ildefonso et al. (in preparation) found two psychosocial factors (subcategories) as pertinent to the psychosocial PFP experience. These include "run by any means necessary" attitude and having an emotional attachment to running, characterized by accomplishment, happiness, and euphoria.

What

The theoretical category *what* refers to participants' perceived psychosocial responses to PFP. In the sample of ten recreational runners, Ildefonso et al. (in preparation) found three pertinent cognitive-affective responses (subcategories) to PFP. These include (a) uncertainty (i.e., unacquaintedness or unknowingness) as to whether training influenced pain or vice versa; (b) worry (i.e., genuine concern, nervousness, and/or anxiousness), often associated with frustration with continuing to run; and (c) perceived pain. The subcategory of perceived pain refers to pain-related perceptions participants described having when continuing to run with PFP. Perceived pain fluctuated between low and high intensities during training and activities of daily living.

How

The theoretical category *how* refers to the means through which participants addressed what they perceived to be the cause of their dominant psychosocial responses (i.e., *what*). In the sample of ten recreational runners, Ildefonso et al. (in preparation) found three pertinent behavioral responses (subcategories) participants' used to address their dominant psychosocial responses to PFP. These include (a) training responses (i.e., training modifications), (b) physical responses (i.e., tapping, icing, over-the-counter anti-inflammatories, footwear, insoles, orthotics, or knee sleeves), and (c) psychological responses. The psychological responses included seeking help from friends, teammates, family, and/or medical professionals; documenting training pace, duration, distance, weather, and/or how runs felt; and engaging in positive self-talk.

Why

The theoretical category *why* refers to the reasons participants responded to their dominant psychosocial responses (i.e., *what*) with the means they did to address the perceived cause (i.e., *how*). In the sample of ten recreational runners, Ildefonso et al. (in preparation) found four pertinent factors (subcategories). These include (a) previous experiences, (b) extrinsic motivation (i.e., externally focused aspirations of achievement), (c) intrinsic motivation (i.e., internally focused aspirations of achievement), and (d) social influences. The social influences included friends, teammates, family, coaches, medical professionals, run-store staff, and Internet/print media.

Psychosocial Outcomes

The theoretical category *psychosocial outcomes* refers to the prominent psychosocial sequelae described by participants as integral to their experiences of recreational running with PFP. In the sample of ten recreational runners, Ildefonso et al. (in preparation) found robust psychosocial outcomes were secondary results that arose from and influenced *who* the participants are, *what* they experienced, *how* they responded, and *why* they responded in the ways they did to PFP. In the sample of recreational runners, Ildefonso et al. (in preparation) found two pertinent psychosocial outcomes (subcategories). These include (a) relatedness (i.e., the level of connectedness participants described having with others) and (b) acceptance (i.e., willingness to make the training accommodations necessary to minimize the discomfort of recreational running with PFP).

Next Steps in Psychosocial Patellofemoral Pain Research

By design, the conceptual framework created by Ildefonso et al. (in preparation) is the first attempt to create a foundational framework for understanding the psychosocial PFP experience of recreational runners. Grounded in empirical evidence, the data-driven and conceptually defined theoretical categories and subcategories provide a foundation for future psychosocial PFP research. The next steps in this line of research would be to design early-stage exploratory research, followed by applied and/experimental research before any evidence-based clinical recommendations can be made.

Conclusion

Patellofemoral pain is a common overuse injury among runners of various competitive levels with poor prognosis. Researchers have suggested that poor prognosis is partially due to lack of understanding of the role of psychosocial factors that influence the PFP experience. This chapter provided an overview of current understanding of the psychosocial aspects of PFP and outlined a conceptual framework that inaugurally explains the psychosocial experiences of recreational runners with patellofemoral pain. In doing so, the chapter hopes to provide a foundational framework for future psychosocial PFP research.

Case study

Katrina is a 26-year-old doctoral student and an avid recreational runner diagnosed with patellofemoral pain nine months ago. She typically runs in excess of 20 km/week, knee willing. For Katrina, running is fun. "I mean, running is a great stress relief from all things PhD. You know, it's the runner's high . . . it's fun. It's addicting," Katrina explains to fellow PhD student Mico, who asked about Katrina's running when he saw her icing her knees in the laboratory for the third day in a row.

Over the past months, Katrina has tried all sorts of things to minimize her knee pain. She has learned that focusing on speed as opposed to distance, adding rest days for recovery, and keeping a positive attitude prevent her from experiencing high levels of pain and allow her to continue running. "I mean . . . I keep telling myself that you are already running, so you can't quit. I'm stubborn . . . haha . . . you know, it's the pride."

For the past four weeks, Katrina has been "secretly" training for a half-marathon, which is now two weeks away. Her knee pain has gradually gotten worse, and a lot of her old tricks that have allowed her to continue running in the past are not working as well. She feels more worried and uncertain about her ability to race the half-marathon. "I don't know . . . I feel like there is this constant worry at the back of my mind . . . and lately, I cannot shake it off. It's this nervousness . . . what if I cannot run?" she tells her run group friend Josh.

Together, Katrina and Josh search the Internet for some advice on how to navigate PFP and continue to run in a way that allows Katrina to run the half-marathon in two weeks. Combining their past experiences with a training plan retrieved from an Instagram page posted by a run group in Switzerland, Katrina and Josh create a custom plan for Katrina. "I cannot thank you enough, Josh. You have helped me reset my expectations. Right now, I'm just trying to very cautiously maintain that running base. So I am in injury-prevention mode."

Josh hugs Katrina and says, "No problem! That's what friends are for. They stick with you, run with you, and help you be logical and rational. We are, you know, accepting what is."

"Yeah, totally," Katrina laughs. "We are being positive and just accept what comes. Bring on more miles!"

Questions

1. How would you describe Katrina's relationship with running?
2. How would you characterize Katrina's coping with her injury?
3. Consistent with the conceptual framework for psychosocial experiences of recreational runners with patellofemoral pain, what theoretical categories and subcategories can you identify from Katrina's case?
4. Considering your (future) profession, how can you help Katrina navigate the injury and desire to continue running despite the pain?

References

Ak, A., & No, N. (2018). Patellofemoral pain syndrome: Prevalence and coping strategies of amateur runners in Lagos state. *Medicina Sportivâ*, *14*(2), 3059–3067. www.medicinasportiva.ro/SRoMS/ english/Journal/No.50/patellofemoral_pain_syndrome_prevalence_coping_strategies_runners. html

Bagheri, S., Naderi, A., Mirali, S., Calmeiro, L., & Brewer, B. W. (2021). Adding mindfulness practice to exercise therapy for female recreational runners with patellofemoral pain: A randomized controlled trial. *Journal of Athletic Training*, *56*(8), 902–911. https://doi.org/10.4085/1062-6050-0214.20

Bandura, A. (1977). Self-efficacy: Towards a unifying theory of behavior change. *Psychological Reviews*, *84*(2), 191–215. https://doi.org/10.1037/0033-295X.84.2.191

Barber, P., Lack, S., Bartholomew, C., Curran, A., Lowe, C., Morrissey, D., & Neal, B. (2022). Patient experience of the diagnosis and management of patellofemoral pain: A qualitative exploration. *Musculoskeletal Science and Practice*, *57*, 102473. https://doi.org/10.1016/j.msksp.2021.102473

Barton, C., de Oliveira Silva, D., Patterson, B., Crossley, K., Pizzari, T., & Nunes, G. (2019). A proximal progressive resistance training program targeting strength and power is feasible in people with patellofemoral pain. *Physical Therapy in Sport*, *38*, 59–65. https://doi.org/10.1016/j.ptsp.2019.04.010

Bosshardt, L., Ray, T., & Sherman, S. (2021). Non-operative management of anterior knee pain: Patient education. *Current Reviews in Musculoskeletal Medicine*, *14*(1), 76–81. https://doi.org/10.1007/ s12178-020-09682-4

Clark, D., Downing, N., Mitchell, J., Coulson, L., Syzpryt, E., & Doherty, M. (2000). Physiotherapy for anterior knee pain: A randomised controlled trial. *Annals of the Rheumatic Diseases*, *59*(9), 700–704. https://doi.org/10.1136/ard.59.9.700

Clark, L., & Watson, D. (1991). Tripartite model of anxiety and depression: Psychometric evidence and taxonomic implications. *Journal of Abnormal Psychology*, *100*(3), 316–336. https://doi. org/10.1037/0021-843X.100.3.316

Corbin, J., & Strauss, A. (2015). *Basics of qualitative research: Techniques and procedures for developing grounded theory* (4th ed.). Sage Publishing.

Crossley, K., Stefanik, J., Selfe, J., Collins, N., Davis, I., Powers, C., . . . Callaghan, M. (2016). 2016 Patellofemoral pain consensus statement from the 4th international patellofemoral pain research retreat, Manchester. Part 1: Terminology, definitions, clinical examination, natural history, patellofemoral osteoarthritis and patient-reported outcome measures. *British Journal of Sports Medicine*, *50*(14), 839–843. https://doi.org/doi.org/10.1136/bjsports-2016-096384

de Oliveira Silva, D., Barton, C., Crossley, K., Waiteman, M., Taborda, B., Ferreira, A., & de Azevedo, F. (2018). Implications of knee crepitus to the overall clinical presentation of women with and without patellofemoral pain. *Physical Therapy in Sport, 33*, 89–95. https://doi.org/10.1016/j.ptsp.2018.07.007

Doménech, J., Sanchis-Alfonso, V., & Espejo, B. (2014). Changes in catastrophizing and kinesiophobia are predictive of changes in disability and pain after treatment in patients with anterior knee pain. *Knee Surgery, Sports Traumatology, Arthroscopy, 22*(10), 2295–2300. https://doi.org/10.1007/s00167-014-2968-7

Doménech, J., Sanchis-Alfonso, V., López, L., & Espejo, B. (2013). Influence of kinesiophobia and catastrophizing on pain and disability in anterior knee pain patients. *Knee Surgery, Sports Traumatology, Arthroscopy, 21*(7), 1562–1568. https://doi.org/10.1007/s00167-012-2238-5

Ellis, A. (1962). *Reason and emotion in psychotherapy*. Stuart.

Eysenck, M., & Fajkowska, M. (2018). Anxiety and depression: Toward overlapping and distinctive features. *Cognition and Emotion, 32*(7), 1391–1400. https://doi.org/10.1080/02699931.2017.1330255

Folkman, S. (1984). Personal control and stress and coping processes: A theoretical analysis. *Journal of Personality and Social Psychology, 46*(4), 839–852. https://doi.org/10.1037/0022-3514.46.4.839

Francis, P., Whatman, C., Sheerin, K., Hume, P., & Johnson, M. (2019). The proportion of lower limb running injuries by gender, anatomical location and specific pathology: A systematic review. *Journal of Sports Science & Medicine, 18*(1), 21–31. www.ncbi.nlm.nih.gov/pmc/articles/PMC6370968/

Glaviano, N., Baellow, A., & Saliba, S. (2017). Physical activity levels in individuals with and without patellofemoral pain. *Physical Therapy in Sport, 27*, 12–16. https://doi.org/10.1016/j.ptsp.2017.07.002

Glaviano, N., Baellow, A., & Saliba, S. (2019). Elevated fear avoidance affects lower extremity strength and squatting kinematics in women with patellofemoral pain. *Athletic Training & Sports Health Care, 11*(4), 192–200. https://doi.org/10.3928/19425864-20181029-01

Glaviano, N., Holden, S., Bazett-Jones, D., Singe, S., & Rathleff, M. (2022). Living well (or not) with patellofemoral pain: A qualitative study. *Physical Therapy in Sport, 56*, 1–7. https://doi.org/10.1016/j.ptsp.2022.05.011

Glaviano, N., & Saliba, S. (2018). Association of altered frontal plane kinematics and physical activity levels in females with patellofemoral pain. *Gait & Posture, 65*, 86–88. https://doi.org/10.1016/j.gaitpost.2018.07.164

Greaves, H., Comfort, P., Liu, A., Herrington, L., & Jones, R. (2021). How effective is an evidence-based exercise intervention in individuals with patellofemoral pain? *Physical Therapy in Sport, 51*, 92–101. https://doi.org/10.1016/j.ptsp.2021.05.013

Holden, S., Matthews, M., Rathleff, M., Kasza, J., & Vicenzino, B. (2021). How do hip exercises improve pain in individuals with patellofemoral pain? Secondary mediation analysis of strength and psychological factors as mechanisms. *Journal of Orthopedic & Sports Physical Therapy, 51*(12), 602–610. https://doi.org/10.2519/jospt.2021.10674

Hott, A., Brox, J., Pripp, A., Juel, N., & Liavaag, S. (2019). Patellofemoral pain: One year results of a randomized trial comparing hip exercise, knee exercise, or free activity. *Scandinavian Journal of Medicine & Science in Sports, 30*(4), 741–753. https://doi.org/10.1111/sms.13613

Hott, A., Brox, J., Pripp, A., Juel, N., & Liavaag, S. (2020). Predictors of pain, function, and change in patellofemoral pain. *The American Journal of Sports Medicine, 48*(2), 351–358. https://doi.org/10.1177/0363546519889623

Hott, A., Brox, J., Pripp, A., Juel, N., Paulsen, G., & Liavaag, S. (2019). Effectiveness of isolated hip exercise, knee exercise, or free physical activity for patellofemoral pain: A randomized controlled trial. *The American Journal of Sports Medicine, 47*(6), 1312–1322. https://doi.org/10.1177/0363546519830644

Hott, A., Pripp, A., Juel, N., Liavaag, S., & Brox, J. (2022). Self-efficacy and emotional distress in a cohort with patellofemoral pain. *Orthopedic Journal of Sports Medicine, 10*(3), 232596712210796. https://doi.org/10.1177/23259671221079672

Ildefonso, K. (2023). *Exploring the perceived psychosocial experiences of recreational runners with patellofemoral pain: A grounded theory approach* (Doctoral dissertation). University of Wisconsin-Milwaukee.

Ildefonso, K., Smith, B., & Arvinen-Barrow, M. (in preparation). Recreational runners' perceived psychosocial experiences with patellofemoral pain: A Grounded Theory Approach. *Journal of Athletic Training.*

James, J., Selfe, J., & Goodwin, P. (2021). Does a bespoke education session change levels of catastrophizing, kinesiophobia and pain beliefs in patients with patellofemoral pain? A feasibility study. *Physiotherapy Practice and Research, 42*(2), 153–163. https://doi.org/10.3233/ppr-210529

Kakouris, N., Yener, N., & Fong, D. T. (2021). A systematic review of running-related musculoskeletal injuries in runners. *Journal of Sport and Health Science, 10*(5), 513–522. https://doi.org/10.1016/j.jshs.2021.04.001

Kinesiophobia. (2007). In R. Schmidt & W. Willis (Eds.), *Encyclopedia of pain.* Springer.

Lazarus, R., & Folkman, S. (1984). *Stress, appraisal, and coping.* Springer. https://doi.org/10.1007/978-3-540-29805-2_2102

Leeuw, M., Goossens, M., Linton, S., Crombez, G., Boersma, K., & Vlaeyen, J. (2007). The fear-avoidance model of musculoskeletal pain: Current state of scientific evidence. *Journal of Behavioral Medicine, 30*(1), 77–94. https://doi.org/10.1007/s10865-006-9085-0

Lethem, J., Slade, P., Troup, J., & Bentley, G. (1983). Outline of a fear-avoidance model of exaggerated pain perception – I. *Behaviour Research and Therapy, 21*(4), 401–408. https://doi.org/10.1016/0005-7967(83)90009-8

Maclachlan, L., Collins, N., Hodges, P., & Vicenzino, B. (2019). Can the provision of written information change the natural course of patellofemoral pain? *Journal of Science and Medicine in Sport, 22*(S44). https://doi.org/10.1016/j.jsams.2019.08.223

Maclachlan, L., Collins, N., Hodges, P., & Vicenzino, B. (2020). Psychological and pain profiles in persons with patellofemoral pain as the primary symptom. *European Journal of Pain, 24*(6), 1182–1196. https://doi.org/doi.org/10.1002/ejp.1563

Maclachlan, L., Matthews, M., Hodges, P., Collins, N., & Vicenzino, B. (2018). The psychological features of patellofemoral pain: A cross-sectional study. *Scandinavian Journal of Pain, 18*(2), 261–271. https://doi.org/10.1515/sjpain-2018-0025

Manojlović, D., Šarabon, N., & Prosen, M. (2022). The influence of an 8-week therapeutic exercise program on the patient experience of patellofemoral pain: A qualitative descriptive study. *Physiotherapy Theory and Practice,* 1–9. https://doi.org/10.1080/09593985.2022.2045410

Mansfield, C., & Selhorst, M. (2018). The effects of fear-avoidance beliefs on anterior knee pain and physical therapy visit count for young individuals: A retrospective study. *Physical Therapy in Sport, 34,* 187–191. https://doi.org/10.1016/j.ptsp.2018.10.008

Martinelli, N., Bergamini, A., Burssens, A., Toschi, F., Kerkhoffs, G., Victor, J., & Sansone, V. (2022). Does the foot and ankle alignment impact the patellofemoral pain syndrome? A systematic review and meta-analysis. *Journal of Clinical Medicine, 11*(8), 2245. https://doi.org/10.3390/jcm11082245

Miller, R. P., Kori, S. H., & Todd, D. D. (1991). The Tampa scale: A measure of kinesiophobia. *Clinical Journal of Pain, 7*(1), 51–52.

Neal, B., Lack, S., Lankhorst, N., Raye, A., Morrissey, D., & Van Middelkoop, M. (2019). Risk factors for patellofemoral pain: A systematic review and meta-analysis. *British Journal of Sports Medicine, 53*(5), 270–281. https://doi.org/10.1136/bjsports-2017-098890

Nicholas, M. (2007). The pain self-efficacy questionnaire: Taking pain into account. *European Journal of Pain, 11*(2), 153–163. https://doi.org/10.1016/j.ejpain.2005.12.008

Pazzinatto, M., Silva, D., Willy, R., Azevedo, F., & Barton, C. (2022). Fear of movement and (re)injury is associated with condition specific outcomes and health-related quality of life in women with patellofemoral pain. *Physiotherapy Theory and Practice, 38*(9), 1254–1263. https://doi.org/10.1080/09593985.2020.1830323

Pincus, T., Smeets, R., Simmonds, M., & Sullivan, M. (2010). The fear avoidance model disentangled: Improving the clinical utility of the fear avoidance model. *The Clinical Journal of Pain, 26*(9), 739–746. https://doi.org/10.1097/AJP.0b013e3181f15d45

Piva, S., Fitzgerald, G., Irrgang, J., Fritz, J., Wisniewski, S., McGinty, G., . . . Delitto, A. (2009). Associates of physical function and pain in patients with patellofemoral pain syndrome. *Archives of Physical Medicine and Rehabilitation, 90*(2), 285–295. https://doi.org/10.1016/j.apmr.2008.08.214

Piva, S., Fitzgerald, G., Wisniewski, S., & Delitto, A. (2009). Predictors of pain and function outcome after rehabilitation in patients with patellofemoral pain syndrome. *Journal of Rehabilitation Medicine, 41*(8), 604–612. https://doi.org/doi.org/10.2340/16501977-0372

Powers, C. M., Witvrouw, E., Davis, I. S., & Crossley, K. M. (2017). Evidence-based framework for a pathomechanical model of patellofemoral pain: 2017 patellofemoral pain consensus statement from the 4th international patellofemoral pain research retreat, Manchester, UK: Part 3. *British Journal of Sports Medicine 51*(24), 1713–1723. https://doi.org/10.1136/bjsports-2017-098717

Priore, L., Azevedo, F., Pazzinatto, M., Ferreira, A., Hart, H., Barton, C., & de Oliveira Silva, D. (2019). Influence of kinesiophobia and pain catastrophism on objective function in women with patellofemoral pain. *Physical Therapy in Sport, 35*, 116–121. https://doi.org/10.1016/j.ptsp.2018.11.013

Rejeski, W., Martin Jr, K., Ettinger, W., & Morgan, T. (1998). Treating disability in knee osteoarthritis with exercise therapy: A central role for self-efficacy and pain. *Arthritis & Rheumatism, 11*(2), 94–101. https://doi.org/10.1002/art.1790110205

Robertson, C., Hurley, M., & Jones, F. (2017). People's beliefs about the meaning of crepitus in patellofemoral pain and the impact of these beliefs on their behaviour: A qualitative study. *Musculoskeletal Science and Practice, 28*, 59–64. https://doi.org/10.1016/j.msksp.2017.01.012

Selhorst, M., Fernandez-Fernandez, A., Schmitt, L., & Hoehn, J. (2020). Adolescent psychological beliefs, but not parent beliefs, associated with pain and function in adolescents with patellofemoral pain. *Physical Therapy in Sport, 45*, 155–160. https://doi.org/10.1016/j.ptsp.2020.07.003

Selhorst, M., Fernandez-Fernandez, A., Schmitt, L., & Hoehn, J. (2021). Effect of a psychologically informed intervention to treat adolescents with patellofemoral pain: A randomized controlled trial. *Archives of Physical Medicine and Rehabilitation, 102*(7), 1267–1273. https://doi.org/10.1016/j.apmr.2021.03.016

Selhorst, M., Hoehn, J., Degenhart, T., Schmitt, L., & Fernandez-Fernandez, A. (2020). Psychologically-informed video reduces maladaptive beliefs in adolescents with patellofemoral pain. *Physical Therapy in Sport, 41*, 23–28. https://doi.org/10.1016/j.ptsp.2019.10.009

Sluijs, E. (1991). Patient education in physiotherapy: Towards a planned approach. *Physiotherapy, 77*(7), 503–508. https://doi.org/10.1016/s0031-9406(10)61855-x

Smith, B., Moffatt, F., Hendrick, P., Bateman, M., Rathleff, M., Selfe, J., . . . Logan, P. (2018). The experience of living with patellofemoral pain – loss, confusion and fear-avoidance: A UK qualitative study. *BMJ Open, 8*(1), 1–9. https://doi.org/10.1136/bmjopen-2017-018624

Smith, B., Moffatt, F., Hendrick, P., Bateman, M., Selfe, J., Rathleff, M., . . . Logan, P. (2019). Barriers and facilitators of loaded self-managed exercises and physical activity in people with patellofemoral pain: Understanding the feasibility of delivering a multicentred randomised controlled trial, a UK qualitative study. *BMJ Open, 9*(6), 1–10. https://doi.org/10.1136/bmjopen-2018-023805

Smith, B., Selfe, J., Thacker, D., Hendrick, P., Bateman, M., Moffatt, F., . . . Logan, P. (2018). Incidence and prevalence of patellofemoral pain: A systematic review and meta-analysis. *PLoS One, 13*(1), 1–18. https://doi.org/10.1371/journal.pone.0190892

Sullivan, M., Thorn, B., Haythornthwaite, J., Keefe, F., Martin, M., Bradley, L., & Lefebvre, J. (2001). Theoretical perspectives on the relation between catastrophizing and pain. *The Clinical Journal of Pain, 17*(1), 52–64. https://doi.org/10.1097/00002508-200103000-00008

Thomeé, P., Thomeé, R., & Karlsson, J. (2002). Patellofemoral pain syndrome: Pain, coping strategies and degree of well-being. *Scandinavian Journal of Medicine & Science in Sports, 12*(5), 276–281. https://doi.org/10.1034/j.1600-0838.2002.10226.x

Van Middlekoop, M., van der Heijden, R., & Bierma-Zeinstra, S. (2017). Characteristics and outcome of patellofemoral pain in adolescents: Do they differ from adults? *Journal of Orthopaedic & Sports Physical Therapy, 47*(10), 801–805. https://doi.org/10.2519/jospt.2017.7326

Vicenzino, B., Rathleff, M., Holden, S., Maclachlan, L., Smith, B., de Oliveira Silva, D., . . . 2019 IPFRN Group Collaborators. (2022). Developing clinical and research priorities for pain and psychological feature in people with patellofemoral pain: An international consensus process with health care professionals. *Journal of Orthopedic & Sports Physical Therapy*, *52*(1), 29–39. https://doi.org/10.2519/JOSPT.2022.10647

Vlaeyen, J., Kole-Snijders, A., Rotteveel, A., Ruesink, R., & Heuts, P. (1995). The role of fear of movement/(re) injury in pain disability. *Journal of Occupational Rehabilitation*, *5*(4), 235–252. https://doi.org/10.1007/BF02109988

Vlaeyen, J., & Linton, S. (2000). Fear-avoidance and its consequences in chronic musculoskeletal pain: A state of the art. *Pain*, *85*(3), 317–332. https://doi.org/10.1016/S0304-3959(99)00242-0

Winters, M., Holden, S., Lura, C., Welton, N., Caldwell, D., Vicenzino, B., . . . Rathleff, M. (2021). Comparative effectiveness of treatments for patellofemoral pain: A living systematic review with network meta-analysis. *British Journal of Sports Medicine*, *55*(7), 369–377. https://doi.org/10.1136/bjsports-2020-102819

Witvrouw, E., Lysens, R., Bellemans, J., Cambier, D., & Vanderstraeten, G. (2000). Intrinsic risk factors for the development of anterior knee pain in an athletic population: A two-year prospective study. *The American Journal of Sports Medicine*, *28*(4), 480–489. https://doi.org/10.1177/03635465000280040701

Wride, J., & Bannigan, K. (2019). Investigating the prevalence of anxiety and depression in people living with patellofemoral pain in the UK: The Dep-Pf Study. *Scandinavian Journal of Pain*, *19*(2), 375–382. https://doi.org/10.1515/sjpain-2018-0347

Part 2

Professional Practice in Sport Injury and Rehabilitation

7 Interprofessional Practice Models in Sport Injury and Rehabilitation

Monna Arvinen-Barrow and Damien Clement

Chapter Objectives

- To outline existing sport injury-specific interprofessional practice models.
- To explain the process of setting up an interprofessional team for sport injury and rehabilitation.
- To summarize the benefits and critical success factors in adopting an interprofessional approach to sport injury.

Introduction

Consistent with the biomedical model of medicine that considers mind and body as separate entities (Straub, 2012), existing theoretical definitions of sports injury (i.e., *what* is sport injury) continue to focus on the physical deficits and functional consequences of trauma to the physical body (Arvinen-Barrow & Clement, 2019a). In a similar manner, operational definitions (i.e., *how* sport injuries happen) continue to focus on the mechanical properties of injury, such as injury location, mechanics of onset, time taken for tissue to become injured, affected tissue type, and severity (Granquist et al., 2014). It is therefore not surprising that many sports medicine professionals (SMPs) continue to treat sport injuries consistent with the biomedical model, by adopting a lone-physician practice approach and using unidimensional treatment modalities and interventions when treating athletes with injuries (Hess et al., 2019).

While existing theoretical and operational definitions of sport injury fail to account for any psychosocial-onset factors and injury consequences (Arvinen-Barrow & Clement, 2019b), over the past 50 years, a growing body of empirical research has been conducted supporting the need to re-define and theorize sport injury as a complex biopsychosocial phenomenon (for more details, see Brewer & Redmond, 2017). A plethora of theoretical models has been developed to explain how biopsychosocial factors influence both sport injury risk (i.e., Appaneal & Perna, 2014; Richardson et al., 2008; Wiese-Bjornstal, 2009, 2010; Williams & Andersen, 1998; see Chapter 2) and a myriad of biopsychosocial consequences resulting from sport injury (e.g., Brewer et al., 2002; Wadey et al., 2018; Wiese-Bjornstal et al., 1998; see Chapter 3). In a similar manner, existing empirical research yields its support to the use of multidimensional injury prevention strategies and treatment modalities (for review and synthesis, see Brewer & Arvinen-Barrow, 2021; Brewer & Redmond, 2017; Faude et al., 2017; Ivarsson et al., 2017; Olmedilla et al., 2015). There is, however, a noticeable gap in the literature informing *how* professionals working with athletes with injuries can adopt an interprofessional approach to sport injury

DOI: 10.4324/9781003295709-9

rehabilitation (Morris et al., 2020). According to Hess et al. (2019), this is problematic for a few of reasons. First, in the absence of clear guidelines on how to set up an interprofessional team, "solo practitioners may attempt to deliver interventions across disciplines without adequate training, thereby increasing the potential for inadequate interventions and harm to the client" (p. 233). Second, the apparent absence of research evidence and clear guidelines on how to operationalize and adopt an interprofessional approach to sport injury rehabilitation could be "part of the multifaceted and systematic challenges contributing to suboptimal rehabilitation outcomes" (p. 233).

The purpose of this chapter is to highlight the importance of interprofessional practice in sport injury rehabilitation. More specifically, this chapter will (a) introduce existing interprofessional practice models proposed as applicable for sport injury rehabilitation, (b) provide a brief summary of research on interprofessional practice models used in sport injury rehabilitation, (c) describe the process of setting up an interprofessional team in sport injury and rehabilitation, (d) highlight the benefits and barriers to interprofessional approach to sport injury rehabilitation, and (e) outline critical success factors in adopting an interprofessional approach to sport injury rehabilitation.

Interprofessional Practice Models

With a goal to provide holistic biopsychosocial care during sport injury rehabilitation, three interprofessional practice models have been proposed in the literature (Hess et al., 2019). Consistent with existing interprofessional terminologies (Barr et al., 2005; Melvin, 1980; Reeves et al., 2010), the models presented in this chapter represent different levels of integration between the sport injury rehabilitation team members. While each of the models has their intricacies, they are all underpinned by the same core philosophy: each athlete with an injury should be evaluated, diagnosed, and treated in a holistic, patient-centered manner (Arvinen-Barrow & Clement, 2019a). This is also consistent with general healthcare – where the patient is seen as central, and the team structures that surround them are shaped by the *people* (i.e., healthcare providers, patients, and families), and numerous *organizational* and *contextual* factors (DiazGranados et al., 2018). What follows here is a brief description of the multidisciplinary approach (Clement & Arvinen-Barrow, 2013), the interdisciplinary approach (Dijkstra et al., 2014), and the transdisciplinary approach (Meyer et al., 2014).

Multidisciplinary Approach

An interprofessional practice model that adopts a multidisciplinary approach is characterized by having a variety of professionals from diverse disciplines "working in a coordinated effort" to meet a desired objective (Karol, 2014, p. 657). In a multidisciplinary approach, professionals provide a viewpoint from their own professional perspective. The team members operate independently within their scope of practice while being aware of other professionals that are also involved in the care of the athlete. This approach often lacks collective communication between the professionals and other significant individuals. Instead, communication is "channeled" through one person, such as the physician or an athletic trainer (Clement & Arvinen-Barrow, 2013; Karol, 2014), or, in some cases, directly from each professional involved.

The multidisciplinary approach to sport injury rehabilitation (Clement & Arvinen-Barrow, 2013) is based on the premise that when injured, an athlete becomes central and is surrounded by a range of professionals and other significant individuals, forming a "dual-layered" approach to care (Arvinen-Barrow & Clement, 2019a). The model by Clement and Arvinen-Barrow (2013) also ascribes to the notion that professionals and individuals whom athletes with injuries rely on during their rehabilitation continue to evolve beyond the traditional physiotherapist, athletic trainer, and physician (Kolt & Andersen, 2004; Wiese-Bjornstal & Smith, 1999). It is common for a variety of professionals (i.e., sport/clinical psychologist, massage therapist, nutritionist, and strength and conditioning coaches) and other significant individuals (e.g., family, coaches, teammates, chaplains) to interact with the athletes during injury rehabilitation (for more details, see Arvinen-Barrow & Clement, 2019b).

Primary and Secondary Rehabilitation Teams

In a multidisciplinary approach, the primary rehabilitation team often consists of SMPs who will work closely with the athlete from the injury onset, through rehabilitation, to return to participation. Typical members of the primary team include primary treatment providers, such as physiotherapist/athletic trainer and/or physician/orthopedic surgeon. The secondary rehabilitation team should consist of all professionals and individuals who are integral in assisting athletes toward successful recovery but may not be directly involved in the physical treatment of the injury. These include, but are not limited to, biomechanist, clinical/counseling psychologist, dentist, friends, parents/family, physical/sport/massage therapist, podiatrist, psychiatrist, sport coaches, sport nutritionist, sport psychologist, sport/exercise physiologist, spouse/partner, strength and conditioning coach, and teammates. The secondary team members often contribute to the rehabilitation experience in a myriad of different ways.

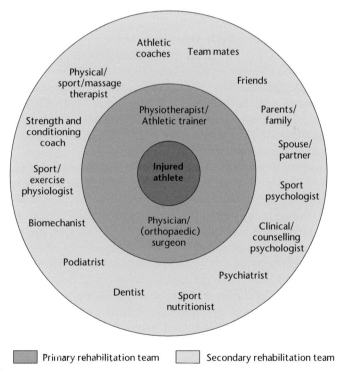

Figure 7.1 The multidisciplinary team approach to rehabilitation.

Primary and Secondary Rehabilitation Team Interactions

Despite the obvious distinction between the primary and secondary rehabilitation teams, the roles of the various members interact and intertwine in a myriad of ways. Some of the roles may be direct (i.e., the ways in which family members and spouse/partner can facilitate recovery), whereas others may be more indirect (i.e., sport psychology professional [SPP] may influence the rehabilitation process through the physiotherapist/athletic trainer). The strength and nature of these relationships may change across the rehabilitation stages (for more on psychological phases of rehabilitation, see Kamphoff et al., 2013), depending on the athlete's personal and/ or situational needs. The type of injury (a personal factor) can influence the extent of tangible support an athlete may need from those close to them. An athlete with recurrent acute/overuse injuries may need direct or indirect involvement from various members of the sports medicine team (a situational factor). As an example, an athlete with recurrent problems with medial tibial stress syndrome (shin splints) and their primary treatment provider may need to consult a podiatrist and/or a biomechanist to ensure the underlying cause for the shin splints will be treated appropriately. The athlete may also require regular consultations with an SPP or a licensed mental health professional to address any psychological concerns that may have been amplified because of the injury. Moreover, access (or lack of) to appropriate support from SPP and SMPs may also change the roles and relationships of those involved in the day-to-day care of the athlete.

Interdisciplinary Approach

An interprofessional practice model that adopts an interdisciplinary approach is characterized by having a variety of professionals from diverse disciplines working together while recognizing the overlap in each other's expertise and clinical focus to meet the desired objective (Karol, 2014). In an interdisciplinary approach, the treatment and rehabilitation outcomes are no longer a simple sum of separate parts but rather an amalgamation of how different disciplines can influence each other and the desired outcomes. The team members operate interdependently and engage in meaningful collective communication, both of which can positively affect both the treatment and the rehabilitation outcomes (Karol, 2014).

The integrated performance health management and coaching model (Dijkstra et al., 2014) ascribes to the philosophy that sport injury and athletic performance are inherently intertwined. The model also recognizes the benefits of considering athlete preferences in the decision-making process, particularly during injury rehabilitation and return to participation. The model focuses on operational integration of two specific yet overlapping departments that are integral to elite sport: performance coaching and performance health management. Led by the head coach/performance director, the performance coaching department focuses on the management of sport performance–related operations, including case management of healthy athletes. The performance health management department is led by a medical director/chief medical officer who oversees the day-to-day functions of the medicine and therapy (e.g., physicians and SMPs) and associated sciences of nutrition, physiology, psychology, biomechanics, and podiatry (Dijkstra et al., 2014).

These departments operate both "in synergy" and at times with "appropriate autonomy" (Dijkstra et al., 2014, p. 525) toward a common performance goal. While both departments focus on specific areas of expertise, it is an expectation that each has an adequate understanding of the other domains. According to Dijkstra and colleagues, "coaches, for instance, should have a working knowledge of important injuries and illnesses, and doctors should have a thorough understanding of the physiological and mechanical demands of the specific sport or event" (p. 525).

Transdisciplinary Approach

An interprofessional practice model that adopts a transdisciplinary approach is characterized by having a variety of professionals from diverse disciplines share the responsibility of addressing the patient concerns in a way that no issue is "owned by a particular discipline" (Karol, 2014, p. 659). In a transdisciplinary approach, the treatment and rehabilitation outcomes are achieved by the different disciplines transcending each other to form a holistic approach to care. The team members are collectively responsible for identifying and prioritizing patient needs, as well as creating and implementing an appropriate treatment plan to ensure successful, holistic treatment and rehabilitation outcomes (Karol, 2014).

The Meyer athlete performance management model (Meyer et al., 2014) ascribes to the philosophy that collaboration between different performance domains (i.e., mental, physical, technical, and senior management operations) surrounding an elite athlete is instrumental to athlete health, well-being, and performance. The model proposes that for optimal elite sport injury rehabilitation and performance outcomes, all performance management team members should work together in a performer-centered, interdependent, and collaborative manner (Meyer et al., 2014).

The Meyer athlete performance management model depicts how different sport performance operations can work collaboratively and engage in continuous communication with a common goal to ensure optimal sport injury rehabilitation and performance outcomes. By spending more time working directly with professionals representing different operations, the interprofessional team is able to intersect different disciplines and maximize the performance outcomes (Meyer et al., 2014).

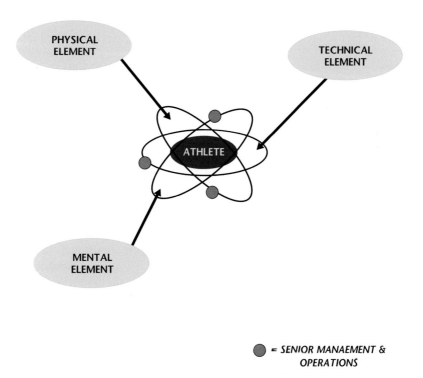

Figure 7.2 The Meyer athlete performance management model.

Source: Copyright ©2014. Reprinted with permission from Andrew M. Lane, *Case Studies in Sport Science and Medicine*. CreateSpace.

Research Evidence on Interprofessional Practice Models

Despite an abundance of research in general healthcare, evidence in support of sport injury–specific interprofessional practice models is sparse. The transdisciplinary approach (Meyer et al., 2014), while based on decades of professional practice evidence in diverse elite sport domains, has only been researched once with a single performance management team through two injury and rehabilitation cases in the lead-up to the 2014 Winter Olympics (Hess & Meyer, 2022). Using interpretative phenomenological analysis (Smith et al., 2009), Hess and Meyer found that when the interprofessional team functioned as a transdisciplinary team (as opposed to multidisciplinary team), their lived experiences of working as part of the team were better, and the observed rehabilitation and return-to-sport outcomes for the athlete with an injury were improved. The interdisciplinary approach (Dijkstra et al., 2014) is based on the experiences of United Kingdom (UK) Athletics in preparation for the 2012 London Olympic and Paralympic Games (Dijkstra et al., 2014) and underpinned the gold medal performances for track-and-field athletes at the London Games. While the model is rooted in the team members' previous experiences of implementing the approach at the Olympic level, it has not been empirically tested. To date, four studies have explicitly explored the views and experiences of different stakeholders of the multidisciplinary approach (Clement & Arvinen-Barrow, 2013). Preliminary investigations with previously injured athletes (Arvinen-Barrow & Clement, 2016; Clement & Arvinen-Barrow, 2020), SPPs (Arvinen-Barrow & Clement, 2017), and SMPs (Arvinen-Barrow & Clement, 2015) have confirmed the dual-layered structure of the multidisciplinary approach to sport injury rehabilitation; however, discrepancies in which professionals should be part of the primary team have also been noted (Arvinen-Barrow & Clement, 2015, 2016, 2017; Clement & Arvinen-Barrow, 2020).

Team Members

Evidence in support of the inclusion of numerous individuals as members of the interprofessional team exists in the literature. Support for the inclusion of general medical professionals (e.g., orthopedic surgeons, physicians), SMPs (e.g., athletic trainers, physiotherapists, sports therapists), SPPs (e.g., mental performance consultants, licensed sport psychologists), mental health professionals (e.g., clinical psychologists, psychiatrists), and other allied health professionals (e.g., chiropractors, nutritionists, podiatrists) as members of the interprofessional team has been found in the literature (Arvinen-Barrow & Clement, 2015, 2016, 2017; Clement & Arvinen-Barrow, 2020; Hess & Meyer, 2022; Kraemer et al., 2019).

The role of sport coaches as members of the interprofessional team has also received some attention in the literature (Arvinen-Barrow & Clement, 2015, 2016, 2017). Among athletes who were injured during high school, sport coaches were among the closest individuals the athletes interacted with while injured (Clement & Arvinen-Barrow, 2020). Sport coaches are also likely to serve multiple roles to athletes (i.e., teachers, parental figures, disciplinarians), therefore, having both a direct and an indirect influence over the injury rehabilitation and subsequent return to participation (Tunick et al., 2009; Yang et al., 2010).

The importance of parents/family, friends, spouses/partners, and teammates as members of the interprofessional team has also been recognized in the literature (Arvinen-Barrow & Clement, 2015, 2016, 2017). Among athletes who were injured during high school, family, along with athletic trainers and athletic coaches, were among the closest individuals the athletes interacted with while injured (Clement & Arvinen-Barrow, 2020). A number of studies have also found family members to be a significant source of different forms of social support during injury rehabilitation, thus warranting their inclusion as members of the interprofessional team (Johnston & Carroll, 1998; Yang et al., 2010).

Primary Professional Contact

Central to an interprofessional team is the identification of a "primary professional contact," also known as a "primary point person," or a "case manager." Recognizing the variability in sport injury rehabilitation teams due to sport type, level, and overall cultural/organizational context, this person could be a professional with expertise in general medicine, sports medicine, (sport) psychology, nutrition, or any other allied health profession (Dijkstra et al., 2014). With *multidisciplinary* approach, existing research with athletes, SPPs, and SMPs has identified primary treatment providers (e.g., athletic trainers and physical therapists) as the typical professionals serving in this role (Arvinen-Barrow & Clement, 2015, 2016, 2017; Clement & Arvinen-Barrow, 2020; Kraemer et al., 2019). As such, they are typically tasked to recruit the relevant and appropriate SPP, SMP, and other significant individuals for the athlete's interprofessional rehabilitation team. This recruitment process should occur in consultation with the athlete with an injury and, in case of minors, include parents/caregivers. With *interdisciplinary* and *transdisciplinary* approaches, it is likely that different members of the team are already in place, and the team leader is tasked to contact the relevant individuals to the athlete's rehabilitation management team.

Setting Up an Interprofessional Team: The Process

Athletes with injuries may or may not have access to SMPs who are intricately involved in their care and rehabilitation from the injury onset. Much like access to healthcare in general (Dawkins et al., 2021), this is likely due to several personal (e.g., age, gender, and socioeconomic status) and numerous sociocultural factors in which the athlete operates (e.g., sport culture, country of domicile, structure of the healthcare system), to name a few. In a similar way, access to an established interprofessional team during sport injury rehabilitation may or may not be available to athletes with injuries. With the exception of those at the elite and/or professional level (Wiese-Bjornstal & Smith, 1993), most athletes are likely to find their treatment providers after the injury has already happened. Many factors go into the selection of relevant individuals, including athletes' individualized rehabilitation needs, professional expertise, socioeconomic status, insurance coverage, availability of different professionals. This process should start by identifying the primary professional contact who will be responsible for generating the list of professionals and individuals who need to be involved in the rehabilitation process. This person is then responsible for contacting the professionals for their availability and willingness to participate. Typically, they also ensure all members of the team are aware of, and have accepted their roles and responsibilities as part of the team. It is advised that a meeting (online or in-person) be organized to formalize, identify, and introduce all members of the rehabilitation team. This meeting will serve three purposes: (1) to introduce members to each other, (2) to educate each member about the possible resources at the athlete's disposal, and (3) to enable all members to establish and come to an agreement on a referral protocol for the athlete with an injury. Finally, it is imperative that the athlete is introduced to all members of the rehabilitation team.

The primary professional contact is also responsible for continuity and consistency of care to ensure rehabilitation efficacy. One way to conceptualize how the team operates is through sociograms. A sociogram is a tool to measure social cohesion by disclosing affiliations and attractions within a group (Weinberg & Gould, 2019). It can be beneficial for establishing and

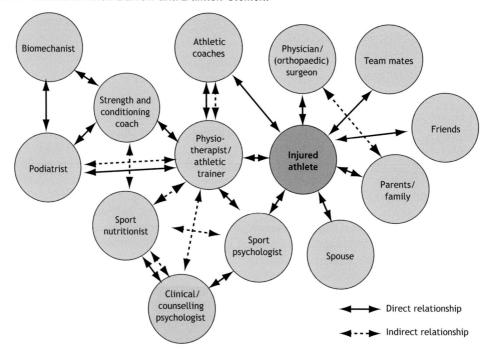

Figure 7.3 An example of a sociogram in injury rehabilitation setting.

Source: Copyright ©2013 from *Psychology of Sport Injury and Rehabilitation* by Monna Arvinen-Barrow and Natalie Walker (eds.). Reproduced by permission of Taylor and Francis Group, LLC, a division of Informa plc. This permission does not cover any third party copyrighted work which may appear in the material requested. User is responsible for obtaining permission for such material separately from this grant.

gaining clarity of the roles, relationships, and interactions between the different team members involved in the rehabilitation process to understand the different interactions the team members have with each other and the athlete. A sociogram can be used to highlight the impact (direct/ indirect) that different members of the team may have on the athlete. This increased awareness can help facilitate improved communication between the team members and consequently build trust and rapport among all those involved in the process.

Benefits of Interprofessional Approach to Sport Injury Rehabilitation

Adopting an interprofessional approach to sport injury rehabilitation has the potential to provide several benefits to both athletes and members of the interprofessional team. Essentially, an interprofessional approach exposes athletes to a holistic approach to injury rehabilitation. Athletes can have access to a rehabilitation protocol that does not focus solely on the physical aspect of injury, but offers opportunities for potentially neglected areas (e.g., psychological, nutritional, and social aspects) to receive attention. Other professionals representing varied fields can bring a new perspective into rehabilitation and offer athletes an alternative outlook. Adopting an interprofessional approach also has the potential to improve comprehensiveness of care (Brandt et al., 2014; Kraemer et al., 2019; Manspeaker & Hankemeier, 2019; Reeves et al., 2017; Sangaleti et al., 2017), facilitate better rehabilitation outcomes (Brandt et al., 2014; Lutfi-yya et al., 2019; Reeves et al., 2017; Sangaleti et al., 2017), and possibly increase the efficiency of a referral processes when necessary.

The use of an interprofessional approach can improve communication between individuals who are concerned about the injured athlete's well-being. Communication between different general medical, sport psychology, SMPs, and other significant individuals close to the athlete, all who have the injured athlete's best interest at heart, can sometimes be difficult – or contradictory even – if each is interacting with the athlete from a solitary view. However, with an interprofessional approach, all rehabilitation team members should be on the "same page." This will inherently provide opportunities to (a) improve collaboration and communication (Kraemer et al., 2019; Manspeaker & Hankemeier, 2019; Ulrich & Breitbach, 2022; Ulrich et al., 2022), (b) learn from other professionals and build understanding of each other's scope of practice (Arvinen-Barrow & Clement, 2015; Kraemer et al., 2019; Manspeaker & Hankemeier, 2019), and (c) increase mutual respect, trust, and understanding between different professionals (Ulrich & Breitbach, 2022; Ulrich et al., 2022), all of which can increase practitioner job satisfaction and experience (Hess & Meyer, 2022; Ulrich et al., 2022).

Barriers to Interprofessional Approach to Sport Injury Rehabilitation

While research with sport psychology and SMPs has highlighted both the importance of and openness to adopt an interprofessional team approach to sport injury rehabilitation (Arvinen-Barrow & Clement, 2015, 2017; Kraemer et al., 2019; Manspeaker & Hankemeier, 2019; Ulrich & Breitbach, 2022), adopting an interprofessional approach comes with its challenges. For example, recent cross-sectional research with sport science and SMPs in Switzerland highlighted systemic barriers to interprofessional collaboration (Ulrich & Breitbach, 2022). Similarly, various contextual differences in interprofessional care team have also been identified across different types of patient care settings (DiazGranados et al., 2018). Lack of (a) understanding of other healthcare professional's role (e.g., Kraemer et al., 2019; Manspeaker & Hankemeier, 2019), (b) communication (Manspeaker & Hankemeier, 2019), and (c) acceptance (Antle et al., 2021) as part of the interprofessional team have been found to be barriers for successful collaboration. For example, the role of SPPs in injury rehabilitation has been highlighted as important but very seldom is utilized to its full capacity (Arvinen-Barrow, Hemmings et al., 2007; Arvinen-Barrow, Penny et al., 2010; Clement et al., 2013; Heaney et al., 2017). Research has also found that many SPPs are struggling to gain entry into the interprofessional team (Arvinen-Barrow & Clement, 2017), sentiment also shared by registered dieticians (Antle et al., 2021).

Critical Success Factors

To date, several interprofessional competency frameworks have been developed to inform and educate healthcare professionals (Brewer & Jones, 2013). While all frameworks vary in their level of integration between the team members, all of them are founded on collective key factors: communication, conflict resolution, shared decision-making, reflective practice, role clarity, and core values and ethics. What follows is a brief description of these core competencies as outlined by McLaney et al. (2022) in the Sunnybrook framework for interprofessional collaboration.

Communication

Defined as "the transmission of information, which may be by verbal (oral or written) or nonverbal means" (American Psychological Association, 2022), *communication* is probably the most important critical success factor in interprofessional practice. The Sunnybrook framework recommends that the interprofessional team members should be "actively providing and seeking information from each other to ensure a thorough understanding of the situation" (McLaney et al., 2022, p. 115). The communication should also be "clear, accurate information at the right time, in the right environment, to the right person, in the right way" (Hayward, 2021, p. 355). Interprofessional team members should also be cognizant of their use of acronyms and/or medical jargon that may or may not be understood by all team members, and provide explanations when necessary (McLaney et al., 2022). Interprofessional communication can be further enhanced through *emotional intelligence*, that is, the ability to be self-aware and regulate behavior as appropriate to the situation (Goleman, 2007; Salovey & Mayer, 1990), as it can further influence positive interactions among team members and lead to improved biological and health outcomes.

Conflict Resolution

Defined as "reduction of discord and friction between individuals or groups, usually through the use of active strategies, such as conciliation, negotiation, and bargaining" (American Psychological Association, 2022), *conflict resolution* is instrumental for the success of an interprofessional team. Much like in any team, conflicts in interprofessional rehabilitation teams can and are likely to occur due to systemic reasons (e.g., lack of resources, power, autonomy), issues in communication (e.g., misinterpreted non-verbal cues, past experiences, conflicting expectations), and/or personal reasons (e.g., locus of control, perceived status, trust, respect; Broukhim et al., 2018). Existing literature suggest that interprofessional teams should be (a) prepared to actively respond to arising conflict "by collaborating to create a range of solutions" (McLaney et al., 2022, p. 11), (b) address conflict by developing and actively using conflict resolution protocols (Brown et al., 2010), and (c) proactively identify and address conflict in a timely manner (McLaney et al., 2022). When attempting to resolve conflict, team members should (a) listen to different ideas with an open mind, (b) communicate in a direct and respectful manner, (c) demonstrate willingness to find a solution, and (d) commit to the process until a mutually agreed-upon solution is reached (Brown et al., 2010; McLaney et al., 2022).

Shared Decision-Making

Defined as "the cognitive process of choosing between two or more alternatives, ranging from the relatively clear cut to the complex" (American Psychological Association, 2022), another critical success factor for interprofessional practice is *decision-making*. First, clear policies and procedures regarding how each team member participates in the decision-making process should be established (Dunn et al., 2018). This is particularly important since many of the team members will represent varied discipline-specific perspectives and differing levels of professional experience and confidence. In general, team members should work collaboratively to make decisions (McLaney et al., 2022). Opportunities should also be created for all team members to interact together (in-person or virtually) to discuss the case and explore all options (Dunn et al., 2018). The process of making decisions should be shared so that the team members can exchange information regarding the pros and cons of treatment option(s), obtain input from the athlete with injuries, and use the information gathered to arrive at a decision(s) (Légaré et al., 2011). The final decision(s) should then be vetted for benefits and potential harm (Elwyn et al., 2009) prior to being presented to the athlete with injuries.

Reflective Practice

Reflective practice, that is, having the ability to reflect on one's actions and performance with a "significant forethought and slow, deliberate examination of available options" (American

Psychological Association, 2022), and a goal to make conscious actionable adaptations to one's practice (Leitch & Day, 2000), should be a stable part of every interprofessional team (McLaney et al., 2022). Dedicating time for individual and team reflection should be founded on a premise where team members have an opportunity to openly and critically reflect on areas that are functioning well and are in need of improvement (McLaney et al., 2022). For effective reflective practice, team members need to be "attentive to optimizing how they interact with one another and the impact their team function may have on patient care" (McLaney et al., 2022, p. 115).

Role Clarity

Role clarity, that is, the degree in which team members have a clear understanding of their tasks, responsibilities, and processes, is another critical success factor for interprofessional teams (McLaney et al., 2022). This can be achieved by ensuring each team member is able to appropriately explain their role and scope of practice within the team and understand each other's role, scope, and expertise within the team (McLaney et al., 2022). Equally, any interdependencies between roles should be optimized to minimize repetition and redundancies, and team members should be cognizant of their personal limitations and willingness to consult with fellow team members as necessary (McLaney et al., 2022). While the aforementioned should facilitate both interprofessional collaboration and patient care (Schmitt et al., 2011), role clarity can be enhanced when team members are given formal and informal opportunities to learn from each other (Ambrose-Miller & Ashcroft, 2016). Interprofessional teams should also implement relationship building, team development, and team dynamics strategies to continually assess and evaluate team functioning (Schmitt et al., 2011).

Core Values and Ethics

According to McLaney et al. (2022), a key factor in interprofessional team functioning is having a climate of "transparency, openness and willingness to collaborate" (p. 115). Some of the core values associated with such climate include mutual respect for each member and their discipline-specific expertise (Schmitt et al., 2011), encouraging everyone to speak up, and demonstrating positive regard to other members of the team and their professions (McLaney et al., 2022). Additionally, all members of the team should be cognizant of any discipline-specific ethical and legal regulations (McLaney et al., 2022), particularly as they relate to patient confidentiality and privacy that may vary between professions.

Conclusion

While the use of a holistic approach to injury rehabilitation has become increasingly common, very little is known on *how* professionals working with athletes with injuries can adopt an interprofessional approach to sport injury rehabilitation (Morris et al., 2020). This chapter presented the reader with three interprofessional practice models proposed as suitable for sport injury rehabilitation and provided a brief synthesis of both benefits and barriers for such practice. While different, all the models are all underpinned by the same core philosophy: each athlete with an injury should be evaluated, diagnosed, and treated in a holistic, patient-centered manner (Arvinen-Barrow & Clement, 2019a). The chapter also described the process of setting up an interprofessional team and outlined six critical success factors in adopting an interprofessional approach during sport injury rehabilitation.

Case Study

Adaeh is a 12-year-old artistic gymnast from Atlanta, Georgia, who suffered a grade 3 hamstring tear two weeks ago at vault practice. "When it happened, I felt a sudden, sharp pain in the back of my leg, and something, like, popped. My butt hurts – it's like something is poking it," Adaeh explained amid tears to her mother following the accident. The coach had provided Adaeh limited first aid as the team does not have an athletic trainer on-site. The next day, Adaeh's father took her to urgent care, and a magnetic resonance imaging (MRI) confirmed a complete tear in her proximal hamstring. A surgery was scheduled for the following week, which was successful. Adaeh was given crutches, advised not to put much weight on the injured leg for the next couple of weeks, and sent home.

A month later, Adaeh and her parents meet with the orthopedic surgeon for her first post-operative evaluation. Dr. Singh confirms that Adaeh is healing well, but notices that she has some stiffness and limited range of motion in her injured knee. "How are your physical therapy sessions going?" Dr. Singh asks.

Adaeh and her parents look at each other, confused. "What physical therapy sessions? She has not been to see a physical therapist [PT]. I am confused. No one told us about seeing one . . . where would we find one?" Adaeh's father responds.

"I am so sorry," responds Dr. Singh, "I thought the nurse gave you instructions and a list of physical therapists that accept the same insurance I do. You should have started Adaeh's PT physical therapy sessions a couple of weeks ago already. I would like her to see one as soon as possible, frequently, for the next three to five months."

Adaeh is devastated and starts crying. "Three to five months? That long? I cannot be away from gymnastics that long. I am going to be so far behind," she whispers to her mother.

Over the next few weeks, Adaeh's father manages to schedule regular physical therapy sessions for Adaeh. Her rehabilitation is progressing well, and her PT is seeing signs of joy and excitement on Adaeh's face when she speaks about gymnastics. However, every time the PT, Adaeh's parents, coach, or friends ask when she can get back to the gym, Adaeh tenses up. "I don't know . . . I am not sure I can anymore. I mean, I am so behind all my teammates, and I worry that I hurt my hamstring again. So many of my friends have also moved up in group, so I would be training with younger girls I do not know."

Questions

1. What personal and situational factors may have influenced Adaeh's rehabilitation and return to participation process?
2. It is clear that Adaeh's rehabilitation has not been interprofessional in nature. Who are (or should be) the key stakeholders in Adaeh's rehabilitation to ensure successful physical and psychosocial return to participation?
3. What would her care look like if her rehabilitation team had adopted a multi-, inter-, or transdisciplinary approach to rehabilitation? What are the potential benefits and barriers of each approach?
4. What critical success factors would be important to consider in Adaeh's case to ensure a successful return to gymnastics?

References

Ambrose-Miller, W., & Ashcroft, R. (2016). Challenges faced by social workers as members of interprofessional collaborative health care teams. *Health & Social Work*, *41*(2), 101–109. https://doi.org/10.1093/hsw/hlw006

American Psychological Association. (2022). *APA dictionary of psychology*. https://dictionary.apa.org/

Antle, L., Beasley, L., & Hardin, R. (2021). The career experiences of female registered dietitians in NCAA division I athletic departments. *Journal of Intercollegiate Sport*, *14*(2), 90–115. https://doi.org/10.17161/jis.v14i2.15007

Appaneal, R. N., & Perna, F. M. (2014). Biopsychosocial model of injury. In R. C. Eklund & G. Tenenbaum (Eds.), *Encyclopedia of sport and exercise psychology* (pp. 74–77). Sage Publishing. https://doi.org/10.4135/9781483332222.n30

Arvinen-Barrow, M., & Clement, D. (2015). A preliminary investigation into athletic trainers' views and experiences of a multidisciplinary team approach to sports injury rehabilitation. *Athletic Training & Sports Health Care*, *7*(3), 97–107. https://doi.org/10.3928/19425864-20150422-05

Arvinen-Barrow, M., & Clement, D. (2016, September 29). *Preliminary investigation into previously injured athletes' views and experiences of a multidisciplinary approach to sport injury rehabilitation.* Association for Applied Sport Psychology 31st Annual Conference.

Arvinen-Barrow, M., & Clement, D. (2017). Preliminary investigation into sport and exercise psychology consultants' views and experiences of an interprofessional care team approach to sport injury rehabilitation. *Journal of Interprofessional Care*, *31*(1), 66–74. https://doi.org/10.1080/13561820.2016.1235019

Arvinen-Barrow, M., & Clement, D. (2019a). A case for interprofessional care. In M. Arvinen-Barrow & D. Clement (Eds.), *The psychology of sport and performance injury: An interprofessional case-based approach* (pp. 1–9). Routledge. https://doi.org/10.4324/9781351111591

Arvinen-Barrow, M., & Clement, D. (Eds.). (2019b). *The psychology of sport and performance injury: An interprofessional case-based approach*. Routledge.

Arvinen-Barrow, M., Hemmings, B., Weigand, D. A., Becker, C. A., & Booth, L. (2007). Views of chartered physiotherapists on the psychological content of their practice: A national follow-up survey in the United Kingdom. *Journal of Sport Rehabilitation*, *16*(2), 111–121. https://doi.org/10.1123/jsr.16.2.111

Arvinen-Barrow, M., Penny, G., Hemmings, B., & Corr, S. (2010). UK chartered physiotherapists' personal experiences in using psychological interventions with injured athletes: An interpretative phenomenological analysis. *Psychology of Sport and Exercise*, *11*(1), 58–66. https://doi.org/10.1016/j.psychsport.2009.05.004

Barr, H., Koppel, I., Reeves, S., Hammick, M., & Freeth, D. (2005). *Effective interprofessional education: Argument, assumption and evidence*. Blackwell Publishing Ltd. https://doi.org/10.1002/9780470776445

Brandt, B., Lutfiyya, M. N., King, J. A., & Chioreso, C. (2014). A scoping review of interprofessional collaborative practice and education using the lens of the Triple Aim. *Journal of Interprofessional Care*, *28*(5), 393–399. https://doi.org/10.3109/13561820.2014.906391

Brewer, B. W., Andersen, M. B., & Van Raalte, J. L. (2002). Psychological aspects of sport injury rehabilitation: Toward a biopsychological approach. In D. L. Mostofsky & L. D. Zaichkowsky (Eds.), *Medical aspects of sport and exercise* (pp. 41–54). Fitness Information Technology.

Brewer, B. W., & Arvinen-Barrow, M. (2021). Psychology of injury and rehabilitation. In Association for Applied Sport Psychology (AASP). In S. C. Sackett, N. Durand-Bush, & L. Tashman (Eds.), *The essential guide for mental performance consultants*. Human Kinetics Custom Content.

Brewer, B. W., & Redmond, C. J. (2017). *Psychology of sport injury*. Human Kinetics.

Brewer, M. L., & Jones, S. (2013). An interprofessional practice capability framework focusing on safe, high-quality, client-centered health service. *Journal of Allied Health*, *42*(2), e45–e49.

Broukhim, M., Yuen, F., McDermott, H., Miller, K., Merrill, L., Kennedy, R., & Wilkes, M. (2018). Interprofessional conflict and conflict management in an educational setting. *Medical Teacher*, *41*(4), 408–416. https://doi.org/10.1080/0142159x.2018.1480753

Brown, J., Lewis, L., Ellis, K., Stewart, M., Freeman, T. E., & Kasperski, M. J. (2010). Conflict on interprofessional primary health care teams – can it be resolved? *Journal of Interprofessional Care*, *25*(1), 4–10. https://doi.org/10.3109/13561820.2010.497750

Clement, D., & Arvinen-Barrow, M. (2013). Sport medicine team influences in psychological rehabilitation: A multidisciplinary approach. In M. Arvinen-Barrow & N. Walker (Eds.), *The psychology of sport injury and rehabilitation* (pp. 156–170). Routledge.

Clement, D., & Arvinen-Barrow, M. (2020). An investigation into former high school athletes' experiences of a multidisciplinary approach to sport injury rehabilitation. *Journal of Sport Rehabilitation, 30*(4), 619–624. https://doi.org/10.1123/jsr.2020-0094

Clement, D., Granquist, M., & Arvinen-Barrow, M. (2013). Psychosocial aspects of athletic injuries as perceived by athletic trainers. *Journal of Athletic Training, 48*(4), 512–521. https://doi.org/10.4085/1062-6050-48.3.21

Dawkins, B., Renwick, C., Ensor, T., Shrinkins, B., Jayne, D., & Meads, D. (2021). What factors affect patients' ability to access healthcare? An overview of systematic reviews. *Tropical Medicine & International Health, 26*(10), 1177–1188. https://doi.org/10.1111/t mi.13651

DiazGranados, D., Dow, A. W., Appelbaum, N., Mazmanian, P. E., & Retchim, S. M. (2018). Interprofessional practice in different patient care settings: A qualitative exploration. *Journal of Interprofessional Care, 32*(2), 151–159. https://doi.org/10.1080/13561820.2017.1383886

Dijkstra, P. H., Pollock, N., Chakraverty, R., & Alonso, J. M. (2014). Managing the health of the elite athlete: A new integrated performance health management and coaching model. *British Journal of Sports Medicine, 48*(7), 523–531. https://doi.org/10.1136/bjsports-2013-093222

Dunn, S. I., Cragg, B., Graham, I. D., Medves, J., & Gaboury, I. (2018). Roles, processes, and outcomes of interprofessional shared decision-making in a neonatal intensive care unit: A qualitative study. *Journal of Interprofessional Care, 32*(2), 284–294. https://doi.org/10.1080/13561820.2018.1428186

Elwyn, G., Frosch, D., & Rollnick, S. (2009). Dual equipoise shared decision making: Definitions for decision and behaviour support interventions. *Implementation Science, 4*, 75. https://doi.org/10.1186/1748-5908-4-75

Faude, O., Rössler, R., Petushek, E. J., Roth, R., Zahner, L., & Donath, L. (2017). Neuromuscular adaptations to multimodal injury prevention programs in youth sports: A systematic review with meta-analysis of randomized controlled trials. *Frontiers in Physiology, 8*. https://doi.org/10.3389/fphys.2017.00791

Goleman, D. (2007). *Social intelligence*. Arrow.

Granquist, M., Hamson-Utley, J. J., Kenow, L. J., & Stiller-Ostrowski, J. (2014). *Psychosocial strategies for athletic training*. F. A. Davis Company.

Hayward, C. (2021). Community specialist practitioner's role in enhancing interprofessional collaboration. *British Journal of Community Nursing, 26*(7), 354–357. https://doi.org/10.12968/bjcn.2021.26.7.354

Heaney, C., Rostron, C. L., Walker, N. C., & Green, A. J. (2017). Is there a link between previous exposure to sport injury psychology education and UK sport injury rehabilitation professionals' attitudes and behaviour towards sport psychology? *Physical Therapy in Sport, 23*(1), 99–104. https://doi.org/10.1016/j.ptsp.2016.08.006

Hess, C. W., Grnacinski, S., & Meyer, B. B. (2019). A review of the sport-injury and -rehabilitation literature: From abstraction to application. *The Sport Psychologist, 33*(3), 232–243. https://doi.org/10.1123/tsp.2018-0043

Hess, C. W., & Meyer, B. B. (2022). Lived experiences of an elite performance management team through injury rehabilitation: An interpretative phenomenological analysis. *Journal of Sport Rehabilitation, 31*(2), 199–210. https://doi.org/10.1123/jsr.2021-0072

Ivarsson, A., Johnson, U., Andersen, M. B., Tranaeus, U., Stenling, A., & Lindwall, M. (2017). Psychosocial factors and sport injuries: Meta-analyses for prediction and prevention *Sports Medicine, 47*(2), 353–365. https://doi.org/10.1007/s40279-016-0578-x

Johnston, L. H., & Carroll, D. (1998). The context of emotional responses to athletic injury: A qualitative analysis. *Journal of Sport Rehabilitation, 7*(3), 206–220. https://doi.org/10.1123/jsr.7.3.206

Kamphoff, C., Thomae, J., & Hamson-Utley, J. J. (2013). Integrating the psychological and physiological aspects of sport injury rehabilitation: Rehabilitation profiling and phases of rehabilitation. In M. Arvinen-Barrow & N. Walker (Eds.), *Psychology of sport injury and rehabilitation* (pp. 134–155). Routledge.

Karol, R. L. (2014). Team models in neurorehabilitation: Structure, function, and culture change. *NeuroRehabilitation, 34*(4), 655–669. https://doi.org/10.3233/nre-141080

Kolt, G. S., & Andersen, M. B. (Eds.). (2004). *Psychology in the physical and manual therapies*. Churchill Livingstone Inc.

Kraemer, E., Keeley, K., Martin, M., & Breitbach, A. P. (2019). Athletic trainers' perceptions and experiences with interprofessional practice. *Health, Interprofessional Practice & Education, 3*(4), eP1171; 1171–1115. https://doi.org/10.7710/2159-1253.1171

Légaré, F., Stacey, D., Gagnon, S., Dunn, S., Pluye, P., Frosch, D., . . . Graham, I. D. (2011). Validating a conceptual model for an inter-professional approach to shared decision making: A mixed methods study. *Journal of Evaluation in Clinical Practice, 17*(4), 554–564. https://doi.org/10.1111/j.1365-2753.2010.01515.x

Leitch, R., & Day, C. (2000). Action research and reflective practice: Towards a holistic view. *Educational Action Research, 8*(1), 179–193. https://doi.org/10.1080/09650790000200108

Lutfiyya, M. N., Chang, L. F., McGrath, C., Dana, C., & Lipsky, M. S. (2019). The state of the science of interprofessional collaborative practice: A scoping review of the patient health-related outcomes based literature published between 2010 and 2018. *PLoS One, 14*(6), e0218578. https://doi.org/10.1371/journal.pone.0218578

Manspeaker, S. A., & Hankemeier, D. A. (2019). Collegiate athletic trainers' perceptions of the benefits and drawbacks of interprofessional collaborative practice. *Journal of Interprofessional Care, 33*(6), 654–660. https://doi.org/10.1080/13561820.2019.1569604

McLaney, E., Morassaei, S., Hughes, L., Davies, R., Campbell, M., & Di Prospero, L. (2022). A framework for interprofessional team collaboration in a hospital setting: Advancing team competencies and behaviours. *Healthcare Management Forum, 35*(2), 112–117. https://doi.org/10.1177/08404704211063584

Melvin, J. L. (1980). Interdisciplinary and multidisciplinary activities and the ACRM. *Archives of Physical Medicine and Rehabilitation, 61*(8), 379–380.

Meyer, B. B., Merkur, A., Ebersole, K. T., & Massey, W. V. (2014). The realities of working in elite sport: What they didn't teach you in graduate school. In A. M. Lane, M. Godfrey, M. Loosemore, & W. G. P (Eds.), *Applied sport science and medicine: Case studies from practice* (pp. 137–142). CreateSpace: Self-published.

Morris, J. H., Bernhardsson, S., Bird, M.-L., Connell, L., Lynch, E., Jarvis, K., . . . Fisher, R. (2020). Implementation in rehabilitation: A roadmap for practitioners and researchers. *Disability and Rehabilitation, 42*(22), 3265–3274. https://doi.org/10.1080/09638288.2019.1587013

Olmedilla, A., Rubio, V. J., & Ortega, E. (2015). Predicting and preventing sport injuries: The role of stress. In G. Hopkins (Ed.), *Sports injuries* (pp. 87–102). Nova Science Publishers Inc.

Reeves, S., Lewin, S., Espin, S., & Zwarenstein, M. (2010). *Interprofessional teamwork for health and social care*. Blackwell-Wiley.

Reeves, S., Pelone, F., Harrison, R., Goldman, J., & Zwarenstein, M. (2017). Interprofessional collaboration to improve professional practice and healthcare outcomes. *Cochrane Database of Systematic Reviews* (6). https://doi.org/10.1002/14651858.cd000072.pub3

Richardson, S. O., Andersen, M. B., & Morris, T. (2008). *Overtraining athletes: Personal journeys in sport*. Human Kinetics.

Salovey, P., & Mayer, J. D. (1990). Emotional intelligence. *Imagination, Cognition and Personality, 9*(3), 185–211. https://doi.org/10.2190/dugg-p24e-52wk-6cdg

Sangaleti, C., Schveitzer, M. C., Peduzzi, M., Zoboli, E. L. C. P., & Soares, C. B. (2017). Experiences and shared meaning of teamwork and interprofessional collaboration among health care professionals in primary health care settings: A systematic review. *JBI Database of Systematic Reviews and Implementation Reports, 15*(11), 2723–2788. https://doi.org/10.11124/jbisrir-2016-003016

Schmitt, M., Blue, A., Aschenbrener, C. A., & Viggiano, T. R. (2011). Core competencies for interprofessional collaborative practice: Reforming health care by transforming health professionals' education. *Academic Medicine, 86*(11), 1351. https://doi.org/10.1097/acm.0b013e3182308e39

Smith, J. A., Flowers, P., & Larkin, M. (2009). *Interpretative phenomenological analysis*. Sage Publishing.

Straub, R. O. (2012). *Health psychology: A biopsychosocial approach*. Worth Publishers.

Tunick, R., Clement, D., & Etzel, E. F. (2009). Counseling injured and disabled student-athletes: A guide for understanding and intervention. In E. F. Etzel (Ed.), *Counseling and psychological services for college student-athletes*. Fitness Information Technology.

Ulrich, G., & Breitbach, A. P. (2022). Interprofessional collaboration among sport science and sports medicine professionals: An international cross-sectional survey. *Journal of Interprofessional Care*, *36*(1), 4–14. https://doi.org/10.1080/13561820.2021.1874318

Ulrich, G., Carrard, J., Nigg, C. R., Erlacher, D., & Breitbach, A. P. (2022). Is healthcare a team sport? Widening our lens on interprofessional collaboration and education in sport and exercise medicine. *BMJ Open Sport & Exercise Medicine*, *8*(e001377). https://doi.org/10.1136/bmjsem-2022-00137

Wadey, R., Day, M. C., Cavallerio, F., & Martinelli, L. A. (2018). Multilevel model of sport injury (MMSI): Can coaches impact and be impacted by injury? In R. C. Thelwell & M. Dicks (Eds.), *Professional advances in sports coaching: Research and practice* (pp. 336–357). Routledge. https://doi.org/10.4324/9781351210980

Weinberg, R. S., & Gould, D. (2019). *Foundations of sport and exercise psychology* (7th ed.). Human Kinetics.

Wiese-Bjornstal, D. M. (2009). Sport injury and college athlete health across the lifespan. *Journal of Intercollegiate Sport*, *2*(1), 64–80. https://doi.org/10.1123/jis.2.1.64

Wiese-Bjornstal, D. M. (2010). Psychology and socioculture affect injury risk, response, and recovery in high-intensity athletes: A consensus statement. *Scandinavian Journal of Medicine & Science in Sports*, *20*, 103–111. https://doi.org/10.1111/j.1600-0838.2010.01195.x

Wiese-Bjornstal, D. M., & Smith, A. M. (1993). Counseling strategies for enhanced recovery of injured athletes within a team approach. In D. Pargman (Ed.), *Psychological bases of sport injuries* (pp. 149–182). Fitness Information Technology.

Wiese-Bjornstal, D. M., & Smith, A. M. (1999). Counseling strategies for enhanced recovery of injured athletes within a team approach. In D. Pargman (Ed.), *Psychological bases of sport injuries* (2nd ed., pp. 125–156). Fitness Information Technologies.

Wiese-Bjornstal, D. M., Smith, A. M., Shaffer, S. M., & Morrey, M. A. (1998). An integrated model of response to sport injury: Psychological and sociological dynamics. *Journal of Applied Sport Psychology*, *10*(1), 46–69. https://doi.org/10.1080/10413209808406377

Williams, J. M., & Andersen, M. B. (1998). Psychosocial antecedents of sport injury: Review and critique of the stress and injury model. *Journal of Applied Sport Psychology*, *10*(1), 5–25. https://doi.org/10.1080/10413209808406375

Yang, J., Peek-Asa, C., Lowe, J. B., Heiden, E., & Foster, D. T. (2010). Social support patterns of collegiate athletes before and after injury. *Journal of Athletic Training*, *45*(4), 372–379. https://doi.org/10.4085/1062-6050-45.4.372

8 Ethical Issues in Sport Injury and Rehabilitation

Brandonn S. Harris, Megan M. Byrd, Kaytlyn Johnson, and Luca Ziegler

---

Chapter Objectives

- To demonstrate the importance of ethics in sport injury.
- To outline specific ethical issues, principles, standards, and virtues pertinent to sport injury rehabilitation.
- To explain the process of ethical decision-making in sport injury.

Introduction

Comprehensive care for athletes with injuries calls for a holistic interprofessional approach (for more details, see Chapter 7). Such approach typically includes professionals representing general medicine, sports medicine, psychology, and other allied professions, each of whom subscribe to their own unique code of ethics guiding their practice in this area (Wiese-Bjornstal et al., 1998). Each professional, although working in different capacities, maintains the responsibility of facilitating the psychological, physical, and emotional health and well-being of athletes. Such responsibility also includes a possibility of making (complicated) decisions and challenges that are unique to the injury rehabilitation setting (Burgess, 2011; Moncier, 2014). With each professional having their own code of ethics guiding their work and the collaborative nature of providing comprehensive care during injury rehabilitation, it is critical that everyone work ethically within their unique "lane" and scope of practice on behalf of the athlete with injuries.

For psychologically trained professionals, a thorough understanding of professional code of ethics is important when working in interprofessional settings. The code of ethics within sport psychology–focused organizations often include guidelines for professional behavior and work as denoted by principles and standards. For example, the principles associated with the Association for Applied Sport Psychology's (AASP) code of ethics (i.e., competence, integrity, professional and scientific responsibility, respect for people's rights and dignity, concern for others' welfare, and social responsibility) all serve to represent more general and aspirational behaviors. Conversely, ethical standards, such as the 26 found within the AASP ethics code, generally seek to "more precisely specify the boundaries of ethical conduct" (Association for Applied Sport Psychology, 2011) as they include proscribed rules of ethical behavior within a number of roles sport psychology professionals (SPPs) frequently work in (e.g., teaching, research, applied practice).

This chapter serves to discuss several ethical areas SPPs are likely to encounter when involved in the provision of services for athletes with injuries. Using codes of ethics from AASP and the

DOI: 10.4324/9781003295709-10

International Society for Sport Psychology (ISSP; Association for Applied Sport Psychology, 2011; Quartiroli et al., 2021) as a guide, this chapter will (a) outline relevant ethical issues, principles, standards, and virtues pertinent to sport injury rehabilitation and (b) explain the process of ethical decision-making and its role in sport injury.

While this chapter utilizes the AASP and ISSP codes of ethics to guide the content covered, the ethical issues covered in this chapter are not unique to these organizations, but quite the contrary. The authors strongly encourage professionals to review the code(s) of ethics and professional practice guidelines of the associations they are affiliated with, as well as any legal implications pertaining to jurisdictions one practices in. Further, it is important to note that a comprehensive review of all ethical issues that may present themselves in injury settings for SPPs is difficult to provide, given these may vary based on setting, training background, credentials, and competencies of the professional (Watson II, Clement et al., 2020).

Ethical Issues, Principles, and Standards in Sport Injury and Rehabilitation

The following section highlights ethical issues that have the potential to exist in sport psychology, sports medicine, or other healthcare service delivery within sport injury and rehabilitation settings. What follows here is a discussion of implications pertaining to confidentiality, harm prevention, competence, multiple-role relationships, and conflicts of interest within sport injury settings.

Confidentiality and Harm Prevention

In psychology, *confidentiality* is defined as the service providers' ethical, and sometimes legal, obligation to protect and refrain from disclosing client information to others outside of the consultation relationship (Koocher & Keith-Spiegel, 2016). For SPPs, maintaining confidentiality is of utmost importance to build a trusting foundation and relationship with athletes and represents the cornerstone of such working relationships (Koocher & Keith-Spiegel, 2016). Indeed, the ethical issue of confidentiality exists in most, if not all, ethical practice guidelines in psychology worldwide (e.g., American Psychological Association, Association for Applied Sport Psychology, Australian Psychological Society, British Psychological Society, Canadian Sport Psychology Association, International Society of Sport Psychology) and can have legal ramifications if not adhered to, depending on licensure, state, and/or country statutes. As such, understanding confidentiality and its limits is imperative prior to beginning a sport psychology consultation.

Right to Privacy

The term *privacy* is often connected to *confidentiality*; however, there is a delineation between the two terms. *Privacy* is "a legal right that allows an individual to talk/behave in a manner that is free from public knowledge and interference" (Watson II, Harris et al., 2020, p. 754). In the United States, the Health Insurance Portability and Accountability Act of 1996 (HIPAA) protects health information and privacy concerns and allows for the transfer of information when necessary (United States Department of Health and Human Services, 1996).

While confidentiality and the right to privacy from the practitioner's perspective may be clear, the nature of sport can challenge adherence to the code of ethics. This is particularly pertinent when working within an organizational or interprofessional team system or when hired by a third party (Moore, 2003). As it relates to athletes with injuries, confidentiality and the right to privacy can become blurred and hard to navigate, particularly as many stakeholders such as coaches, parents/guardians, and sports medicine personals (SMPs) are involved in the injury rehabilitation and return to participation protocols. Additionally, it is common for information about athletes' injuries to be shared with multiple stakeholders and even the media (Bell et al., 2008). Based on HIPAA, athlete health information can only be shared with authorization from the athlete (Magee et al., 2003), which is often required as part of their participation in sport.

Regardless, if an athlete has waived their HIPAA protections, this does not mean that SPPs are free to share information an athlete has shared in a consultancy session, or to share personal health information of the athlete. At times, as part of a triangulation of care, it may be advantageous to obtain a release of information form so that the SPPs and the sports medicine professionals (SMPs) can discuss specific aspects of the athlete's injury care as part of an interprofessional collaboration. Any information shared between SPPs and SMPs would need to be discussed with the athlete prior to any sharing taking place. The athlete should also be aware of the parameters and limits of disclosure (Brown & Cogan, 2006). To ensure confidentiality and the right to privacy are upheld and maintained, it is important to establish clearly delineated roles and responsibilities for all members of the interprofessional rehabilitation team from the beginning of the relationship. It may also be beneficial to consistently revisit confidentiality parameters and who maintains the rights to the information gathered with the members of the interprofessional team (Moncier, 2014). Loubert (1999) suggests fully disclosing all roles that one holds that may involve the athlete directly or indirectly, including (a) being employed by the athlete's team or organization, (b) social or legal obligations, (c) referrals, and/or (d) responsibilities to other teams/team members.

Location of Service

Another consideration for upholding confidentiality is the location of service delivery. As SPPs tend to work where athletes are, such as athletic training rooms or sport fields, the work can be visible to others. If an athlete with an injury approaches an SPP in a public place, they should take precautions to create as confidential a space as possible, upholding the confidentiality of the discussion content, and record session notes later (Etzel & Watson II, 2007). If the SPP professional's office is in a hallway where athletes travel to other sport spaces, teammates may notice someone coming or going from the office, thus potentially violating confidentiality or the right to privacy. These and other potential instances that may result in compromising confidentiality should be discussed with the athlete to collectively determine how to best handle the breach of confidentiality.

Client Rights and Dignity

As an addendum of upholding confidentiality, principle 2 of the ISSP Ethical Code for Sport Psychology Practice and principle D of the AASP Ethics Code is respect for people's rights and dignity. This principle states that SPPs act in

> a manner that exemplifies respect for the dignity and worth of all people, and an individual's right to privacy, confidentiality, self-determination and justice. In particular, they take special safeguards that may be necessary to protect the rights and welfare of persons or communities they serve whose vulnerabilities could impair autonomous decision-making.
> (Quartiroli et al., 2021; ISSP ethics code, p. 3)

This principle can further guide SPPs' decision-making when faced with challenges from other stakeholders or third party, particularly when they press for information about an athlete's injury and recovery process. The rehabilitation process can be a vulnerable time for athletes (Brewer, 2017), and although some stakeholders may feel privy to an athlete's personal health information, SPPs need to ensure they are the information gatekeepers.

Harm Prevention

There are limits to confidentiality that are in place to keep athletes safe, most notably when there is a potential threat of harm to oneself or others, and when the athlete is a minor (i.e., under the age of 18 in the United States). Unfortunately, there have been cases in all levels of sport where athletes with an injury have been harmed by those in positions of power and responsible for the health and safety of the athlete. If such information is shared to an SPP, it would be necessary for them to break confidentiality and make a report to the appropriate authorities. This further illustrates the need for SPPs to uphold athletes' rights and dignity, as too many athletes have had their trust violated by someone who was purported to provide care. In the case of minor athletes, they cannot legally consent to service provision, thus requiring a parent or guardian to consent on their behalf. This means that parents and/or guardians could have access to information divulged in session, limiting confidentiality between SPP and the athlete. Parents and/or guardians may also choose to play more of an active role in the athlete's rehabilitation and recovery and seek to gain knowledge of the athlete's personal health information.

Competence

Many SPPs work in varied settings and, as a result, may find themselves working with an increasingly diverse group of athletes, highlighting the importance of competency in practice. According to Koocher and Keith-Spiegel (2016), *competency* includes both intellectual and emotional elements. The former highlights the acquisition of clinically and scholarly informed knowledge regarding practice and client care, as well as an awareness of the information or area(s) which professionals may *not* be knowledgeable about. The latter addresses the ability of practitioners to emotionally manage the session content of their clients while remaining aware of their own biases and well-being in the process as a service provider.

The importance and complexity of competence are also underscored in both the principles and standards of the AASP ethics code (Association for Applied Sport Psychology, 2011) and the standards of the ISSP Ethical Code for Sport Psychology Practice (Quartiroli et al., 2021). Within the AASP's ethics code, the notion of ethical and competent care is embedded within principle C ("integrity and professional responsibility") and principle E ("concern for others' welfare"), highlighting its significance for both service delivery and concern for the welfare of the athlete. Both the principle C and the principle E also acknowledge the SPPs' responsibility in ensuring athletes' best interests are being served while concurrently minimizing harm. Relative to sport injury, these considerations are particularly important, given SMPs have previously identified SPPs as the most appropriate service provider to address many of the psychological and emotional concerns associated with injury and rehabilitation (Wiese-Bjornstal et al., 1991). Following sport injury, numerous biological, psychological, and social factors interact and influence athletes' biopsychosocial responses to the injury, rehabilitation, and return to participation process (Brewer & Redmond, 2017). To provide competent care to athletes with injuries, it is important for SPPs to understand the psychological sequelae of sport injury (Wiese-Bjornstal et al., 2020) and how it interacts with the physical aspects of injury (Brewer & Redmond, 2017).

Competency in Sport Injury Psychology within Sports Medicine

With the variability of experiences and training included in sport psychology graduate pro-grams worldwide, it is likely that not all students and professionals have received specific and in-depth training in sport injury psychology (e.g., Heaney et al., 2012). Competent integration of sport injury psychology into applied practice requires mastery of theoretical and empirical knowledge within sport psychology. Competent practitioner also possesses mastery of theoreti-cal and empirical understanding of multicultural and biopsychosocial sport injury risk factors, psychosocial responses to injury, rehabilitation, and return to participation process. They also have theoretical and empirical understanding of the efficacy of implementing psychosocial strat-egies with injured athletes and how to make referrals to other professionals when necessary (Brewer & Arvinen-Barrow, 2021). To competently work with athletes with injuries and vari-ous medical professionals in an interprofessional manner, Brewer and Arvinen-Barrow (2022, March 18) suggested that those serving this population in a competent manner should seek out continuing educational resources, such as webinars, workshops, relevant research, and other sport psychology–specific sources, including this textbook.

Across all contexts and types of sport psychology consultations, it is imperative for the prac-titioner to reflect on their own competencies – as they themselves serve as the immediate deter-minant of the boundaries of ethical and competent practice. Building on the work of Watson II, Clement et al. (2020), the present authors suggest that competent sport psychology service pro-vision to athletes with injuries minimally includes unique knowledge of (a) sport injury–related biopsychosocial theory and terminology; (b) psychosocial injury risk factors, challenges, and responses to injury and rehabilitation; and (c) how and when to mobilize a referral protocol (for assessment and referral, see Chapter 10).

To do competent work with athletes with injuries and their medical providers, it is also rec-ommended to have, at minimum, a basic understanding of common medical terminology and the physical rehabilitation process. Listening to and collaborating with medical professionals is one such way to learn about the process and help build trust and rapport. It is also recommended to gain an understanding of how to set up and work as a member of an interprofessional reha-bilitation team. Thus far, three interprofessional practice models (Clement & Arvinen-Barrow, 2013; Dijkstra et al., 2014; Meyer et al., 2014) have been proposed as suitable for sport injury rehabilitation. While these models vary in memberships and level of interprofessional integra-tion, all of them place the athlete at the center of the care, with a number of professionals and significant individuals supporting the rehabilitation and return to participation process (for more details, see Chapter 7).

Referrals and Boundaries of Competence

Both theoretical and empirical evidence has provided support for a variety of psychological, emotional, and behavioral responses to injury (Evans & Brewer, 2022; Watson II, Clement et al., 2020) (for more details, see Chapters 3–6). For example, Tunick et al. (2009) noted that when an athlete is injured, common psychosocial responses include (a) changes in athletes' perception of their social status, (b) feelings of isolation, (c) withdrawal from their team and others, (d) shock and uncertainty associated with injury, (e) changes in mood (anger, depression, anxiety), and (f) grieving the loss of status and identity as a competitive athlete.

From an ethical perspective, the challenge for SPPs is the accurate identification and con-ceptualization of the injured athletes' needs and if addressing them is within the boundaries of professional competence of the service provider. Many psychosocial responses can be managed effectively utilizing various non-clinical mental skills interventions as a part of the rehabilitation process by the SPP or the SMP. However, with such variability in psychosocial responses experienced and numerous coping mechanisms used by athletes (for more on coping, see Chapter 12), some athletes may require more specialized attention from a clinically trained and licensed mental health provider. Moreover, existing research has consistently found that athletes are at risk for experiencing clinical concerns (i.e., psychopathology) following injury and during rehabilitation (e.g., Appaneal et al., 2009; Brewer & Petrie, 1995; Byrd et al., 2022; Leddy et al., 1994; Manuel et al., 2002).

The first step in providing an injured athlete with ethical, competent, and appropriate care is determining their individual needs. This requires having a mastery of signs and symptoms of psychopathology. The use of clinical screening assessments for depression, anxiety, and mental well-being would be advantageous to detect psychopathology-related concerns, provided the person administering and interpreting the results is appropriately trained and/or licensed/certified. If a concern for psychopathology exists, a referral to a clinically trained and appropriately licensed mental health professional would be the appropriate course of action. The referral process, which is detailed in the ISSP Ethical Code for Sport Psychology Practice (standard 11), aims to provide the athlete appropriate support when their psychological needs are beyond the competency of the practitioner. It is important to note that making a referral does not mean that the practitioner lacks competency but, rather, awareness of limits to their professional competency. Making a referral indicates that the practitioner is competent in knowing what services they can and cannot provide within their scope of practice. Prior to initiating a referral, the SPP should ensure the athlete is aware of their options and the reasons for the referral. A referral should be discussed as a facilitative action aimed to provide the athletes with the best possible support, and not as something punitive, or as a response to something "bad" the athlete did. An ethically competent practitioner will develop a referral network of professionals they trust and can have confidence in their work (for more details on assessment and referral, see Chapter 10).

Multiple-Role Relationships and Conflict of Interests

Multiple-role relationships also represent an important ethical consideration when working within a sport injury rehabilitation setting and as a part of an interprofessional team (Moncier, 2014). Multiple-role relationships materialize when the SPP, whose specific role is a mental health and/or mental skills service provider, also assumes an additional role relative to the athlete as a coach, teacher, mentor, friend, or other stakeholder (Makarowski, 1999a). When assuming the additional role increases the likelihood of potential harm to the athlete, most psychology ethics codes generally discourage assuming secondary roles, given the conflict(s) of interest, exploitation, or dependency that can result (e.g., Makarowski, 1999b; Moncier, 2014; Watson II, Clement et al., 2020; Watson II, Harris et al., 2020). The Principles and Standards of the AASP Ethics Code (Association for Applied Sport Psychology, 2011) and the Standards of the ISSP Ethical Code for Sport Psychology Practice (Quartiroli et al., 2021) address potential consequences of multiple role conflict within standards 4 and 9, respectively, and provide similar guidance specific to sport psychology.

Within sport injury setting specifically, SPPs may find multiple-role relationships to occur and become problematic when evaluating their service obligations and responsibilities to various stakeholders invested in the injured athlete's progress and well-being. For example, aside from providing care to the athlete with injuries as a member of the support staff or interprofessional team, SPPs may also have obligations to coaches' (inter)national governing bodies, team owners/organization, and/or athletic department supervisors (Watson II, Clement et al., 2020). Should the SPPs' obligations to various stakeholders conflict with one another (e.g., what may be in the best interest of the athlete with injury might not be in the best interest of the team or organization), the potential for harm for the athlete is enhanced. Unique to sport injury settings, Moncier (2014) also noted that some SPPs who work in a private practice setting or are affiliated with a physical therapy/rehabilitation facility may also be working within a university athletic department. Should the SPP find themselves working with a team that includes an individual athlete the SPP works with as part of the private practice/rehabilitation facility, the potential for a multiple-role relationship also presents itself.

Within many university systems in the United States in particular, SPPs who are employed as faculty and also provide mental skills or mental health services to student-athletes on the same campus have the potential to have a multiple-role relationship with a student-athlete. Some SPPs may also hold certification and/or licensure as an athletic trainer (ATC, LAT), creating another potential multiple-role relationship. In the aforementioned and other similar multiple-role relationship situations, it is important to discuss the roles and associated boundaries that surround each role occupied (i.e., professor/athletic trainer/SPP, student-athlete). It is also important to both establish and implement necessary safeguards to maintain a safe and appropriate professional arrangement between the professional and the athlete – to ensure risks of harm, exploitation, and conflict of interests are minimized for both the student-athlete and the practitioner (Makarowski, 1999b; Watson II et al., 2006; Watson II, Clement et al., 2020).

Ethical Decision-Making

Given the nuances associated with the ethical practice of sport psychology with injured athletes, SPPs are likely to find themselves having to navigate ethical dilemmas that extend into sports medicine. Understanding professional ethics codes is of utmost importance, as they provide professional guidance, convey values, and allow for autonomy and professionalism of a scientific field (Whelan et al., 2002; Zeigler, 1987). However, while ethics codes attempt to provide guidance and support practitioners in the field, a code of ethics may also prove difficult to navigate when encountering an ethical dilemma. In such instances, individuals may rely on ethical decision-making models for guidance. Ethical decision-making models provide practitioners with a structured approach to (a) analyze an ethical dilemma and (b) make practical decisions that lead to the most appropriate course of action consistent with the underlying ethics code. In case the professional organization an SPP is affiliated with does not have an ethical decision-making model and working with injured athletes can overlap with other professional domains, at times it may be advantageous to consider appropriate ethical decision-making models from other fields. This can be particularly beneficial since the field of sport psychology is closely embedded and/or related to other social sciences.

In recent years, AASP has developed an ethical decision-making tree (see https://applied-sportpsych.org/site/assets/files/1035/basic_ethics_decision_tree_for_aasp_members.pdf) to guide its members and AASP Certified Mental Performance Consultants (CMPC®) toward a personal commitment to ethical conduct as outlined by the AASP ethics code (Association for Applied Sport Psychology, 2011). Different from other decision-making models, the ethical decision-making tree (Association for Applied Sport Psychology) comprises six distinct questions, followed by recommended actions for the SPP to follow based on the specific circumstances of the ethical concern. The ethical decision-making tree is aimed to broadly guide practitioners, rather than providing a step-by-step process on how to proceed.

Specific decision-making models have been developed in related fields and often applied to sport and exercise psychology profession. For example, a model by Hadjistavropoulos and Malloy (2000) has been identified as an appropriate aid for the field of sport and exercise psychology

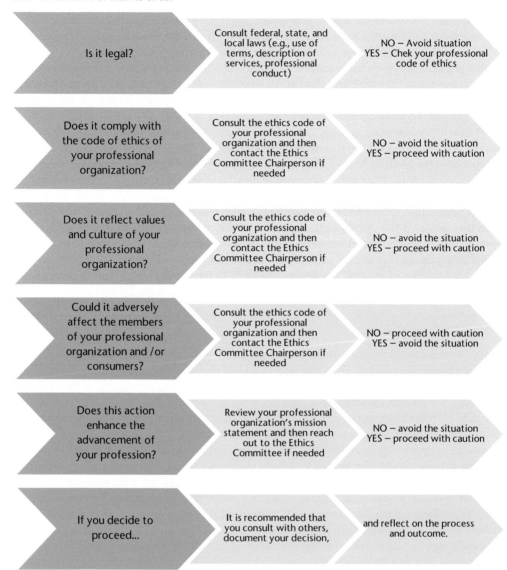

Figure 8.1 An introductory ethical decision-making tree.

Source: Adapted from *Basic Ethics Decision Tree* for AASP members https://appliedsportpsych.org/site/assets/files/1035/basic_ethics_decision_tree_for_aasp_members.pdf, Association for Applied Sport Psychology.

(Harris et al., 2009). The model aligns with the Canadian Psychological Association's (CPA) Canadian Code of Ethics and consists of seven steps that allow practitioners to analyze an ethical dilemma and make ethical choices. The seven steps include identifying ethical concerns, developing and choosing an appropriate course of action, taking responsibility for potential consequences, and evaluating the results of the decision.

While decision-making models provide structure to the resolution of an ethical dilemma, even if practitioners use well-developed models like Hadjistavropoulos and Malloy (2000), it is likely that additional points need to be considered for comprehensive analysis. All models have unique strengths and weaknesses; therefore, utilizing multiple models may provide a more holistic approach to the ethical dilemma, allowing comprehensive analysis lending to more effective decision-making abilities. Combing the ethical decision-making tree (AASP) with established decision-making models might also be beneficial, as it encourages practitioners to consult with other practitioners, a step not specified in other decision-making models (Hadjistavropoulos & Malloy, 2000). It is also important to note that, at times, ethical dilemmas may be difficult to navigate for SPPs, particularly as they are usually a complex process dependent on the professional's situation (i.e., professional career, responsibilities, level of experience, personal values). Ethical decision-making models may help SPPs in navigating these challenges in an ethical manner.

Conclusion

Many injured athletes have access to comprehensive care to ensure their needs and well-being are attended to in a holistic manner. While all service providers have an obligation to provide unique and specialized care to the athletes, each group also faces complicated decisions and challenges that are unique to the sport injury setting (Burgess, 2011; Moncier, 2014). For SPPs, working within sports injury and rehabilitation, particularly when working as a member of an interprofessional team, requires great attention to ethical issues to ensure confidential and competent care. Within this chapter, the authors have addressed some of the most pertinent ethical issues, principles, standards, and virtues pertinent to sport injury rehabilitation.

Case Study

Isla, a 23-year-old Australian native on a professional women's rugby team in the United States, where she attended college, reaches out to meet with the sport psychology consultant. The consultant is a Certified Mental Performance Consultant (CMPC®), employed by the rugby organization and tasked with providing mental performance services to the team and its members. From regularly attending team practices, the consultant observes that Isla is one of the top throwers on the team. Throwers are crucial to a rugby team, requiring high levels of concentration and accuracy.

Isla was the captain of her college team and described her four years of collegiate athletics as highly successful, earning All-American honors and winning one national championship. After developing a trusting relationship during individual sessions, Isla opens up to talk about a rotator cuff injury she experienced prior to her senior year in college. Trying to help her team succeed and secure a professional contract, Isla returned to play before feeling physically and psychologically ready. Isla was offered a professional contract following graduation, despite struggling with severe soreness in her shoulder during competition. She still does not fully trust her shoulder, because it does not feel like it did before the injury occurred.

During the contract negotiations, Isla downplayed the lingering effects of her injury and denied its impact on her performance. After joining the professional team, Isla realized that the higher intensity and physicality at this level lead to increased soreness and impaired mobility during her overhead throws at the end of the game. Because of the pain and immobility, Isla sometimes hesitates before throwing the ball, which leads to inaccuracy, mistiming, and double-clutching, making it difficult for her teammates to catch the ball. Being unable to throw as well as she is capable of has negatively affected her athletic performance.

In the latest session, she confides that she does not want the coaches to know about the severity of her injury because she fears losing her position on the team. Knowing the terms of her professional contract, she understands that the organization has the power to dismiss her from the team, potentially without paying her. Due to the culture of rugby, particularly in her home country of Australia, she also does not feel that it is acceptable to quit, because it is "all in her head." Her college coach constantly discussed the importance of toughness: "Rugby is only for tough athletes. Those who are not tough enough can quit." Given this, Isla feels she has no other option but to play through the pain.

In the most recent staff meeting, the coach mentions Isla's throwing performance during recent games and practices. He is sure that Isla is struggling with the "yips." To the consultant's knowledge, the yips affect muscle movement, particularly with repetitive skills. The consultant also knows that there is a stigma associated with the yips and coaches typically avoid the word entirely. During the meeting, the coach warns that if Isla's performance continues to dwindle, she will become a danger to their reputation as "the toughest team in the league." He is also worried that other players might start to notice it and "catch the yips" as well. During the meeting, he suggests the consultant meet with Isla to "confirm she has the yips." He hopes to utilize this information to add to the organization's case for dismissing Isla from the team and using her open spot for a new recruit, who has been performing well at the college level. The coach also addresses the financial constraints of the organization and emphasizes that they do not have room on the team for underperformers.

Isla has recently exhibited some depressive symptoms associated with the reality of her situation, including excessive sleeping and lack of motivation. The consultant is aware that Isla's inability to throw is due to severe soreness caused by the residual effects of her previous injury, rather than the yips. She is reluctant to seek sports medicine services because she fears the coaches do not want to keep her on the team and will cut her. In this case, her rugby career may be over. Isla feels torn between taking a break from rugby or continuing to play and hoping that her symptoms will get better. She feels her shoulder "should feel much better" after more than a year of rehabilitation. The emphasis on upholding a tough demeanor creates pressure for Isla to continue playing through the pain, even if it is not to her full potential. Feeling like she cannot talk about her struggles with anyone, she seeks the CMPC® consultant out for advice.

Questions

1. If you were the CMPC®, what additional information would you need before deciding how to proceed?
2. What ethical concerns associated with confidentiality and competence would you need to be aware of?
3. What ethical issues, if anything, might be different if the CMPC® were not employed by the organization but rather by the individual client (Isla)?
4. What multicultural factors may influence Isla's case?
5. How would you apply Isla's case to the ethical decision-making model?

References

Appaneal, R. N., Levine, B. R., Perna, F. M., & Roh, J. L. (2009). Measuring postinjury depression among male and female competitive athletes. *Journal of Sport & Exercise Psychology*, *31*(1), 60–76. https://doi.org/10.1123/jsep.31.1.60

Association for Applied Sport Psychology. *Introductory ethical decision-making tree for AASP members.* https://appliedsportpsych.org/site/assets/files/1035/basic_ethics_decision_tree_for_aasp_members.pdf

Association for Applied Sport Psychology. (2011). *Ethics code: AASP ethical principles and standards.* https://appliedsportpsych.org/about-the-association-for-applied-sport-psychology/ethics/ethics-code/

Bell, R., Ratzlaff, S. E., & Murray, S. R. (2008). The impact of the HIPAA privacy rule on collegiate sport professionals. *The Sport Journal*, *24*, 1–7. https://thesportjournal.org/article/the-impact-of-the-hipaa-privacy-rule-on-collegiate-sport-professionals/

Brewer, B. W. (2017). Psychological responses to injury. In *Oxford research encyclopedia of psychology*. Oxford University Press.

Brewer, B. W., & Arvinen-Barrow, M. (2021). Psychology of injury and rehabilitation. In Association for Applied Sport Psychology (AASP). In S. C. Sackett, N. Durand-Bush, & L. Tashman (Eds.), *The essential guide for mental performance consultants*. Human Kinetics Custom Content.

Brewer, B. W., & Arvinen-Barrow, M. (2022, March 18). Comment on SIG spotlight: "Does the CMPC credential apply to sport injury?" *AASP Newsletter*. https://appliedsportpsych.org/members/newsletters/march-2022/comment-on-sig-spotlight-does-the-cmpc-credential-apply-to-sports-injury/

Brewer, B. W., & Petrie, T. A. (1995). A comparison between injured and uninjured football players on selected psychological variables. *The Academic Athletic Journal*, *10*, 11–18.

Brewer, B. W., & Redmond, C. J. (2017). *Psychology of sport injury*. Human Kinetics.

Brown, J. L., & Cogan, K. D. (2006). Ethical clinical practice and sport psychology: When two worlds collide. *Ethics & Behavior*, *16*(1), 15–23. https://doi.org/10.1207/s15327019eb1601_3

Burgess, T. L. (2011). Ethical issues in return-to-sport decisions. *South African Journal of Sports Medicine*, *23*(4), 138–139. https://doi.org/10.17159/2078-516X/2011/v23i4a327

Byrd, M., Kontos, A. P., Eagle, S. R., & Zizzi, S. (2022). Preliminary evidence for a relationship between anxiety, anger, and impulsivity in collegiate athletes with a sport-related concussion. *Journal of Clinical Sport Psychology*, *16*(2), 89–108. https://doi.org/10.1123/jcsp.2020-0003

Clement, D., & Arvinen-Barrow, M. (2013). Sport medicine team influences in psychological rehabilitation: A multidisciplinary approach. In M. Arvinen-Barrow & N. Walker (Eds.), *The psychology of sport injury and rehabilitation* (pp. 156–170). Routledge.

Dijkstra, P. H., Pollock, N., Chakraverty, R., & Alonso, J. M. (2014). Managing the health of the elite athlete: A new integrated performance health management and coaching model. *British Journal of Sports Medicine*, *48*(7), 523–531. https://doi.org/10.1136/bjsports-2013-093222

Etzel, E. F., & Watson II, J. C. (2007). Ethical challenges for psychological consultations in intercollegiate athletics. *Journal of Clinical Sport Psychology*, *1*(3), 304–317. https://doi.org/10.1123/jcsp.1.3.304

Evans, L., & Brewer, B. W. (2022). Applied psychology of sport injury: Getting to – and moving across – The valley of death. *Journal of Applied Sport Psychology*, *34*(5), 1011–1028. https://doi.org/10.1080/10413200.2021.2015480

Hadjistavropoulos, T., & Malloy, D. (2000). Making ethical choices: A comparative decision-making model for Canadian psychologists. *Canadian Psychologist*, *41*(2), 104–115. https://doi.org/10.1037/h0086860

Harris, B., Visek, A. J., & Watson II, J. C. (2009). Ethical decision-making in sport psychology: Issues and implications for professional practice. In R. Schinke (Ed.), *Contemporary sport psychology* (pp. 217–232). Nova Science Publishers, Inc.

Heaney, C., Green, A. J. K., Rostron, C. L., & Walker, N. (2012). A qualitative and quantitative investigation of the psychology content of UK physiotherapy education programs. *Journal of Physical Therapy Education*, *26*(3), 24–56.

Koocher, G. P., & Keith-Spiegel, P. (2016). *Ethics in psychology and the mental health professions* (4th ed.). Oxford University Press.

Leddy, M. H., Lambert, M. J., & Ogles, B. M. (1994). Psychological consequences of athletic injury among high-level competitors. *Research Quarterly for Exercise and Sport*, *65*(4), 347–354. https://doi.org/10.1080/02701367.1994.10607639

Loubert, P. (1999). Ethical perspectives in counseling. In R. Ray & D. M. Wiese-Bjornstal (Eds.), *Counseling in sports medicine*. Human Kinetics.

Magee, J. T., Almekinders, L. C., & Taft, T. N. (2003). HIPAA and the team physician. *Sports Medicine Update*, 4–7.

Makarowski, L. M. (1999a). Ethical and legal issues for sport professionals counseling injured athletes. In D. Pargman (Ed.), *Psychological bases of sport injuries* (pp. 29–47). Fitness Information Technology.

Makarowski, L. M. (1999b). Ethical and legal issues for sports professionals counseling injured athletes. In D. Pargman (Ed.), *Psychological bases of sport injuries* (pp. 29–47). Fitness Information Technology.

Manuel, J. C., Shilt, J. S., Curl, W. W., Smith, J. A., DuRant, R. H., Lester, L., & Sinal, S. H. (2002). Coping with sports injuries: An examination of the adolescent athlete. *The Journal of Adolescent Health*, *31*(5), 391–393. https://doi.org/10.1016/s1054-139x(02)00400-7

Meyer, B. B., Merkur, A., Ebersole, K. T., & Massey, W. V. (2014). The realities of working in elite sport: What they didn't teach you in graduate school. In A. M. Lane, M. Godfrey, M. Loosemore, & W. G. P (Eds.), *Applied sport science and medicine: Case studies from practice* (pp. 137–142). CreateSpace: Self-published.

Moncier, J. C. (2014). Sports medicine: The ethics of working as part of a university medical team. In E. F. Etzel & J. Watson II (Eds.), *Ethical issues in sport, exercise, and performance psychology* (pp. 99–111). Fitness Information Technology.

Moore, Z. E. (2003). Ethical dilemmas in sport psychology: Discussion and recommendation for practice. *Professional Psychology: Research and Practice*, *34*(6), 601–610. https://doi.org/10.1037/0735-7028.34.6.601

Quartiroli, A., Harris, B. S., Brückner, S., Chow, G. M., Connole, I. J., Cropley, B., . . . Zito, M. (2021). The international society of sport psychology registry (ISSP-R) ethical code for sport psychology practice. *International Journal of Sport and Exercise Psychology*, *19*(6), 907–928. https://doi.org/10.1080/1612197X.2020.1789317

Tunick, R., Clement, D., & Etzel, E. F. (2009). Counseling injured and disabled student-athletes: A guide for understanding and intervention. In E. F. Etzel (Ed.), *Counseling and psychological services for college student-athletes*. Fitness Information Technology.

United States Department of Health and Human Services. (1996). *Health insurance portability and accountability act of 1996*. https://aspe.hhs.gov/reports/health-insurance-portability-accountability-act-1996

Watson II, J. C., Clement, D., Harris, B. S., Leffingwell, T., & Hurst, J. (2006). Teacher-practitioner dual role issues in sport psychology. *Ethics & Behavior*, *16*(1), 41–59. https://doi.org/10.1207/s15327019eb1601_5

Watson II, J. C., Clement, D., & Hilliard, R. (2020). Ethical issues for sport psychology professionals consulting with injured athletes. In A. Ivarsson & U. Johnson (Eds.), *Psychological bases of sport injuries* (4th ed., pp. 153–167). Fitness Information Technology.

Watson II, J. C., Harris, B. S., & Baillie, P. (2020). Ethical issues impacting the profession of sport psychology. In G. Tenenbaum & R. C. Eklund (Eds.), *Handbook of sport psychology* (4th ed., pp. 751–772). John Wiley & Sons, Inc.

Whelan, J. P., Meyers, A. W., & Elkins, T. D. (2002). Ethics in sport and exercise psychology. In J. L. Van Raalte & B. W. Brewer (Eds.), *Exploring sport and exercise psychology* (pp. 503–523). American Psychological Association. https://doi.org/10.1037/10465-024

Wiese-Bjornstal, D. M., Smith, A. M., Shaffer, S. M., & Morrey, M. A. (1998). An integrated model of response to sport injury: Psychological and sociological dynamics. *Journal of Applied Sport Psychology*, *10*(1), 46–69. https://doi.org/10.1080/10413209808406377

Wiese-Bjornstal, D. M., Weiss, M. R., & Yukelson, D. P. (1991). Sport psychology in the training room: A survey of athletic trainers. *The Sport Psychologist*, *5*(1), 15–24. https://doi.org/10.1123/tsp.5.1.15

Wiese-Bjornstal, D. M., Wood, K. N., & Kronzer, J. R. (2020). Sport injuries and psychological sequelae. In G. Tenenbaum & R. C. Eklund (Eds.), *Handbook of sport psychology* (4th ed., pp. 751–772). John Wiley & Sons, Inc.

Zeigler, E. F. (1987). Rationale and suggested dimensions for a code of ethics for sport psychologists. *The Sport Psychologist*, *1*(2), 138–150. https://doi.org/10.1123/tsp.1.2.138

9 Counseling Skills in Sport Injury and Rehabilitation

Jonathan Katz and Julie A. Waumsley

Chapter Objectives

- To outline key theoretical and applied counseling models.
- To summarize foundational interpersonal counseling skills deemed beneficial for sport injury.
- To explain the process of working with injured athletes, highlighting both benefits and critical success factors.

Introduction

McLeod (2011) offers that *counseling* is "an activity that takes place when someone who is troubled invites and allows another person to enter into a particular kind of relationship with them" (p. 12). Given that athletes with injuries are often "troubled" by the changes their injury imposes on them, the philosophy and underpinning of the professional applied work with this population may need to be broader or different from that of a cognitive behavioral approach to mental skills (skills) straining, which is often the adopted approach by sport psychology professionals (SPPs; Katz & Hemmings, 2009). Within counseling, the psychodynamic, cognitive behavioral, and humanistic approaches are generally recognized as the three main theoretical models. The applied work of a licensed/accredited/registered counsellor or psychologist will often be underpinned by one such approach, although it is true to say that the integrative approach, where several models integrate to form one theory (Katz & Hemmings, 2009), has been adopted by many mental health practitioners. It is also worth saying that the past decade has seen an increasing contribution of neurobiological approaches (Van der Kolk, 2015), which may be too complex for the sport professional to apply but for which referral to an appropriately trained counsellor may be necessary.

While many sport psychology (SPP; Watson II et al., 2017) and sports medicine professionals (SMPs; Heaney et al., 2015) are not trained in counseling or clinical psychology, some foundational interpersonal counseling skills can be beneficial during the sport injury rehabilitation process (Brewer & Redmond, 2017). Many athletes with injuries can experience psychosocial responses that require the SPPs and SMPs to look beyond the visible and the obvious and possibly assess the athlete's psychological functioning and need for referral (for more details on assessment and referral, see Chapter 10). This process can be enhanced by foundational interpersonal counseling skills. The purpose of this chapter is to demonstrate the usefulness of using a psychological model and counseling skills in sport injury and rehabilitation. The chapter will (a) offer a summary of key theoretical and applied models that underpin a counseling approach,

DOI: 10.4324/9781003295709-11

(b) introduce foundational interpersonal counseling skills deemed useful in sport injury rehabilitation, (c) outline the process of working within sport injury and rehabilitation environment,
and (d) discuss some athlete and practitioner factors to consider when using counseling skills
with injured athletes.

To enhance clarity within this chapter, the term "practitioner" is generically used in places
to avoid confusion between the terms "sport psychologist," "counsellor," or "therapist." In
addition, the term "athlete" will be used to avoid confusion between "patient" or "client." The
concept of "relationship" in this chapter is twofold. It refers to the therapeutic element where
there is an unconditional, non-judgmental, and congruently empathic respect for the athlete and
where the "process" occurs in the space in between the content of what is being verbally articulated and what is being experienced by the athlete internally. Lastly, while this chapter discusses
both psychological models and foundational interpersonal counseling skills, it is imperative for
SPPs and SMPs to work ethically within their scope of practice and only use skills and strategies
in which they are appropriately trained.

Theoretical Approaches

The Psychoanalytical/Psychodynamic Approach

Psychoanalysis is defined as a theory of the mind or personality, a method of investigation of
unconscious processes, and a method of treatment (Freud, 1949). Much of Freud's theorizing
was on the development of personality and of the consequences of what he regarded as abnormal development, with the emphasis on the unconscious motivations and needs having a role in
determining behavior. Freud's theory can be divided into three main parts: a description of the
mind or psyche, a description of the development of the psyche, and a description of the way in
which the psyche defends itself. The topographic model of the psyche views the mind as having three levels of consciousness: the conscious, the pre-conscious, and the unconscious. Freud
saw the conscious as everything we are aware of, and the pre-conscious as the area of the mind
containing thoughts and ideas available to recall but are currently "at the back of one's mind."
This is quite different from the unconscious, which Freud saw as holding all the early thoughts
and feelings that might cause anxiety, conflict, or (emotional) pain and which are the motivating
factors, out of awareness and not generally accessible, that drive behavior. The id functions at an
unconscious level, driving primitive needs, and is "controlled" by the ego. The superego brings
a moral sense to behavior. Freud's complex view of the "inner self" describes the ego as battling
against the id and the superego, the "three aspects of 'self'" (Jacobs, 1991). Freud believed that
personality develops through a stage theory of psychosexual development as shown in Table 9.1.

In Freud's stages of psychosexual development, various crises are resolved at each stage,
with the respective quality of crisis resolutions leading to a more healthy or unhealthy personality. If these crises get "stuck" at a specific stage, they will be apparent and manifest in adult
behavior. Consistent with this, the concept of anxiety is central to Freud's theory. According to
Freud, the dynamics of all human behavior were conflicts between the expression of and inhibi-
tion of desires and needs. To deal with and explain this conflict between inhibitions and desires
and needs, Freud developed a series of defense mechanisms, such as denial, repression, projec-
tion, regression, which would prevent immediate goal gratification and resolve the conflict by
transferring it into a socially acceptable form. Thus, when anxiety cannot be dealt with by realistic methods that are socially acceptable, the ego calls on various defense mechanisms to release
the resultant build-up of tensions. These defense mechanisms defy, alter, or falsify reality, work
unconsciously, and are not immediately obvious to us or other people.

Table 9.1 Freud's Stages of Psychosexual Development

Psychosexual Stage	Time Frame	Behavior
Oral Stage	Birth to 12–18 months	Child is focused on oral pleasures (sucking).
Anal Stage	12–18 months to 3 years	Pleasure is on eliminating and retaining faces, learning control, and stimulation.
Phallic Stage	3–6 years	Pleasure zone becomes the genitals. Oedipus complex develops (boys develop unconscious desires for their mother). More recent psychoanalysis describes the same process for girls as the Electra complex.
Latency Stage	7–12 years	Sexual urges remain repressed. Children interact mostly with same-sex peers.
Genital Stage	12–18 years	The primary focus of pleasure is genitals, and sexual urges are awakened. Adolescents direct their sexual urges to opposite-sex peers.

Adopting a psychoanalytical approach will involve working with the unconscious drives through free association and dreamwork, when the practitioner interprets what is being said to make sense of it to the athlete. Central to this approach are the concepts of transference and countertransference. *Transference* refers to the way athletes relate to the practitioner based on their experiences with those who cared for them in their formative years. Thus, they bring with them expectations and assumptions based on their experiences of life that will influence the way they perceive the practitioner (Gray, 2007). The practitioner can begin to learn about these previous experiences by listening to the athlete and by noticing the ways in which they relate to them. *Countertransference* can be useful in learning about how athletes relate to others, but the practitioner must be sufficiently skilled and self-aware to, sometimes painfully, recognize some feelings within a therapeutic alliance do not belong to the athlete but to the practitioner's own unresolved difficulties (Gray, 2007).

The Cognitive Behavioral Approach

The primary role of cognition in understanding mental health and well-being has led to the cognitive behavioral approach to counseling, which is founded on the core tenet that cognition mediates emotion and behavior. Consequently, the idea that dysfunctional thinking, which guides a person's mood and behaviors, is a common factor for all psychological disturbances (Beck, 2011). Dating back to the 1950s, Ellis (1913–2007) and Beck (1921–2021), who both started their careers as psychoanalysts, came to believe that cognitions (thoughts, attitudes, beliefs, and so on) played an important role in emotional and behavioral consequences or outcomes. Ellis's approach, currently known as rational emotive behavior therapy, is operationalized using the A-B-C model, with A being the activating event, B being the belief, and C being the emotional and behavioral consequence. Ellis argued that emotional difficulties are a consequence of "distorted thinking" and problems occur when people's interpretation of situations and events around them is excessively biased from the "reality" of those situations or events. More rational (realistic) belief statements allow a person to cope with relationship difficulties in a more constructive and balanced fashion, with their interpretation being consistent with "the facts."

Beck (1976) suggests some commonalities between cognitive and behavioral approaches: "both employ a structured, problem solving or symptom reduction approach with a highly active therapy style and both stress the 'here-and-now' rather than making speculative reconstruction of the patient's childhood relationships and early family relationships" (p. 321). The cognitive behavioral approach concentrates on the stimulus, the cognitions, the emotions, and the behavioral outcome. Three key features of this approach are its problem-solving delivery style, with a change in focus from interpretative in the psychoanalytic model to working collaboratively with clients, a respect for scientific values, and a close attention to the cognitive processes through which people monitor, control, and mediate their behavior.

A cognitive theorist, Kelly (1905–1967) sought to investigate the world as constructed by the individual. Personal construct psychology is concerned with the ways in which clients represent or view their own experiences rather than seeing them (experiences) as victims of impulses and defenses. Kelly's therapeutic process is concerned with helping the client find appropriate or useful constructs rather than to be concerned with diagnosis and categorization. This approach aims to help clients expand and articulate meaning(s) by which they construct a sense of self. Becoming aware of their personal constructs, and thereby of their ways of thinking and feeling, leads to modifying behavior in a similar way to the aims of cognitive behavioral therapy (CBT).

Adopting a cognitive behavioral approach will often involve establishing rapport and building a therapeutic alliance, explaining the rationale for treatment, assessing the problem, setting goals and targets primarily for cognitive and behavioral change, and monitoring progress. Some ways of executing this might be through challenging irrational beliefs, reframing issues using cognitive restructuring techniques, scaling feelings, in vivo exposure, and homework assignments (for more details on how CBT has been applied in the sport injury context, see the integrated models presented in Chapters 3 and 5, and Chapters 13–18 on psychosocial strategies).

The Humanistic Approach

The emphasis of the humanistic approach is on the athlete's perceptions as determinants of their actions. Carl Rogers (1902–1987) adopted a view where individual's functioning is an organized whole. He suggested that:

> [T]here is one central force of energy in the human organism; that is a function of the whole organism rather than some portion of it; and that is perhaps best conceptualized as a tendency toward fulfilment, toward actualization, toward the maintenance and enhancement of the organism.
>
> (Rogers, 1963, p. 6)

According to Rogers, people who are self-actualizing are fully functioning individuals, open to new experiences, and trust their feelings rather than being threatened by them. Within this approach, self-actualization is seen as the fundamental motivation and underpins the notion that athletes have the necessary resources for dealing with their own problems effectively. Thus, athletes are encouraged, in a non-directive way, to explore their own solutions to their issues and/or problems.

Adopting a humanistic approach with athletes will be underpinned by what Rogers called the "core conditions" of empathy, unconditional positive regard, and congruence, without which self-actualization will not be achieved. The core conditions allow a therapeutic relationship of trust and non-judgment to develop, within which the process of work between athlete and practitioner allows the space for self-actualization to be realized. The development of this therapeutic relationship requires the use of various counseling skills, which are highlighted in the next section of this chapter.

The Integrative Approach

There are many integrative approaches that underpin work with athletes (see for example Clarkson, 2007; Lapworth et al., 2007; Moursund & Erskine, 2004). Integrating the three primary models as outlined earlier is suggested as one way of working with injured athletes. Adopting this approach allows working with presenting issues while also gaining a better understanding of why past experiences impact current mechanisms of coping and behavior. This approach also affords the development of a relationship or "working alliance" that is conducive to positive change.

The integrated approach provides practitioners with a systematic understanding of athletes' presentations, which is helpful as it assists with case conceptualizations and intervention formulations. The model is designed to be viewed as three-dimensional, with the bottom level being most superficial and relating to what is being experienced in the current situation, the "here and now." This bottom level comprises of environmental and psychological factors and the interactions between them. The psychological factors, represented within the rectangles, are further made up of cognitions, emotions, and interactions between them. The psychological factors are layered from current to historical. Each layer has specific types of experience associated with it, and the more general or global an athlete experiences something, the more important it is to

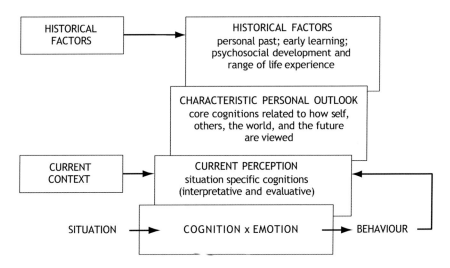

Figure 9.1 Integrated theoretical and applied model of stress and coping.

Source: Copyright ©2009 from *Counselling Skills Handbook for the Sport Psychologist* by Jonathan Katz and Brian Hemmings. The British Psychological Society, Figure 6, Page 46. Reproduced with permission of The Licensor through PLSclear.

them as a person, not "just as an athlete." Each of the layers is also located with the context in which that experience occurred.

It is sometimes argued that the theories and techniques of counseling are delivered through the presence and "being" of the counsellor as a person (McLeod, 2011). No matter what the theoretical approach, research suggests that the usefulness of the intervention of counseling comes from the quality of the relationship between the athlete and the practitioner (e.g., Clarkson, 2007; Erskine et al., 1999; McLeod, 2011; Moursund & Erskine, 2004). This relationship will usually convey trust and a deep sense of being special in the presence of another who demonstrates deep caring. Within an integrative approach, this is a safety that is felt where transference and countertransference are often played out between two people. It is also safety where understanding over specific behaviors and emotions can be mediated through thought, words, and "being" in an environment of unconditional positive regard, acceptance, and congruence.

Foundational Interpersonal Counseling Skills

Each practitioner – be it counseling, sport psychology, or sports medicine – faces the challenge of translating their chosen theoretical approach into practice. The application of theory into practice is achieved by using a set of techniques or skills. The "doing" of counseling, as opposed to the "being" of counseling, can be seen as the skills used to build rapport and a strong working alliance with athletes. The main foundational counseling skills recognized by practitioners of humanistic and integrative approaches are attending, observing, active listening, reflecting, probing, and immediacy.

Attending Skills

Attending skills refer to the set of skills a practitioner adopts to ensure an effective professional relationship. Attending acts as a basis for listening to and observing athletes, the means by which the practitioner communicates "non-verbally" that they are "with" their athlete and interested in them (Culley & Bond, 2007). Attending communicates acceptance and congruence. Attending and listening are interrelated; it is not possible to fully attend to athletes without listening to them. Attending to athletes allows verbal and non-verbal messages, and their contradictions between these verbal messages and behavior, to be noticed (Egan, 2002). An open, upright, and relaxed posture and good eye contact, without staring, are important (Culley & Bond, 2007).

Observing

Observing is the set of skills the practitioner uses to better understand the athlete's non-verbal behavior and how it correlates, or not, with the athlete's verbal expression. Athletes communicate non-verbally through their dress, tone of voice, facial expressions, gestures, postures, and so on, all of which inform the practitioner of inconsistencies between what athletes verbalize and their behaviors. These observations offer opportunities for the practitioner and athlete to further explore inconsistencies for better understanding of presenting issues.

Active Listening

Listening actively means listening with explicit purpose, using silences appropriately, and communicating that you have listened and understood. It is about listening to, receiving, and understanding messages whilst clarifying and organizing information that is heard, checking what to respond to, and asking for clarity on what is unclear (Culley & Bond, 2007). Active listening enables the practitioner to gain an empathic understanding of the athlete's situation from their perspective. It provides a useful insight into both what the athlete thinks and feels and the process of how these thoughts and feelings arise.

Using silences to further inform the process between practitioner and athlete is a necessary active listening skill that necessitates practitioners to be "tuned in" to their athlete's emotional state. Listening to silences informs greatly about what is happening in the moment. Breaking silences should be for the client's benefit, used purposefully by the practitioner with a view to enhancing the therapeutic session, not to ease the practitioner's feelings of discomfort with silence or because of a lack of skill in working effectively with silence (Culley & Bond, 2007).

Reflective Skills

The three reflective skills are restating, paraphrasing, and summarizing, and these offer a way for the practitioner to construct how they communicate their empathic understanding (that is, from the athlete's perspective). Reflective skills help in the building of trust and empathy by offering to the athlete the practitioner's empathic understanding through active listening. This takes place with the professional relationship that provides "time and space" within a safe environment and without imposing direction from the practitioner's frame of reference (Culley & Bond, 2007).

Restating involves repeating single key words or phrases back to the athlete to emphasize a point or an emotion. Paraphrasing lets the athlete know that the practitioner understands what they are saying by communicating back to them, in the practitioner's own words, the main message expressed by the athlete. Summarizing organizes the athlete's sometimes-disorganized content by bringing together the salient aspects of their story (Culley & Bond, 2007). The consequence for athletes by practitioners using these skills is that they feel that they have been "listened to," with their "story" being valued, appreciated, and understood.

Probing Skills

Practitioners are sometimes required to question or gently challenge what athletes express, and these actions are collectively referred to as "probing skills." Practitioners should use these skills with care; we may be going into areas where we "have not been invited" (Culley & Bond, 2007, p. 42). Probing offers opportunities for the athlete to explore issues that the practitioner thinks are important. The most helpful type of probing questions often begin with "what," "how," "when," "where," and "who," because they offer opportunity for open dialogue from the client rather than providing one-word responses.

Immediacy

Immediacy is a skill that involves listening to one's own reactions as the practitioner and using this to invite the athlete to look at what is happening between you and them. It is a very powerful tool because it invites immediate exploration of the athlete's feelings, thoughts, and somatic responses. Using the skill of immediacy often feels risky for the practitioner because it involves verbalizing a "hunch" and, in so doing, inviting the client in to clarify what they are feeling or thinking in light of their immediate behavior. Thus, it can be described as a coming together of the practitioner's feelings in the moment and the athlete's behavior in the moment to make sense of what is going on in the relationship in that moment.

In much the same way as understanding transference and countertransference does within the psychodynamic approach, immediacy offers a way of interpreting what is going on in the therapeutic relationship. In relation to the humanistic approach, it is a way of focusing on the here and now of the practitioner and athlete. When relating it to a cognitive behavioral approach, it may be interpreted as using constructs to address patterns of relating between practitioner and athlete. Of all the skills discussed, immediacy is a more advanced skill that tends to be used by more experienced practitioners, who will rely on their own highly tuned and acute self-awareness to provide valuable information to aid understanding of the athlete.

A Process of Working

When injured, an athlete's physical injury is given primary attention, with the objective of providing diagnosis and subsequent medical and/or physical treatment. This is followed by a process of treatment and recovery consisting of structured rehabilitation and appropriate return to participation protocols. While viewed predominantly as sequential, this process is generally not linear, whereby the athlete's biopsychosocial responses typically include a variety of fluctuations associated with how the treatment and rehabilitation process meanders with the ups and downs of recovery over time.

The continuous medical focus on the injury can mask or hide underlying psychosocial responses, including feelings of doubt and associated anxiety. Over time, the athlete can experience a disassociation between medical care and psychological feelings about the impact and consequences of injury. When injury-related anxiety coincides with a pre-existing anxiety, there may be a pattern of unhelpful behavior that presents as challenging, as confusing, and appears non-responsive to the more traditional mental skills work of sport psychology professionals. When an athlete's sense of identity is strongly associated with their sporting prowess, serious injury can also be experienced as threatening to who they are as an individual and not just as athletes. Consequently, psychological recovery post-injury needs to support the athlete in re-establishing a sense of worth and value as a person before restoring their "sporting confidence."

Becoming injured can interrupt the usual physical and psychological homeostasis of the athlete. As discussed earlier, the physical aspect of the injury is the initial focus. Having identified potential long-term and significant psychological consequences to injury for some athletes, it is important to introduce psychological support as early in the process as is practical, preferably as part of an interprofessional team (for more on interprofessional practice, see Chapter 7). The earlier the practitioner can get involved within the treatment and rehabilitation process, the sooner the psychological and emotional needs of the athlete can be met, resulting in a more holistic process for the athlete. In this way, the professionals behind the athlete are also receiving support, as it offers an environment within which the athlete can discuss the difficulties that their injury presents without fear of judgment and separate from the aspects of sporting performance within their rehabilitation. This type of psychological support places significance and importance of practitioner observation to ensure the practitioner is aware of the complete impact that the injury has had on the person behind the athlete and on their broader lifestyle. Further, good observation provides the opportunity for the practitioner to explore with athletes any potential secondary or underlying issues that may arise consequent to the physical injury and/or to psychosocial responses to the injury, rehabilitation, or simply managing change.

The ideal one-on-one counseling scenario requires a beginning, middle, and an end to both the whole process and to each individual session. Typically, within the counseling relationship, the beginning of the whole process involves making an assessment, negotiating a contract, establishing boundaries, building trust and a working alliance, and clarifying and defining difficult areas to explore together. The middle aspect of the process of counseling largely follows the contract negotiated at the beginning, maintains the working relationship, and reassesses difficulties and concerns as they are worked through. Any end to the work, or part thereof, requires planning with mutual consent between practitioner and athlete. It is important to discuss the way in which this will occur, given that there may be consequences of ending the bond developed throughout working together. Thus, the process of emotional disengagement between practitioner and athlete requires respect within the work of "ending" with an athlete.

Some basic assumptions within this process are that people (a) deserve acceptance and understanding, (b) are capable of change, (c) are experts on themselves, (d) demonstrate behavior that is purposeful, and (e) will work harder to achieve goals that are meaningful to them (Culley & Bond, 2007). Within all this, the individual, rather than their injury, is at the forefront of the work, and this thereby allows for recognition of the athlete behind the injury. An important aspect of working with athletes is the recognition of attachment issues within the journey of eventual self-empowerment. Attachment can be seen as a bond between two people that involves a desire for regular contact with that person and experiencing discomfort when separated from that person (Ainsworth, 1989; Bowlby, 1979). An athlete's attachment style may present as dependency, and some knowledge of how and when to gradually encourage them to regain control of their own choices about their treatment is a necessity for the aware practitioner.

There may also be a myriad of contextual factors to be aware of. First, the beginning of psychological support may be untimely if it conflicts with the need for physical rehabilitation activities. At times, the athlete's readiness to address psychosocial needs is superseded with more immediate needs to address (physical) pain and discomfort associated with injury. Timely psychological support is sometimes sought contingent to an athlete expressing anxiety during return to sport. Second, practitioners may need to consider and coordinate psychological support delivery with other members of the sports medicine team. Having all members of the team on the "same page" has implications for how the athlete "hears, understands, and responds" to the psychological support when faced with multiple "channels" of support. Third, psychological support delivery needs to be considered within the wider organizational context and how the associated organizational structures, demands, and pressures may impact the athlete in general and their response to psychological support in particular.

Key Considerations: Athlete Factors

While athletes with injuries respond to the injury and its consequences in myriad ways, three key athlete factors are worth noting. These are likely to influence all athletes and the subsequent need for psychosocial support during rehabilitation and the return to participation process. These are perceived lack of control, accepting help from others, and self-image and identity.

Perceived Lack of Control

Experiencing an injury can leave some athletes feeling "powerless" or "not in control." This perceived lack of control is often in contrast with their preferred self-image and may result in a range of unpleasant emotional responses, including anxiety, anger/frustration, resentment, and hurt. Please note that the aforementioned is not a comprehensive list, as athletes may experience additional and/or a subset of emotions other than the ones stated. Practitioners assisting athletes to regain a sense of "power and feeling in control" can be assisted by focusing on "mastery," that is, a subjective perception of one's own ability to influence their situation and circumstances.

Accepting Help from Others

Depending on the injury severity and location, a major consequence can be a "loss" of physical independence and the need to rely on others for assistance with daily activities. This can have psychosocial consequences for the athlete, and the role of early life experience in the formation of secure or insecure attachment is important here as it influences the degree of perceived sense of feeling "safe, secure, and trusting." Practitioners need to be aware of the aforementioned and focus on supporting the athlete in their quest to both tolerate and accept help from others.

Self-Image and Identity

The degree to which an athlete who utilizes subjective appraisal of their "physical prowess" to inform their global psychological and emotional well-being is important for practitioners to appreciate. All individuals have an "ideal self-image" and a (perceived) "self-image." The degree of harmony or difference between one's "ideal self-image" and "self-image" influences well-being, with enhanced well-being associated with a close correlation between the two. Appreciating how the consequences and associated practical implications of experiencing an injury interact with this relationship is important for practitioners to understand in order to assist with forming effective therapeutic relationship (Katz & Keyes, 2020).

Key Considerations: Practitioner Factors

Supporting athletes who have experienced an injury can be challenging. Several key factors are consistent with the psychological models presented earlier that are worthy of noting. These include understanding the injury and appreciating the person, timing of psychosocial support, therapeutic relationship/alliance, empathic understanding, facilitating active participation, and promoting constructive change.

Understanding the Injury and Appreciating the Person

When an athlete experiences an injury, it can subjectively feel as though they are responded to "as the injury" rather than a person, particularly when the medical and physical management needs take precedence. It is important to appreciate that the athlete's psychosocial responses to the injury are concurrent with the physical and medical responses. As such, practitioners need to appreciate the need to provide opportunities for support to the person along with the injury as soon as is appropriate and that it is coordinated with medical, physical, and other logistical support provision.

Timing of Psychosocial Support

It may be that (a) the athlete views their circumstance exclusively through an injury lens – "this is a medical/physical issue that needs to be treated accordingly" – (b) the primary intervention may need to be medical that supersedes other needs, and (c) lack of appreciation of the psycho-social impact and how psychology support can assist. In short, practitioners should appreciate the "timing" of providing support and "being present" on the athlete's psychological radar, building rapport as a foundation to facilitate when required.

Therapeutic Relationship/Alliance

Athletes tend to respond more favorably to psychological support when it happens in the context of helpful therapeutic relationship. Defined as "a cooperative working relationship between client and therapist" (American Psychological Association, 2022) and characterized by the athlete feeling "safe, secure, and trusting," this subjective psychological climate builds on the quality of the therapeutic relationship, particularly from the athlete's perspective. Practitioners need to be mindful of how to proactively and explicitly "work with" establishing, maintaining, and repairing (if needed) the quality of the bond within the therapeutic relationship. Additional resource to support the therapeutic relationship can be found from the working alliance framework (see Bordin, 1979, and Katz and Hemmings, 2009, for additional information).

Empathic Understanding

Using a range of active listening skills effectively will enhance the practitioner's empathic understanding, which then creates and facilitates the (a) quality of the therapeutic relationship and (b) appreciation of the athlete's experience and (c) reinforces a psychological climate to encourage athlete growth and change. Practitioners need to tune into their own felt sense of what they feel when with the athlete and emotionally "reach" the athlete with their own genuine sense of empathy. This forms a congruent connection between two human beings where trust can be built.

Facilitating Active Participation

An important therapeutic principle is to ensure that because of receiving effective psychological support, athletes with injuries are able "to choose their reaction and response" to situations and circumstances, thereby facilitating mastery in general and to their injury in particular. One way to facilitate active participation is through the relational model, based on "five aspects of your life experience" by Greenberger and Padesky (1995). As shown in Figure 9.2., the relational model describes how the "five aspects" of an athlete's experience interact. First, in each situation or circumstance, the remaining four factors will be experienced. It is important to note that an athlete may not be consciously aware of the content of one or more of the four factors. Second, the content of each factor interacts with the other three. Third, influencing the content of any one factor can also influence the content of the other three because of the interaction. It is through the intentional navigation of this series of processes and interactions that an athlete can proactively influence "how they choose" to react, respond, and subsequently cope in a given circumstances.

Promoting Constructive Change

Coping with change is a frequent consequence for an athlete to manage following an injury and how the associated different psychological and emotional experiences progress with varying speeds, both within and between athletes (Katz & Hemmings, 2009). For example, an athlete may accept their injury at a relatively superficial intellectual level quite quickly, while appreciating the emotional consequences and implications for their appraisal of "ideal self-image" with "(perceived) self-image" may take considerably longer. For practitioners, it is therefore helpful to view change as a process that may need several iterations to negotiate that facilitates increasing "depths" to the change process.

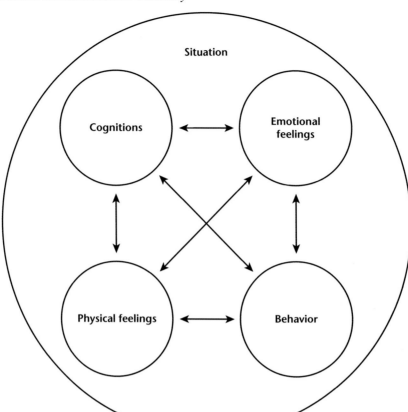

Figure 9.2 Graphical representation of the relational model.

Source: Adapted from Katz and Hemmings (2009). *Counselling skills handbook for the sport psychologist.* The British Psychological Society, Figure 2, Page 27. This figure is an adaptation from Greenberger, D., & Padesky, C. A. (1995). *Mind Over Mood: A Cognitive Therapy Treatment Manual for Clients.* Guilford Press.

As shown in Figure 9.3, constructive change can be supported with clear "tasks" associated with stages of recovery and change that need to be negotiated between practitioner, athlete, and relevant stakeholders. The emphasis of appreciating the change process is to support the practitioner in facilitating constructive change in the athlete. Importantly, the aim is for the athlete to arrive at their bespoke solution/resolution for each task, through a collaborative goal-setting process, within the context of both who they are as individuals and within their specific sporting context. What follows is an explanation of each of the factors presented in the change cycle.

Event or Situation

It is important for the practitioner to understand how the current injury relates to the athlete's "injury history," as some injuries may be perceived as being greater or lesser in terms of feeling "subjective traumatic stress." It is imperative for the practitioner to ask, Is this a first "significant" injury or one of several? What role does the mechanism and/or context of the cause of injury play?

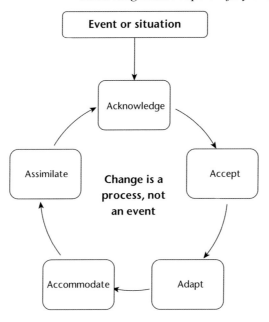

Figure 9.3 Change cycle.

Acknowledge and Accept

It is helpful for the practitioner to provide "time and space" for the athlete to share their experience. This supportive, or nondirective, discussion creates an opportunity for the athlete to recognize and appreciate what has happened at deeper psychological and emotional levels, best summarized as the process of "coming to terms" with what's happened, how it happened, and what it means going forward. Practitioners are encouraged to support athlete ownership of the experience by *acknowledging* that what has happened has happened to them because it happened, whether or not the athlete "likes, wants, or agrees with what happened." Additionally, practitioners are encouraged to facilitate athlete awareness and appreciation to differentiate between "the facts" of what happened and how they "feel, experience internally" about what happened. This is to support athlete *acceptance* and "psychological/emotional mastery" described previously.

Adapt, Accommodate, and Assimilate

These tasks collectively are related to practitioners facilitating athlete change. Please note here that *change* refers to either or both covert and/or overt change. *Covert change* refers to an athlete creating an internal narrative that enables them to manage the pressures and demands associated with injury recovery, rehabilitation, and return to training. *Overt change* refers to an athlete demonstrating observable behavior, verbal and physical, that supports constructive coping with their injury and then recovery process. Practitioners need to support the implicit task of athletes who are recognizing the need to change and become supportive of this process. *Adapting* can be viewed as an outcome to these three tasks by working through the other two. There can be a need for an athlete to create new or different ways of thinking, feeling, and doing, consequent to experiencing an injury. *Accommodation* is the process of creating "psychological and emotional space" for new behaviors. This is metaphorically similar to needing to remove old, unwanted, or redundant files on a computer disc drive to facilitate space to save new and preferred information. *Assimilation* is the process of integrating this new information into existing knowledge, experience, understanding, and awareness, with a net result of "updating" and "upgrading" one's coping resources.

Conclusion

This chapter has highlighted a way of working with an athlete following injury that departs from the more traditional mental skills training approach adopted to injury rehabilitation. The main aim of this chapter has been to offer an overview of some theoretical approaches and skills to inform the practitioner when carrying out applied work with an injured athlete, and as such, it has suggested an alternative approach based on a counseling psychology model. To this end, the importance of "professional relationship" is paramount since it bears the fruit of renewed hope for an athlete whose future has often been put in jeopardy through injury. This "professional relationship," underpinned by an integrative theoretical approach within which specific skills can operate, is the framework within which practitioners might work should they be faced by an athlete who is either not responding to a mental skills approach or whose more complex range of underlying psychological issues requires a greater understanding through in-depth work.

Case Study

George is a well-known young professional soccer player. When playing for his country, he tears his anterior cruciate ligament during a televised match. This is the first serious injury George has experienced and, therefore, the first time he has been in the spotlight for reasons beyond his control. George is gay, but he has not "come out" and keeps his "secret" guarded from family, friends, and colleagues because of his fear of homophobia within and beyond his sport. George's family are religious, and he fears their response to his sexuality should they find out.

George's serious injury has meant he is in the news headlines constantly. The media, particularly the tabloids, are inquisitive about his personal life. Despite the seriousness of his physical injury, George presents himself as upbeat, courageous, and non-emotional. His sports medicine team is praising him for his attitude. His coach and teammates are similarly impressed by his disposition. However, the sport psychologist within the management team "felt" something was incongruent about sustaining his injury and George's behavior and decides to reach out and arranges a meeting with George.

Questions

1. How might the theoretical and applied models described in this chapter conceptualize George's observable and non-observable responses to his injury?
2. When reading George's case study, how do you think counseling might be beneficial over and above mental skills training?

3. Discuss what is meant by "relationship." Notice what emotions and physical feelings are evoked within you as you discuss this topic.
4. What skill(s) do you think the sport psychologist was inadvertently using when she "felt" George's incongruence?

References

Ainsworth, M. (1989). Attachment beyond infancy. *American Psychologist*, *44*, 709–716.

American Psychological Association. (2022). *APA dictionary of psychology*. https://dictionary.apa.org/

Beck, A. T. (1976). *Cognitive therapy and the emotional disorders*. Penguin.

Beck, J. S. (2011). *Cognitive behavior therapy: Basics and beyond* (2nd ed.). The Guilford Press.

Bordin, E. S. (1979). The generalizability of the psychoanalytic concept of the working alliance. *Psychotherapy: Theory, Research and Practice*, *16*(3), 252–260. https://doi.org/10.1037/h0085885

Bowlby, J. (1979). *The making and breaking of affectional bonds*. Tavistock.

Brewer, B. W., & Redmond, C. J. (2017). *Psychology of sport injury*. Human Kinetics.

Clarkson, P. (2007). *The therapeutic relationship*. Whurr Publishers.

Culley, S., & Bond, T. (2007). *Integrative counselling skills in action* (2nd ed.). Sage Publishing.

Egan, G. (2002). *The skilled helper: A problem-management and opportunity-development approach to helping* (7th ed.). Brooks/Cole.

Erskine, R., Moursund, J., & Trautmann, R. (1999). *Beyond empathy: A therapy of contact-in-relationship*. Routledge.

Freud, S. (1949). *An outline of psychoanalysis*. Hogarth Press.

Gray, A. (2007). *An introduction to the therapeutic frame*. Routledge.

Greenberger, D., & Padesky, C. A. (1995). *Mind over mood: Change how you feel by changing the way you think*. The Guildford Press.

Heaney, C., Walker, N., Green, A. J., & Rostron, C. L. (2015). Sport psychology education for sport injury rehabilitation professionals: A systematic review. *Physical Therapy in Sport*, *16*(1), 72–79. https://doi.org/10.1016/j.ptsp.2014.04.001

Jacobs, M. (1991). *Psychodynamic counselling in action*. Sage Publishing.

Katz, J., & Hemmings, B. (2009). *Counselling skills handbook for the sport psychologist*. The British Psychological Society.

Katz, J., & Keyes, J. (2020). Person-centred approaches. In D. Tod & M. Eubank (Eds.), *Applied sport, exercise and performance psychology: Current approaches to helping clients* (pp. 31–52). Routledge.

Lapworth, P., Sills, C., & Fish, S. (2007). *Integration in counselling and psychotherapy: Developing a personal approach*. Sage Publishing.

McLeod, J. (2011). *An introduction to counselling* (4th ed.). McGraw Hill.

Moursund, J. P., & Erskine, R. G. (2004). *Integrative psychotherapy: The art and science of relationship*. Thomson: Brooks/Cole.

Rogers, C. (1963). The concept of the fully functioning person. *Psychotherapy: Theory, Research and Practice*, *1*, 17–26.

Van der Kolk, B. A. (2015). *The body keeps the score: Brain, mind, and body in the healing of trauma*. Penguin Books.

Watson II, J. C., Hilliard, R., & Way, W. (2017). Counseling and communication skills in sport and performance psychology. In *Oxford research encyclopedia of psychology*. Oxford University Press.

10 Psychosocial Assessment and Referral in Sport Injury and Rehabilitation

Annamari Maaranen*, Hailey A. Chatterton, and Britton W. Brewer

---

Chapter Objectives

- To examine targets and methods of psychosocial assessment during sport injury rehabilitation.
- To outline a process for referring athletes with injury to sport psychology professionals and mental health providers.

Introduction

Given the importance of psychosocial factors in sport injury rehabilitation, ongoing psychosocial assessment can contribute to gaining a holistic perspective on the progress and well-being of athletes during rehabilitation. Under certain circumstances, a referral to professionals with psychological training can be helpful in addressing the needs of athletes with injuries where these are not already available to them as part of their support team. In surveys of sports medicine professionals (SMPs) across nations and disciplines (Arvinen-Barrow et al., 2007; Clement et al., 2013; Heaney et al., 2017; Larson et al., 1996), 17–68% of respondents indicated that they had made one or more psychological referrals of athletes with injuries. There is, however, no evidence that such referrals are routine or commonplace. Consequently, the purpose of this chapter is to examine issues associated with psychosocial assessment and referral of athletes during sport injury rehabilitation. In particular, this chapter (a) examines targets and methods of psychosocial assessment during sport injury rehabilitation and (b) outlines a process for referring athletes with injury to sport psychology professionals (SPPs) and licensed mental health providers (LMHPs).

Although SMPs are the practitioners most likely to assess and refer athletes with injury for psychological assistance, the term "sport professional (SP)" is used frequently in this chapter to acknowledge that practitioners who are not technically SMPs (e.g., administrators, coaches) may also be well-positioned to assist athletes with injuries in obtaining support for their mental health (e.g., Mazzer & Rickwood, 2015; Murphy & Sheehan, 2021). It is also worth noting that there is overlap among the credentials of practitioners who may offer psychological assistance to injured athletes. Some, but not all, SPPs have credentials in a mental health profession (e.g., clinical or counseling psychology, social work), and some, but not most, mental health professionals have credentials in sport psychology. Thus, there are circumstances when an SPP may need to refer an injured athlete to an LMHP (e.g., psychiatrist)

DOI: 10.4324/9781003295709-12

or vice versa, depending on the nature of the athlete's concerns and the credentials of the professionals involved.

Psychosocial Assessment in Sport Injury Rehabilitation

In the context of sport injury rehabilitation, *psychosocial assessment* refers to gathering information about athletes with injuries and their situations for the purposes of describing their current status and projecting where their rehabilitation might be headed from a psychosocial perspective (American Psychological Association, 2022). From the beginning of rehabilitation through to discharge, psychosocial assessment is an ongoing process that can be seamlessly integrated into the more traditional rehabilitation tasks. In this section, targets (i.e., what should be assessed) and methods (i.e., how assessment should be conducted) of psychosocial assessment during sport injury rehabilitation are described.

Targets of Psychosocial Assessment

According to the integrated model of psychological response to sport injury (Wiese-Bjornstal et al., 1998; see Chapter 3), athletes' emotional and behavioral reactions to an injury are shaped by the way they think about the injury and their ability to cognitively cope with it (i.e., cognitive appraisals). These appraisals are thought to be affected by a variety of personal and situational factors. Because of their posited influence on psychosocial and physical rehabilitation outcomes (Wiese-Bjornstal et al., 1998), personal and situational factors and cognitive, emotional, and behavioral responses constitute useful targets for psychosocial assessment during sport injury rehabilitation.

Personal Factors

No two people appraise stressors, including sport injury, in precisely the same manner. Several personal factors, such as injury characteristics, personality, demographics, and personal life history, including the culture in which people were brought up, are thought to shape people's unique cognitive appraisals (Wiese-Bjornstal et al., 1998). Personal characteristics that have been found to have a positive correlation with emotional disturbance after sport injury include injury severity, athletic identity, and neuroticism (Brewer, 2017). Strong athletic identity has also been found to be a risk factor of depression among athletes outside of the injury context, along with high self- and/or other-imposed performance expectations (Wolanin et al., 2015). Smith and Milliner (1994) identified competitive athletes who were highly invested in their sport, had required surgery to treat their injuries, had been successful in their sport pre-injury, and failed to return to their pre-injury level of sport participation to be at the highest risk of attempting suicide after injury.

Situational Factors

Sport-related factors, such as the type of sport, level of competition, and time of the sport season, as well as social influences from coaches, teammates, and other important people in the athletes' lives, are all posited to affect athletes' cognitive appraisals of their injuries and coping abilities (Wiese-Bjornstal et al., 1998). All these factors operate within the broader sociocultural context of sport. Athletes are socialized at a young age into the "culture of risk," in which ignoring pain and injury is seen as normal and expected and unwillingness to pay such a price to strive for excellence is seen as a deficiency of character (Frey, 1991; McGannon & McMahon, 2020). These cultural values and beliefs may contribute to adverse rehabilitation outcomes through problematic cognitive, emotional, and behavioral responses to sport injury and the rehabilitation process, such as delaying treatment of injuries, under-reporting symptoms, and prematurely increasing activities (Brewer & Redmond, 2017). Level of general life stress and quantity, quality, and type of social support available to athletes with injuries are additional situational factors of relevance in the assessment process (Brewer, 2017).

Cognitive Responses

According to stress and coping theory (Lazarus & Folkman, 1984), appraisals of stressful events and situations, such as sport injury, fall into three categories: threat, harm/loss, and challenge. When athletes appraise an injury as a threat, they tend to view it as something that will likely cause harm to their health or self- or social esteem, potentially leading to stress, anxiety, fear, and anger responses. When athletes appraise an injury as a harm/loss, they may believe that the damage has already been sustained, potentially leading to feelings generally associated with grief, such as depression or defeat. When an athlete appraises an injury as a challenge, their focus tends to be on the opportunity for gain or growth, such as thoughts about the way in which they could make the most out of the situation, potentially leading to feelings of commitment and even eagerness or excitement (Lazarus & Folkman, 1984). These appraisal styles are not mutually exclusive, and athletes' perceptions of their injury and coping abilities can change throughout the rehabilitation as a response to their progress and acquired information. Athletes may appraise many things after injury, such as the cause of the injury, injury characteristics, meaning of various signs and symptoms such as pain, implications of the injury for future sport involvement, and recovery status (Brewer & Redmond, 2017). Because predominantly threat and/or harm/loss appraisals can contribute to negative emotional and behavioral responses (Lazarus & Folkman, 1984), listening for athletes' appraisal style throughout the rehabilitation process can provide important indications of their adjustment.

> After receiving my MRI results of a torn ACL and meniscus, I felt so depressed and defeated. I remembered the stories my uncle had told me about his experiences with a similar injury and never being able to fully return to playing soccer. He was only 44 and already had arthritis on his knee. All I had wanted for as long as I could remember was to play basketball in college. What was the point of going to college at all if I could not play? What was the point of working hard at school if I wasn't going to go to college?
>
> *Khalil, a high school freshman, talks about his initial harm/loss appraisals of his knee injury that had been shaped by a variety of personal and situational factors.*

For many athletes, sport serves as a major source of identity and self-worth (Brewer et al., 1993). Consequently, a participation-limiting injury can lead to negative appraisals in these areas. Recurrent thoughts pertaining to worthlessness, having no purpose in life, being a burden to others, letting one's team or family down, and in the extreme, dying or committing suicide are of particular concern. Perceptions of physical self-worth, which may be diminished after sport injury, are inversely related to post-injury depression (Brewer, 1993). Further, sport injury and the resulting activity restrictions may serve to trigger or increase excessive concerns about changes in appearance, such as gaining weight or losing muscle mass, and may contribute to disordered eating patterns or behavior (Sundgot-Borgen, 1994).

Injury- and recovery-related cognitions are a particularly important area of assessment, as athletes' post-injury mood disturbance is associated with their perceptions of recovery (McDonald & Hardy, 1990). Uncertainty and misunderstandings about injury-related information are common and can create unnecessary emotional turmoil for the athlete and complicate rehabilitation progress. In addition to the possibility of misinterpreting information given by SMPs, athletes may obtain inaccurate information from a variety of sources, including the Internet and important people in their lives, such as parents, teammates, and coaches (American College of Sports Medicine et al., 2017). Therefore, athletes' understanding of their injury, treatment (and its rationale), and prognosis, including the likely timeline of return to participation, are some of the key areas that require ongoing assessment as athletes progress in their rehabilitation.

Pain-related cognitions are also of potential importance for assessment. In particular, pain catastrophizing is a cluster of cognitive appraisals that has been associated with increased pain experience (Spanos et al., 1979), persistence of pain (Theunissen et al., 2012), and increased fear of reinjury (Tripp et al., 2004). Cognitions of concern may include magnification of pain (e.g., "I become afraid that the pain will get worse"), rumination about pain (e.g., "I keep thinking about how much it hurts"), and expression of helplessness related to the pain (e.g., "There is nothing I can do to reduce the intensity of the pain"; Sullivan et al., 1995).

Athletes' thoughts relating to their ability to cope with injury and the resulting rehabilitation process, as well as their perceptions of their social support system, are important areas of assessment. Athletes who perceive themselves as unable to cope with their injuries (Albinson & Petrie, 2003) and perceive that their social support system lacks in quality or quantity (Malinauskas, 2010) have reported elevated levels of post-injury emotional disturbance.

Emotional Responses

Emotional responses to injury are generally strongest immediately post-injury, tend to become less intense with the passage of time and progress in rehabilitation, and occasionally intensify when return to play gets near (Brewer, 2017). Although having an emotional response to a sport injury (e.g., sadness, depression, anxiety, fear, anger) is not a problem in and of itself, an emotional response that (a) does not resolve, (b) worsens over time, (c) appears excessive, or (d) significantly impairs the athlete's functioning in important areas of life (e.g., school, work, social relationships) signals a possible psychological problem that may require further assessment and treatment (American College of Sports Medicine et al., 2017; American Psychiatric Association, 2013).

Not all athletes experiencing emotional turmoil after injury directly report (or even have awareness of) their emotional reactions (Neal et al., 2015). Instead, reports of new or increased somatic complaints, such as fatigue, headaches, changes in appetite, and gastrointestinal problems, may signal poor emotional adjustment (Tahtinen et al., 2021). Tahtinen et al. (2021) found that among athletes scoring in the range of "moderate depression" or higher, approximately 50% did not report the core symptoms of depression (i.e., depressed mood or little interest or pleasure in doing things). Whereas female athletes tended to report fatigue more frequently (i.e., feeling tired or having little energy), male athletes tended to report psychomotor issues (i.e., noticeable slowing of their speech and movements or increased fidgeting and restlessness).

Behavioral Responses

Behavioral responses to injury are an important area of assessment and overall health because they can directly affect sport injury rehabilitation outcomes (Wiese-Bjornstal et al., 1998). For example, poor adherence or over-adherence to rehabilitation may interfere with recovery. Social withdrawal, decreased interest in previously enjoyable activities, neglect of personal hygiene, increased fidgeting and restlessness, and excessive avoidance of certain situations, places, activities, or people are additional examples of potential behavioral/appearance indications of underlying psychological difficulties and should be noted (American Psychiatric Association, 2013).

> Samantha was a young gymnast who had required an extensive reconstructive surgery after an elbow dislocation as a result of a fall off the uneven bars in a competition. Samantha's mother had told me that prior to her injury, Samantha had been eagerly waiting to watch the Olympic gymnastics on TV. As an attempt to cheer her up during rehab, I decided to turn the TV on to the channel that showed the gymnastics event finals at the Olympics. Instead of cheering up, Samantha got really upset with me and demanded that I turn off the TV. I did not think much of it at that time, but when Samantha started reporting increasing pain and problems with her elbow as she was slowly returning back to training on the uneven bars, I realized that further assessment of her psychological state was needed.
>
> *Dr. Majumder, Samantha's physical therapist, discusses the signs of Samantha's psychological difficulties as a sequela of her elbow injury.*

Any dramatic changes in behavior or physical appearance are important targets of further inquiry. Major changes in eating patterns, unexplained weight loss or gain, or continued excessive exercise despite injury or other medical complications are possible behavioral indications of psychological difficulties. Athletes in sports emphasizing aesthetics, endurance, and weight classifications are at particular risk for eating concerns (Chang et al., 2020). It is worth noting that disordered eating occurs on a spectrum, ranging from calorie and/or food group/macronutrient restriction and other pathogenic weight control measures (e.g., diet pills, self-induced vomiting, excessive exercise) to diagnosable eating disorders, such as anorexia nervosa and bulimia nervosa (American College of Sports Medicine et al., 2017).

Quality and quantity of sleep are also important aspects of ongoing assessment. Changes in sleeping patterns and excessive daytime sleepiness are behavioral indications of potential sleep-related concerns. The overall prevalence of poor quality of sleep among athletes has been estimated to be as high as 50% (Swinbourne et al., 2016). Sport injury can serve to worsen already-existing sleep difficulties or trigger new ones. Sudden reductions in activity due to injury can worsen sleep quality and quantity, and worry and anxiety relating to one's injury can further exacerbate sleep disruption (Chang et al., 2020). Proper amount and quality of sleep are central to athletes' health and performance. Sleep decrements have been linked to decreased pain tolerance, cognitive performance, and immune functioning, as well as increased risk of sport injury and mental health problems (Walker, 2017).

Some athletes may continue experiencing pain that lasts beyond the expected healing time, appears disproportionate to their injury and stage of healing, or gets triggered by stimuli typically considered benign (e.g., light touch to surgical scar). Such pain is known to result from abnormal processing of the nociception in the central nervous system (Watson & Sandoni, 2016). Behavioral indications of a potential pain-processing problems include poor rehabilitation compliance, decreased activity (or a slower increase in activity than expected), active avoidance of movement, and increased or prolonged use of pain medications (American College of Sports Medicine et al., 2017).

Methods of Psychosocial Assessment

One of the best ways to limit the negative consequences of most mental health conditions is early detection and treatment. Unfortunately, the stigma of mental illness, confidentiality concerns, anticipated perceptions of others, and expectation for "mental toughness" inherent in sport culture might lead athletes to minimize psychological distress and avoid asking for and accepting help for mental health concerns (American College of Sports Medicine et al., 2017; Chang et al., 2020). SPs who spend a considerable amount of time with athletes after injury are in an ideal position to detect emerging psychological problems. In this section, an overview of methods that SPs can use to engage in psychosocial assessment is presented, including (a) building rapport, (b) watching and listening for signs of poor adjustment, (c) using screening tools, and (d) asking questions about cognitions, emotions, and behavior.

Building Rapport

Developing an effective working alliance based on trust, caring, and understanding is vitally important for successful assessment of athletes' psychosocial functioning. An effective working alliance depends on SPs' ability to communicate empathy, acceptance, and genuineness (Petitpas & Cornelius, 2004). This can be accomplished by using basic counseling skills, such as (a) asking open-ended questions, which can help build rapport by conveying that athletes' input is valued in the rehabilitation process; (b) listening actively by making a conscious effort to understand what athletes are saying, rather than merely hearing them, and communicating that effort back to them; and (c) demonstrating unconditional positive regard by showing respect for athletes regardless of what they do, think, or feel (Petitpas & Cornelius, 2004; for more on counseling skills, see Chapter 9).

Respecting the confidentiality of athletes, with the exception of circumstances where athletes pose a danger to themselves or others or have given permission to disclose information to others, is a cornerstone of rapport building (American College of Sports Medicine et al., 2017). The importance of educating athletes about their injury in terms that they can understand (e.g., treatment, treatment rationale, prognosis) and confirming understanding by asking for athletes' interpretation of the information cannot be overstated. Uncertainty and misunderstandings of such information not only create unnecessary emotional turmoil but can also negatively affect the working alliance (American College of Sports Medicine et al., 2017; for more on patient education, see Chapter 13).

In addition to ensuring an adequate exchange of rehabilitation-related information, inquiring how athletes are getting along in activities of daily living and engaging in conversation about topics unrelated to injury convey a sense of genuine caring about athletes as people beyond their physical injury (Brewer & Redmond, 2017). SPs should also attempt to normalize and demystify mental health concerns and convey that symptoms of mental health concerns are as important to recognize and address as physical symptoms (American College of Sports Medicine et al., 2017). When athletes volunteer personal information, SPs should avoid minimizing or invalidating athletes' feelings (e.g., "At least it's not . . ." or "It could be worse"), giving advice as an attempt to fix the problem, and offering clichés in an attempt to make athletes feel better (Neal et al., 2015).

Watching and Listening for Signs of Poor Adjustment

An overview of cognitive, emotional, and behavioral responses that could signify poor adjustment to sport injury was provided earlier in this chapter. Although observations can provide invaluable information in the psychosocial assessment process, they are rarely adequate by themselves and thus should be used merely to steer the direction of further inquiry. Substantial incongruence between SMPs' observations and self-reports of distress of athletes with injuries have been documented in the literature (Brewer et al., 1995). Additionally, it is important to note that not all athletes with injury experiencing psychological distress display signs that are observable by others, and at times, the signs that athletes do display might not have anything to do with their psychological adjustment to injury.

> After my season ended due to an injury, I was having a pretty hard time remaining motivated in any aspect of my life. Only when my AT asked if I was doing okay, because he had noticed my weight loss and unusually low effort during rehab, did I realize that my lack of motivation and fatigue were no longer just normal reactions to a stressful event. After we discussed further how I had been feeling, he offered to help me schedule an appointment at the student counseling center. Had my AT not brought up his concerns, I would have never known that my symptoms were something that could be treated.
>
> *Jia discusses how her athletic trainer's observations led to her getting the support she needed.*

Using Screening Tools

Assessment instruments can be used in many ways throughout rehabilitation, such as at the beginning and the end of rehabilitation, when transitioning from one phase of rehabilitation to another, or periodically across the rehabilitation process (Arvinen-Barrow et al., 2018). Several considerations should be taken into account when choosing whether to use assessment instruments and which instruments to use. Some mental health assessments require specific qualifications to administer and interpret (e.g., clinical training or licensure), and thus, SPs should ensure they possess the appropriate credentials for each instrument they plan to use (Arvinen-Barrow et al., 2018). Further, although symptom checklists and questionnaires can provide useful information, they should be used with caution, keeping their limitations in mind. For example, because screening tools may overestimate the rate of psychological problems (Levis et al., 2020), a clinically significant score alone should not be used as a reason for a mental health referral. Prematurely jumping into action by initiating mental health referrals based on assessment scores alone may not only alienate athletes but may also teach them that it is better not to disclose any symptoms on such questionnaires in the future. On the other hand, athletes who do not present with clinically significant scores may, nevertheless, be experiencing symptoms that cause substantial distress and impairment in their functioning (Tahtinen et al., 2021).

SPs who are considering the use of screening tools might find the International Olympic Committee's recently published Sport Mental Health Assessment Tool-1 (SMHAT-1) a helpful place to start. The SMHAT-1 is a standardized questionnaire designed for early identification of athletes who are already experiencing, or are at risk of developing, mental health concerns. The SMHAT-1 is available online, can be freely copied to be used with individuals, teams, and organizations, and can be administered by sports medicine physicians and other licensed/registered health professionals (Gouttebarge et al., 2021).

The first step of the SMHAT-1 involves a ten-item self-report questionnaire (Athlete's Form 1) that athletes fill out either at pre-determined time intervals (e.g., prior to the start of the season, mid-season, and end of the season) or at the occurrence of any significant event (e.g., injury). A score above a specific threshold suggests an elevated risk for psychological distress and an indication to continue with the assessment protocol. In the second step, athletes fill out six additional self-report questionnaires that assess the symptoms of specific mental health concerns (Athlete's Form 2). If the athlete produces an elevated score in any of the six questionnaires, they should be referred for a clinical assessment by a licensed/registered mental health professional and/or sports medicine physician. In the absence of any elevated scores, a brief intervention and continued monitoring with Athlete Form 1 is recommended (Gouttebarge et al., 2021).

Asking Questions about Cognitions, Emotions, and Behavior

Due to the inherent limitations of observations and screening tools, additional inquiry about any concerning observations and questionnaire responses or scores is an imperative part of the assessment process. If SPs have been successful in building a trusting working alliance with athletes, inquiring about psychological symptoms and coping follow more naturally. Examples of topics that SPs should inquire about are provided in Table 10.1.

Table 10.1 Examples of Topics That Sport Professionals Should Ask Athletes about and Ways of Asking Such Questions

Topics in Need of Further Inquiry	*Example Questions*
Athletes' understanding of their injury, including the prescribed treatment, the rationale for the treatment, and the prognosis (American College of Sports Medicine et al., 2017)	*"What is your understanding of what the surgeon told you about the . . . ?"* *"What are your thoughts on the importance of X exercise/ activity limitation?"*
Any individual symptoms endorsed in questionnaires in order to get a better understanding of what athletes meant by their responses (Tahtinen et al., 2021)	*"You marked in the questionnaire that you have had little interest or pleasure in doing things. Could you tell me more about that?"*
Observations of thoughts, emotions, and behaviors of concern (American College of Sports Medicine et al., 2017)	*"You mentioned that if you don't recover fast enough to play at Nationals, your life will be over. What did you mean by that?"* *"I have noticed that you have been hesitating on progressing to X exercise. What are your concerns?"*

(Continued)

Table 10.1 (Continued)

Topics in Need of Further Inquiry	Example Questions
The impact that athletes' symptoms have on their life	*"It must be difficult to feel so low in energy and concentration. How has that affected your schoolwork?"*
	"It sounds like you are still having a lot of pain. How is that affecting your day-to-day life? "
Athletes' coping with their symptoms	*"Many athletes have similar feelings after an injury. What have you done to try to cope with those feelings? How has that been working for you?"*
Athletes' perceived level of social support (Yang et al., 2014)	*"Who in your life can you talk to about your injury and how you are feeling?"*
Athletes' safety, if appropriate	*"Have you wished you were dead or wished you could go to sleep and not wake up?"*
	"Have you actually had any thoughts of killing yourself?" (Posner et al., 2011). Questions of this sort will NOT plant the idea in athletes' heads; knowledge of local emergency mental health procedures is essential for determining how to proceed with an affirmative answer (American College of Sports Medicine et al., 2017).

Psychosocial Referral in Sport Injury Rehabilitation

In the context of sport injury rehabilitation, psychosocial referral occurs when SPs facilitate a process in which athletes with injuries are directed to psychology-trained professionals who can assist them in addressing issues associated with their mental health. Due to the extensive amount of direct contact they have with athletes after injury, SPs are in a unique position to provide referral to mental health services (Brewer et al., 1999). This section of the chapter provides a roadmap for tackling the referral process, developing a referral network, and considering important issues along the way.

Reasons for Referral

Referral to an SPP or LMHP may be warranted for several reasons. In general, referral is indicated when the challenges athletes with injury face exceed the professional roles or competencies of SPs (Van Raalte & Andersen, 2014). This may be the case when athletes are experiencing issues related to psychopathology (Tod & Andersen, 2015); difficulty functioning in school, work, or social life (Henderson & Carroll, 1993; Makarowski, 2007); or psychological difficulties related to their injury rehabilitation, including significant rehabilitation setbacks, chronic pain, somatizing, over-adhering to the rehabilitation program, or "bothering" staff (Heil, 1993b; Kane, 1984; Petitpas & Danish, 1995). Referral may also be indicated in cases where intentional injury or malingering is suspected (Heil, 1993b; Kane, 1984).

Referral may also be indicated if more subtle "red flags" occur. This might include spending excessive time in the sports medicine facility or demonstrating attachment to the SP (Henderson & Carroll, 1993; Makarowski, 2007; Petitpas & Danish, 1995). Other examples include obsessing over when return to sport will be possible, denying adverse consequences associated with injury, expressing guilt related to being unable to help their team succeed, withdrawing from others, and boasting about past successes (Petitpas & Danish, 1995).

Jacques was a college basketball player undergoing rehabilitation after an ACL reconstruction. He always seemed to be in a positive mood during our appointments, reported being diligent about completing his home exercises, and even remarked that he appreciated having some extra time for his schoolwork without the pressures of basketball. However, when the new season started to approach and he still wasn't cleared to play, Jacques told me that his coach and teammates seemed very disappointed, and I noticed some slight changes in his behavior. Although Jacques still seemed to be in a positive mood, he often quickly changed the topic whenever I mentioned basketball, and he started coming into the athletic training room nearly every day to get ice for his knee and talk with the staff. Despite his seemingly positive mood, these behaviors struck me as being a bit unusual for Jacques, so I decided to consult with the team sport psychologist about the best course of action.

Jacques's athletic trainer discusses some subtle signs he noticed that Jacques was struggling to cope with his injury.

Athletes themselves may request a referral if they have identified a personal concern that they would feel most comfortable discussing with a different professional (e.g., in counseling or psychotherapy; Brewer et al., 1999). Referral may also be mandated, such as when SMPs and SPPs have a legal, ethical, and/or professional obligation to refer athletes to appropriate mental health resources (Kane, 1984; Makarowski, 2007; National Athletic Trainers' Association, 2011; Whelan, 2011), and therefore should be familiar with the rules and regulations of their specific region. Consequences for a failure to provide appropriate referrals when indicated may range from a record of ethical violation to criminal penalties and civil suits (Makarowski, 2007). Situations involving a conflict between the interests of representatives of a sport organization and those of athletes with injuries, such as when an SP's rewards for a team's short-term competitive success are at odds with the long-term health of an athlete, may also warrant referral (Makarowski, 2007).

Referral Process

Referral of athletes with injury to an SPP or LMHP can be a complex process, requiring significant time and sound judgment and decision-making (Brewer & Redmond, 2017). A five-phase model of the referral process (Brewer & Arvinen-Barrow, 2021; Brewer et al., 1999) offers guidance to SPs navigating the challenges of referral of athletes with injury.

Phase 1: Assessment

As detailed earlier in this chapter, the goal of the assessment phase is to evaluate the athletes' psychological status (Brewer & Redmond, 2017) by observing and evaluating their response to their injury throughout rehabilitation (Brewer et al., 1999). When evaluating the psychological status of athletes with injuries, SPs should consider (a) athletes' thoughts, emotions, and behaviors; (b) the composition and quality of athletes' social support systems; (c) environmental and situational factors that may influence athletes' well-being; and (d) effects of athletes' behavior on themselves and others (Brewer & Redmond, 2017).

Table 10.2 Possible Outcomes of Consultation with a Licensed Mental Health Provider

Urgency of Referral	Action
If the situation is *urgent* . . .	. . . immediate referral to an LMHP may be initiated.
If the situation is *complex or unclear* . . .	. . . the LMHP may decide that additional assessment would be useful.
If the situation is *non-urgent* . . .	. . . SPs may be encouraged to conduct a trial intervention with the athlete and potentially avoid the need for referral at that time.

Phase 2: Consultation

If the assessment phase reveals findings that indicate that referral may be needed, SPs should reach out to an SPP or an LMHP, describe their concerns in general terms, and request a recommendation regarding the best course of action (Brewer & Redmond, 2017). Consultation can be informal if the SPP or LMHP is a core part of the SP's team, or formal if an outside source is contacted (Brewer et al., 1999). Several possible outcomes following consultation (Brewer et al., 1999) are outlined in Table 10.2.

Phase 3: Trial Intervention

The purpose of a trial intervention is to offer athletes new or additional coping skills (Heil, 1993a). Trial interventions are generally simple and do not require advanced training to implement (e.g., introducing relaxation techniques). SPs should inform the SPP or LMHP of the outcome of the intervention. If the intervention is successful, referral may not be necessary (Brewer et al., 1999). If the intervention is not successful, referral or additional consultation are likely to occur next (Brewer et al., 1999).

> When my athletic trainer asked how I was managing my first semester of college, I confessed that I had been feeling very overwhelmed, and that the pressure of so many deadlines had made it difficult to take extra time out of my schedule to complete my home exercises. I told her that I was worried this was prolonging the healing of my injury. She really listened to my concerns, and then she demonstrated how to practice a simple box breathing exercise to help me relax when I'm feeling overwhelmed. She also showed me how to contact academic counseling services on campus to learn strategies for managing my workload. These suggestions helped a lot and allowed me to make time for my home rehab, and I also knew that if I needed more support, she would help me make an appointment at the counseling center.
>
> *A first-year college athlete describes the trial intervention that her athletic trainer successfully implemented.*

Phase 4: Referral

If referral is indicated, SPs should be careful to conduct the referral in a way that is respectful of the possible concerns and fears the athlete may have about the referral process. This process can be made more comfortable by:

- Explaining in simple terms why the referral is indicated and what will happen after the referral is made. It may be helpful to describe past situations where other athletes received a similar referral (Brewer et al., 1999).
- Normalizing referral by emphasizing that injury rehabilitation can be very stressful and explaining how psychological factors can influence injury recovery and physical functioning (Heil, 1993a).
- Helping athletes arrange their first appointment (Neal et al., 2013), as this initial step can be intimidating.

Athletes who receive a referral to an LMHP in the community and plan to pay for services using their parents' or guardians' insurance should be informed that their parents/guardians may receive information about their mental health treatment from the insurance company, if relevant under local health insurance policies (Brewer et al., 1999). SPs may also want to encourage, but not require, the athlete to inform their coach about the referral (Neal et al., 2013).

For young athletes (the specific age range may vary across jurisdictions), the athletes' parent(s) or guardian(s) should be included in the discussion of the referral, because they will need to provide consent for the athlete to receive mental health services. To respect the privacy of athletes, sensitive details should be kept confidential to the extent possible, and only a general rationale for the mental health referral should be furnished (Brewer et al., 1999).

After athletes accept the referral, when possible, SPs can ease the nerves of athletes and initiate relationship-building by introducing athletes and SPPs or LMHPs face-to-face (i.e., "referring in"; Van Raalte & Andersen, 2014) and/or arranging for the SP to be present for the initial appointment (Brewer et al., 1999). Prior to disclosing any sensitive information to SPPs or LMHPs, SPs may need to obtain written consent from the athletes (Strein & Hershenson, 1991). After referrals, athletes may occasionally feel like they have been "passed on" to someone else. Consequently, the SPs involved in the athlete's injury rehabilitation should reassure the athletes that their physical rehabilitation work will continue (Heil, 1993a). When the athletes do not accept the referral, an additional trial intervention can be introduced, and the possibility of referral can be revisited in the future (Heil, 1993a).

Phase 5: Follow-Up

In this final phase, when possible, lines of communication should remain open regarding the athlete's progress in counseling or psychotherapy (Brewer et al., 1999). Athletes may sign a "release of information" form that allows their SPP or LMHP to share general information about their progress with SPs (Strein & Hershenson, 1991). SPs should maintain appropriate documentation of any follow-up consultations and ensure athletes' privacy is respected, by sharing only the information necessary for the care coordination (Brewer et al., 1999). SPs and athletes may also choose to talk informally about athletes' progress. After referrals, to monitor athletes' progress, SPs should continue their ongoing psychosocial assessment, as discussed earlier in this chapter.

Referral Networks

A *referral network* is a group of professionals to whom athletes with injuries can be referred (Brewer et al., 1999). This network should ideally include professionals who have prior experience, or at least interest, in working with athletes and are appropriately qualified (Van Raalte & Andersen, 2014). Developing a referral network is a crucial step for SPs whose team does not already include an SPP or an LMHP (Brewer et al., 1999). In the interest of creating a group of professionals who can address the full range of issues an athlete might encounter, it is important to consider which type(s) of professionals to include in the referral network. Descriptions of professionals who may provide relevant expertise are provided in Table 10.3, although it should be noted that professional titles and roles often vary across different geographic regions. A process for developing a referral network is described in Table 10.4.

Table 10.3 Referral Network Professionals

Clinical and counseling psychologists	Clinical and counseling psychologists may have experience with issues such as compliance, pain management, eating disorders, substance use, interpersonal relationships, and career counseling (Brewer et al., 1999). Counselors can often address many of these same issues, but psychologists often hold a PhD, PsyD, or EdD and are typically licensed at the doctoral level (in the United States).
Psychiatrists	Psychiatrists are medical doctors who have completed residency in a mental health setting. In some regions, they are the only LMHPs who can prescribe medications and administer treatments such as electroconvulsive therapy (Brewer et al., 1999). They typically see clients with more serious mental health diagnoses.
Psychiatric social workers	Psychiatric social workers often have skills in interviewing, family evaluation, psychotherapy, and treatment. They often hold an MSW and see clients with more serious mental health diagnoses.
Counselors	Counselors, such as clinical mental health counselors, academic athletic counselors, and substance abuse counselors, are available to address a wide variety of issues that athletes face. Depending on their training, counselors may address mental health, academic, career, substance use, and other concerns. Many types of counselors will have earned a master's degree, and some are required to obtain masters-level licensure. Training for substance abuse counselors varies greatly, and licensure is not required.
Sport psychology professionals	SPPs, such as sport psychologists, performance psychologists, mental performance consultants, and mental skills coaches, are certified to provide athletes with mental skills training and mental performance enhancement tools. Some may have masters- or doctoral-level education in sport or performance psychology, and others may have additional training in clinical or counseling psychology. Some, but not all, SPPs are also LMHPs. In cases where athletes have mental health concerns, it is important to confirm that an SPP has also obtained mental health licensure prior to making a referral.

Table 10.4 How to Develop a Referral Network

Step 1	*Identify practitioners to include in the network.* Ideally, select a group of practitioners who are diverse in gender, ethnicity, professional background, and theoretical orientation (Brewer et al., 1999).
Step 2	*Contact the practitioners to confirm that they are interested in providing consultation and receiving referrals* (Brewer et al., 1999). It may be helpful to include practitioners who offer a sliding scale (Van Raalte & Andersen, 2014) or a range of fees that may be affordable.
Step 3	*Develop working relationships with the practitioners.* Become familiar enough with the practitioners' expertise, approach, preferred referral process, and typical procedures (e.g., appointment scheduling) that you can give athletes a clear idea of what to expect following referral. This reduces anxiety and increases the odds of the relationship being successful (Heil, 1993a). It may be useful to create a consultation and referral plan outlining how to contact the practitioner and how to approach communication in a way that protects athletes' confidentiality (Brewer et al., 1999).
Step 4	*Continually modify the referral network* (Kane, 1984). SPs may want to add practitioners to the network who represent new specialties or remove practitioners if they move to a new location or are no longer available for consultation and referrals, if SPs do not work well with them, or if athletes are continually dissatisfied with their work or relationship with the practitioners.

Financial Considerations

Most health insurance policies offer mental health coverage with varying associated out-of-pocket costs and limits to the length of treatment. To receive insurance coverage, however, athletes may need to receive a formal diagnosis that goes in their medical record. Alternatively, depending on the country or region, some LMHPs allow clients to pay fees on a sliding scale based on their income. Prior to making a referral, SPs should discuss insurance coverage, fees, and payment options with athletes (Brewer et al., 1999; Van Raalte & Andersen, 2014).

Conclusion

Sport injury rehabilitation presents athletes with physical and psychological challenges that can be accompanied by emotional and behavioral disturbances. Professionals in close contact with athletes during the rehabilitation process can assess their psychosocial status. This can be achieved through building rapport, watching and listening for signs of poor adjustment, using screening tools, and asking questions about cognitions, emotions, and behavior. Based on the psychosocial assessment of athletes during rehabilitation, it may be appropriate for SPs to refer athletes for psychological assistance. In this chapter, a framework for making referrals for psychological assistance and suggestions for developing a referral network are provided. Coupled with thorough and ongoing psychosocial assessment, timely referrals for psychosocial assistance during injury rehabilitation can help SPs better serve the athletes with whom they work.

Case Study

Alex is a 19-year-old college baseball player who recently underwent surgery to repair a torn meniscus. He was moving ahead as expected in rehabilitation until he was supposed to progress to plyometric exercises. At that time, he complained about sharp pain, clicking, and catching in his knee. Re-evaluation of the knee revealed no concerns about the integrity of the repair. Alex's progress continued to be minimal, and he appeared increasingly tired and distractible. His typically warm and calm demeanor seemed to turn irritable and emotionally reactive. During one of his manual therapy sessions, his athletic trainer decided to inquire about these observations. Alex revealed that he had been unable to sleep well or focus at school due to feeling increasingly anxious about his parents' upcoming visit, because he had not told them about his knee surgery. He explained that due to their cultural background, his parents would have strongly advised against the surgery. It also became evident that Alex had a very poor understanding of his injury, the rationale for the surgery, and his expected rehabilitation outcome. He was misinterpreting all new sensations in his knee as signs of irreversible damage and had started to regret the surgery, believing that he would never be able to return to baseball, which only exacerbated his anxiety.

Questions

1. Based on the case description, what psychosocial and sociocultural factors may have contributed to Alex's situation?
2. Based on your (future or current) professional competencies, how would you approach the topic of Alex's behavior and mood changes with the athlete?
3. What additional areas and/or methods of assessment should be considered for Alex?
4. What factors should you take into consideration when determining whether to proceed with a trial intervention or a referral to an LMHP for Alex?

Note

* **Disclaimer:** The views expressed in this chapter are solely those of the authors and do not reflect the official policy or position of the Department of the Air Force, the Special Warfare Human Performance Squadron, the Department of Defense, or the US government.

References

Albinson, C. B., & Petrie, T. A. (2003). Cognitive appraisals, stress, and coping: Preinjury and postinjury factors influencing psychological adjustment to sport injury. *Journal of Sport Rehabilitation, 12*(4), 306–322. https://doi.org/10.1123/jsr.12.4.306

American College of Sports Medicine, American Academy of Family Physicians, American Academy of Orthopaedic Surgeons, American Medical Society for Sports Medicine, American Orthopaedic Society for Sports Medicine, & Medicine, A. O. A. o. S. (2017). Psychological issues related to illness and injury in athletes and the team physician: A consensus statement-2016 update. *Medicine and Science in Sports and Exercise, 49*(5), 1043–1054. https://doi.org/10.1249/MSS.0000000000001247

American Psychiatric Association. (2013). *Diagnostic and statistical manual of mental disorders*. https://doi.org/10.1176/appi.books.9780890425596

American Psychological Association. (2022). Psychological assessment. In *APA dictionary of psychology*. https://dictionary.apa.org/psychological-assessment

Arvinen-Barrow, M., Hamson-Utley, J. J., & DeFreeze, J. D. (2018). Sport injury, rehabilitation, and return to sport. In J. Taylor (Ed.), *Assessment in applied sport psychology* (pp. 183–198). Human Kinetics. https://doi.org/10.5040/9781492595236.ch-013

Arvinen-Barrow, M., Hemmings, B., Weigand, D. A., Becker, C. A., & Booth, L. (2007). Views of chartered physiotherapists on the psychological content of their practice: A national follow-up survey in the United Kingdom. *Journal of Sport Rehabilitation, 16*(2), 111–121. https://doi.org/10.1123/jsr.16.2.111

Brewer, B. W. (1993). Self-identity and specific vulnerability to depressed mood. *Journal of Personality, 61*(3), 343–364. https://doi.org/10.1111/j.1467-6494.1993.tb00284.x

Brewer, B. W. (2017). Psychological responses to injury. In *Oxford research encyclopedia of psychology*. Oxford University Press.

Brewer, B. W., & Arvinen-Barrow, M. (2021). Psychology of injury and rehabilitation. In Association for Applied Sport Psychology (AASP). In S. C. Sackett, N. Durand-Bush, & L. Tashman (Eds.), *The essential guide for mental performance consultants*. Human Kinetics Custom Content.

Brewer, B. W., Linder, D. E., & Phelps, C. M. (1995). Situational correlates of emotional adjustment to athletic injury. *Clinical Journal of Sport Medicine, 5*(4), 241–245. https://doi.org/10.1097/00042752-199510000-00006

Brewer, B. W., Petitpas, A. J., & Van Raalte, J. L. (1999). Referral of injured athletes for counseling and psychotherapy. In R. Ray & D. M. Wiese-Bjornstal (Eds.), *Counseling in sports medicine* (pp. 127–141). Human Kinetics.

Brewer, B. W., & Redmond, C. J. (2017). *Psychology of sport injury*. Human Kinetics.

Brewer, B. W., Van Raalte, J. L., & Linder, D. E. (1993). Athletic identity: Hercules' muscles or Achilles' heel? *International Journal of Sport Psychology, 24*(2), 237–254.

Chang, C., Putukian, M., Aerni, G., Diamond, A., Hong, G., Ingram, Y., . . . Wolanin, A. (2020). Mental health issues and psychological factors in athletes: Detection, management, effect on performance and prevention: American medical society for sports medicine position statement-executive summary. *British Journal of Sports Medicine, 54*(4), 216–220. https://doi.org/10.1136/bjsports-2019-101583

Clement, D., Granquist, M. D., & Arvinen-Barrow, M. (2013). Psychosocial aspects of athletic injuries as perceived by athletic trainers. *Journal of Athletic Training, 48*(4), 512–521. https://doi.org/10.4085/1062-6050-48.3.21

Frey, J. H. (1991). Social risk and the meaning of sport. *Sociology of Sport Journal, 8*, 136–145.

Gouttebarge, V., Bindra, A., Blauwet, C., Campriani, N., Currie, A., Engebretsen, L., . . . Budgett, R. (2021). International Olympic committee (IOC) sport mental health assessment tool 1 (SMHAT-1) and sport mental health recognition tool 1 (SMHRT-1): Towards better support of athletes' mental health. *British Journal of Sports Medicine, 55*(1), 30–37. https://doi.org/10.1136/bjsports-2020-102411

Heaney, C., Rostron, C. L., Walker, N. C., & Green, A. J. K. (2017). Is there a link between previous exposure to sport injury psychology education and UK sport injury rehabilitation professionals' attitudes and behaviour towards sport psychology? *Physical Therapy in Sport, 23*(1), 99–104. https://doi.org/10.1016/j.ptsp.2016.08.006

Heil, J. (1993a). Conducting assessment and intervention. In J. Heil (Ed.), *Psychology of sport injury* (pp. 113–136). Human Kinetics.

Heil, J. (1993b). Mental training in injury management. In J. Heil (Ed.), *Psychology of sport injury* (pp. 151–174). Human Kinetics.

Henderson, J., & Carroll, W. (1993). The athletic trainer's role in preventing sport injury and rehabilitating injured athletes: A psychological perspective. In D. Pargman (Ed.), *Psychological bases of sport injuries* (pp. 15–31). Fitness Information Technology.

Kane, B. (1984). Trainer counseling to avoid three face-saving maneuvers. *Athletic Training, 19*(3), 171–174.

Larson, G. A., Starkey, C., & Zaichkowsky, L. D. (1996). Psychological aspects of athletic injuries as perceived by athletic trainers. *The Sport Psychologist, 10*(1), 37–47. https://doi.org/10.1123/tsp.10.1.37

Lazarus, R. S., & Folkman, S. (1984). *Stress, appraisal, and coping*. Springer Publishing Company.

Levis, B., Benedetti, A., Ioannidis, J. P. A., Sun, Y., Negeri, Z., He, C., . . . Thombs, B. D. (2020). Patient health questionnaire-9 scores do not accurately estimate depression prevalence: Individual participant data meta-analysis. *Journal of Clinical Epidemiology, 112*, 115–128. https://doi.org/10.1016/j.jclinepi.2020.02.002

Makarowski, L. M. (2007). Ethical and legal issues for sports professionals counseling injured athletes. In D. Pargman (Ed.), *Psychological bases of sport injuries* (3rd ed., pp. 289–303). Fitness Information Technology.

Malinauskas, R. (2010). The associations among social support, stress, and life satisfaction as perceived by injured college athletes. *Journal of Social Behavior and Personality, 38*(6), 741–752. https://doi.org/10.2224/sbp.2010.38.6.741

Mazzer, K. R., & Rickwood, D. J. (2015). Mental health in sport: Coaches' views of their role and efficacy in supporting young people's mental health. *International Journal of Health Promotion and Education, 53*(2), 102–114. https://doi.org/10.1080/14635240.2014.965841

McDonald, S. A., & Hardy, C. J. (1990). Affective response patterns of the injured athlete: An exploratory analysis. *The Sport Psychologist, 4*(3), 261–274. https://doi.org/10.1123/tsp.4.3.261

McGannon, K. R., & McMahon, J. (2020). Sport media research: Examining the benefits for sport injury psychology and beyond. In R. Wadey (Ed.), *Sport injury psychology: Cultural, relational, methodological, and applied considerations* (pp. 33–40). Routledge.

Murphy, G. P., & Sheehan, R. B. (2021). A qualitative investigation into the individual injury burden of amateur rugby players. *Physical Therapy in Sport, 50*, 74–81. https://doi.org/10.1016/j.ptsp.2021.04.003

National Athletic Trainers' Association. (2011). *Athletic training education competencies*. www.nata.org/sites/default/files/competencies_5th_edition.pdf

Neal, T. L., Diamond, A. B., Goldman, S., Klossner, D., Morse, E. D., Pajak, D. E., . . . Welzant, V. (2013). Inter-association recommendations for developing a plan to recognize and refer student-athletes with psychological concerns at the collegiate level: An executive summary of a consensus statement. *Journal of Athletic Training, 48*(5), 716–720. https://doi.org/10.4085/1062-6050-48.4.13

Neal, T. L., Diamond, A. B., Goldman, S., Liedtka, K. D., Mathis, K., Morse, E. D., . . . Welzant, V. (2015). Interassociation recommendations for developing a plan to recognize and refer student-athletes with psychological concerns at the secondary school level: A consensus statement. *Journal of Athletic Training, 50*(3), 231–249. https://doi.org/10.4085/1062-6050-50.3.03

Petitpas, A. J., & Cornelius, A. (2004). Practitioner-client relationships: Building working alliances. In G. S. Kolt & M. B. Andersen (Eds.), *Psychology in the physical and manual therapies* (pp. 57–70). Churchill Livingstone.

Petitpas, A. J., & Danish, S. J. (1995). Caring for the injured athletes. In S. Murphy (Ed.), *Sport psychology interventions* (pp. 255–281). Human Kinetics.

Posner, K., Brown, G. K., Stanley, B., Brent, D. A., Yershova, K. V., Oquendo, M. A., Currier, G. W., Melvin, G. A., Greenhill, L., Shen, S., & Mann, J. J. (2011). The Columbia-Suicide Severity Rating Scale: Initial validity and internal consistency findings from three multisite studies with adolescents and adults. *The American Journal of Psychiatry, 168*(12), 1266–1277. https://doi.org/10.1176/appi.ajp.2011.10111704

Smith, A. M., & Milliner, E. K. (1994). Injured athletes and the risk of suicide. *Journal of Athletic Training, 29*(4), 337–341.

Spanos, N. P., Radtke-Bodorik, H. L., Ferguson, J. D., & Jones, B. (1979). The effects of hypnotic susceptibility, suggestions for analgesia, and utilization of cognitive strategies on the reduction of pain. *Journal of Abnormal Psychology, 88*(3), 282–292. https://doi.org/10.1037/0021-843X.88.3.282

Strein, W., & Hershenson, D. B. (1991). Confidentiality in nondyadic counseling situations. *Journal of Counseling & Development, 69*(4), 312–316. https://doi.org/10.1002/j.1556-6676.1991.tb01512.x

Sullivan, M. J. L., Bishop, S., & Pivik, J. (1995). The pain catastrophizing scale: Development and validation. *Psychological Assessment, 7*(4), 524–532. https://doi.org/10.1037/1040-3590.7.4.524

Sundgot-Borgen, J. (1994). Risk and trigger factors for the development of eating disorders in female elite athletes. *Medicine and Science in Sports and Exercise*, *26*(4), 414–419. https://doi.org/10.1249/00005768-199404000-00003

Swinbourne, R., Gill, N., Vaile, J., & Smart, D. (2016). Prevalence of poor sleep quality, sleepiness and obstructive sleep apnoea risk factors in athletes. *European Journal of Sport Science*, *16*(7), 850–858. https://doi.org/10.1080/17461391.2015.1120781

Tahtinen, R., Kristjansdottir, H., Olason, D. T., & Morris, R. (2021). What lies beneath: Exploring different depressive symptoms across selected risk factors in Icelandic team sport athletes. *Journal of Clinical Sport Psychology*, *15*(1), 54–79. https://doi.org/10.1123/jcsp.2020-0040

Theunissen, M., Peters, M. L., Bruce, J., Gramke, H. F., & Marcus, M. A. E. (2012). Preoperative anxiety and catastrophizing a systematic review and meta-analysis of the association with chronic postsurgical pain. *The Clinical Journal of Pain*, *28*(9), 819–841. https://doi.org/10.1097/ajp.0b013e31824549d6

Tod, D., & Andersen, M. B. (2015). When to refer athletes for counseling or psychotherapy. In J. M. Williams & V. Krane (Eds.), *Applied sport psychology: Personal growth to peak performance* (7th ed., pp. 405–420). McGrawHill.

Tripp, D. A., Stanish, W. D., Coady, C., & Reardon, G. (2004). The subjective pain experience of athletes following anterior cruciate ligament surgery. *Psychology of Sport and Exercise*, *5*(3), 339–354. https://doi.org/10.1016/S1469-0292(03)00022-0

Van Raalte, J. L., & Andersen, M. B. (2014). Referral processes in sport psychology. In J. L. Van Raalte & B. W. Brewer (Eds.), *Exploring sport and exercise psychology* (3rd ed., pp. 337–350). American Psychological Association.

Walker, M. P. (2017). *Why we sleep: Unlocking the power of sleep and dreams.* Scribner.

Watson, J. C., & Sandoni, P. S. (2016). Central neuropathic pain syndromes. *Mayo Clinic Proceedings*, *91*(3), 372–385. https://doi.org/10.1016/j.mayocp.2016.01.017

Whelan, J. (2011). *Ethics code: AASP ethical principles and standards.* Association for Applied Sport Psychology. https://appliedsportpsych.org/about-the-association-for-applied-sport-psychology/ethics/ethics-code/

Wiese-Bjornstal, D. M., Smith, A. M., Shaffer, S. M., & Morrey, M. A. (1998). An integrated model of response to sport injury: Psychological and sociological dynamics. *Journal of Applied Sport Psychology*, *10*(1), 46–69. https://doi.org/10.1080/10413209808406377

Wolanin, A., Gross, M., & Hong, E. (2015). Depression in athletes: Prevalence and risk factors. *Current Sports Medicine Reports*, *14*(1), 56–60. https://doi.org/10.1249/jsr.0000000000000123

Yang, J., Cheng, G., Zhang, Y., Covassin, T., Heiden, E. O., & Peek-Asa, C. (2014). Influence of symptoms of depression and anxiety on injury hazard among collegiate American football players. *Research in Sports Medicine*, *22*(2), 147–160. https://doi.org/10.1080/15438627.2014.881818

11 Multicultural Considerations in Sport Injury and Rehabilitation

Shameema M. Yousuf

Chapter Objectives

- To define and explain culture, multiculturism, and intersectionality.
- To summarize sociocultural characteristics found to influence sport injury.
- To outline strategies that can be used to develop multicultural competence, with a goal to ensure holistic care during sport injury.

Introduction

With a recent shift toward equity, diversity, inclusion, and belonging in leadership and organizational settings (Kennedy, 2021), adopting a multicultural biopsychosocial practice in healthcare is necessitated. This is particularly important for those working with athletes – injured or not – as athletes have intersectional or hybrid cultural identities that influence their thoughts, feelings, beliefs, values, and practices, both in and out of sport. Recently, a growing interest in examining the intersectional experiences of multiple stakeholders in sport from a transnational perspective has taken place (Ryba, 2017), though there has been limited focus on injury management and recovery from an intersectional lens.

So far, the literature has addressed a few cultural factors that affect the sport injury rehabilitation and recovery process. Research has identified racial and ethnic differences in both athlete pain perceptions (e.g., Dover Wandner et al., 2011) and how healthcare providers interpret them (e.g., Johnson et al., 2004). Research has also highlighted cultural differences in athlete expectations of their healthcare providers (Arvinen-Barrow et al., 2016), emphasizing the importance of providing culturally sensitive care. Additionally, literature has proposed religion and spirituality as a protective and resilience factor in sport injury recovery (Wiese-Bjornstal, 2019) and put forth best practice guidelines for practitioners to consider when integrating spirituality and religion into sport injury rehabilitation (Clement et al., 2019). It has also been argued that although influential in recovery, systemic inequalities related to sociocultural identities and contextual forces are prevalent in non-physical aspects of injury management and recovery (Truong et al., 2021). The purpose of this chapter is to provide an overview of multicultural considerations in sport injury rehabilitation. More specifically, this chapter will (a) define culture and multiculturism, (b) introduce multicultural psychology paradigm (Pedersen, 1990) and intersectionality (Crenshaw, 1989) as two guiding frameworks, (c) introduce sociocultural characteristics that have been found to influence sport injury rehabilitation, (d) discuss the ways culture of pain varies across cultures, (e) introduce strategies that can be used to develop multicultural

DOI: 10.4324/9781003295709-13

competencies in practice, and (f) make recommendations for sport psychology professionals (SPPs) and sports medicine professionals (SMPs) to ensure holistic support during sport injury rehabilitation through a multicultural psychological lens.

Culture and Multiculturism: Definitions

In the context of this chapter, *culture* is defined as "any group that shares a theme or issues (s)" (Sue et al., 1996, p. 16). This chapter will also adopt a broad view of culture, incorporating ethnographic, demographic, status, and affiliation factors, such as "language, gender, ethnicity/ race, spirituality, sexual preference, age, physical issues, socioeconomic status, and survival after trauma" (Mio et al., 2016). The chapter ascribes to the notion that culture is both complex and dynamic (Pedersen, 1990), encompassing a wide diversity that comprises numerous socially meaningful differences (Cunningham, 2019; Schinke & Hanrahan, 2009) that influence the ways in which people view the world and "perceive their relationship to nature, institutions and other people, and things" (Sue, 1978, p. 458).

Multiculturism, on the other hand, is a term used to describe a condition of diversity in settings where more than one culture exists. According to Clayton (2020), multiculturalism refers to the existence of difference and uneven power relations among populations in terms of racial, ethnic, religious, and geographical distinctions and other cultural markers that deviate from dominant, often racialized, "norms" (p. 211). Clayton argues that it is not simply about focusing on how individuals experience "difference, otherness, and exclusion" (p. 218) but on how "environments, objects, and certain atmospheres" (p. 218) may produce identities and inequalities.

Multicultural Psychology Paradigm

While there are many ways to conceptualize the role of culture and multiculturism, this chapter adopts the multicultural psychology paradigm (Pedersen, 1990) as its theoretical framework for understanding multicultural factors in sport injury rehabilitation. Declared as the "fourth force in psychology" (Pedersen, 1990, 1991), multicultural psychology is founded on a premise that "all behaviors are learned and displayed in a cultural context" (Pedersen, 2008, p. 15), and that culture should be regarded as the center of all human thoughts, emotions, and behaviors (David et al., 2014). Multicultural psychology, as a paradigm, examines human behavior through an inclusive lens and is the investigation of identity development, stereotyping, prejudice, discrimination and racism, acculturation and assimilation, development of cultural competence and humility, and health and mental health disparities among other cultural barriers to belonging (Mio et al., 2016). Utilizing multicultural psychology as a theoretical framework when working with injured athletes enables SPPs and SMPs to consider the impact of personal, contextual, and social influences alongside physical recovery. It provides a basis for SPPs and SMPs to self-reflect and examine their personal worldview when engaging with athletes from various cultural backgrounds. As a core tenet of one's practice, multicultural psychology allows for a candid evaluation of the appropriateness of existing monocultural approaches while seeking to dismantle inequitable practices. The SPPs and SMPs who lack multicultural competence rely on monocultural and Eurocentric approaches, normed by Western white middle-class values and thus unaligned with all stakeholder values (Parham, 2005). These values are also further amplified by research and theoretical assumptions of science, where Western Eurocentric practices are dominant, such that even in Eastern monocultural environments, certain Western values and practices are held superior. The SPPs and SMPs may therefore both ignore cultural differences and misinterpret culturally normed behaviors, overgeneralizing and stereotyping those they serve (Parham, 2005). Indeed, Pedersen (2008) posits that when SPPs and SMPs recognize the impact of the cultural context on learned behavior, it also "makes possible accurate assessment, meaningful understanding, and appropriate intervention relative to that cultural context. Interpreting behavior out of context is likely to result in misattribution" (p. 15).

Intersectionality

When working from a multicultural paradigm and seeking to dismantle inequitable practices, another key theoretical framework to understand is intersectionality (Crenshaw, 1989). Defined as the complex interconnected nature of social categorizations (i.e., race, class, and gender) and multiple identities, intersectionality explains how interlocking systems of inequity and power within society empower and disempower individuals. Intersectionality was omitted in early feminist work as it failed to consider the unique intersectional experiences of women of color, non-heterosexual working class, and/or disabled women (Buffington & Lai, 2011). Black feminist philosophy (Collins, 1998, 2005; hooks, 1981) offered an alternative to early feminism, by providing a framework for understanding race and racism through different intersecting social identity characteristics (e.g., women, race, class).

Given that research has identified racial, ethnic, cultural, spiritual, and systemic inequalities relevant to sport injury and rehabilitation experience (e.g., Arvinen-Barrow et al., 2016; Dover Wandner et al., 2011; Johnson et al., 2004; Truong et al., 2021), an understanding of the intertwined nature of an individual's varied and complex identities and how they influence the manifestation of privilege and discrimination (Crenshaw, 1989) is required. Considering intersectional identities when working with athletes with injuries provides SPPs and SMPs an opportunity to examine significant disparities in social group experiences that exist both in sport and in sport injury. Recognizing such disparities also allows the SPPs and SMPs an opportunity to minimize the dominance of commonly adopted Eurocentric practices.

While intersectionality is important to consider alongside multicultural psychology paradigm, there remains limited praxis that examines the intersectional experiences of racial and ethnic individuals that intertwine with other cultural identities. The impact of individual athlete's intersectional experiences on their health, well-being, and performance in sport has also largely gone unexplored. Both sports medicine and sport psychology practices have traditionally ignored the importance of these intertwined and culturally hybrid social and contextual constructs and forces. Despite the lack of research evidence, it is important for both SPPs and SMPs to recognize that nuanced experiences within a sport injury and rehabilitation context cannot be described through a single variable or identity characteristic. The goal is to be better equipped to provide holistic, person-centered care to athletes with injuries. Therefore, when working with athletes with injuries, SPPs and SMPs are urged not to treat all athletes with injuries the same or with a race-blind approach (Butryn, 2002; Schinke & Hanrahan, 2009). They are also challenged to consider stereotypes and stigmas through a sociocultural and sociopolitical lens as sport injury and rehabilitation experiences of certain individuals/groups may be shaped differently by historical political ideologies of national regions around the globe (Yousuf & Owens, 2023).

Intersecting Sociocultural Characteristics in Sport Injury Rehabilitation

Consistent with the multicultural psychology paradigm (Pedersen, 1990) and intersectionality (Crenshaw, 1989), this section of the chapter will introduce key sociocultural characteristics that have been found to influence sport injury rehabilitation. What is presented herein is not intended to be an exhaustive account. Instead, it is intended to prompt the reader to reflect on the complexities of varied sociocultural characteristics, and how they intersect to influence sport injury considerations in systems that may privilege or marginalize and subsequently influence rehabilitation.

Intersectional Identities

Athletes enter the injury rehabilitation environment with multiple intersecting identities, and as such, the ways in which they interpret their injury and approach their rehabilitation are impacted by their cultural worldview, values, and beliefs. These intersectional identities will also affect their rehabilitation behaviors and their experience of being in the rehabilitation environment. This can be particularly pertinent if the injury rehabilitation environment is characterized by homogeneity and dominance of factors that posit the athlete as "other," thus producing inequalities that may influence and shape their intersecting identities.

Scholars have acknowledged the importance of intersectional identities of athletes. They have also acknowledged the numerous systems in which these identities are fluidly developing, interacting, and adapting across different environments, contexts, and cultures, given cross-border movements (Ronkainen et al., 2016; Stambulova & Ryba, 2020). To illustrate, an individual's multiple intersectional identities may provide an athlete with cultural beliefs that act as protective factors during injury while also rendering them more susceptible to trauma in environments that marginalize (Mio et al., 2016). Paradoxically, in an environment that supports individuals' agency to create and choose their own identities (Eubank et al., 2020), one must also recognize the presence of power and privilege of dominant groups as marginalizing forces that may stemmy the very freedom and agency of minoritized intersectional identities. To illustrate, Yousuf and Owens (2023) demonstrated how hegemonic neoliberal ideologies dominate society and sport without consideration of other aspects of intersectional identities. Citing the experiences of two female athletes of color – Naomi Osaka and Simone Biles – during a double pandemic (Addo, 2020), Yousuf and Owens (2023) pointed out how media discussions around these two athletes' withdrawal from competition due to mental health and medical reasons centered on certain aspects of their identities while ignoring others. They highlighted that discussions also failed to consider possible experiences of racial and sexualized trauma. They also posited that assumptions made of Osaka and Biles demonstrated that women of color are often marginalized by idealized behaviors bestowed by those holding neoliberal values, illustrating that individualism above collective and communal responsibility are prized, even within sport psychology and sports medicine. While the author posits that SPPs and SMPs must always consider stakeholders' intersecting identities, this chapter continues to provide operational understanding of social constructs to enable meaningful working relationships with athletes.

Athletic Identity

Described as an "individual's sense of self defined by (a) a set of physical, psychological, and interpersonal characteristics that is not wholly shared with any other person and (b) a range of affiliations (e.g., ethnicity) and social roles" (American Psychological Association, 2022), *identity* has been found to be a factor affecting sport injury rehabilitation. Previous literature has asserted that having a strong athletic identity may impact an athlete during sport injury rehabilitation both positively and negatively. A Strong athletic identity can have both a damaging impact on an athlete's well-being during an injury and benefits, such as commitment and motivation to the rehabilitation and recovery process (Brewer & Petitpas, 2017). Athletic identity may also be impacted by global cultural differences in motivation for sport engagement and affiliation.

American athletes' competitive winning mentality, praise, and publicity that come with such honor (Eitzen & Sage, 2009) may drive a strong athletic identity, whereas transnational athletes may treat sport participation simply as a sporting endeavor and focus more on non-athletic pursuits (Popp et al., 2009).

Strong athletic identity may also affect health-seeking behaviors and adherence to rehabilitation by athletes with injuries. For example, domestic and international athletes competing in the American collegiate athletics system with an athletic scholarship may be driven by increased chances of a professional career (Danylchuk & Grbac, 2016), thus affecting their approach to injury management behaviors. Equally, a fear of losing playing time or a scholarship due to injury can have both short- and long-term financial, physical, and legal ramifications to the athlete that can alter their life journey (Beth, 2021, April 6), hence impacting their athletic identity and rehabilitation behaviors.

Disability

Having a disability can influence sport injury and rehabilitation in several ways. While every effort may be taken to provide inclusive injury rehabilitation spaces, environments designed predominantly for able-bodied athletes may hinder engagement in the rehabilitation process for athletes with physical disabilities (Davis & Ferrara, 1995). For athletes with learning disabilities, previous concussions may go unreported, thus impacting assessment baselines (McKay et al., 2014). Equally, the types of injuries presented by athletes with disabilities may vary, depending on their sport and specific disability (Bohling et al., 2022). When compared to able-bodied athletes, athletes with disabilities experience greater loss in training time due to injuries and disability-related illnesses (Davis & Ferrara, 1995) and shortened careers (Martin, 2005), impacting well-being.

Much like able-bodied athletes, having good social support throughout the injury journey is paramount to injury management and sport longevity (e.g., McFadden, 2022, October 26–29). Both SPPs and SMPs supporting injured athletes with disabilities have been encouraged to assist athletes in developing qualities of self-esteem, self-determination, and self-awareness, with a goal to drive motivation, to distinguish between pain and discomfort resulting from injury and disability, and to monitor levels of fatigue to help limit time loss in shortened careers (Martin, 2005). While the aforementioned is considered important for disabled athlete self-development, SPPs and SMPs are urged to consider how the centering of "self" when working with an athlete of intersectional disability and collective cultural identity also underpins hegemonic neoliberal ideology. With a goal to enhance personal development and growth during sport injury, SPPs and SMPs may also consider exploring various approaches with the athlete, including communal and social support, and spiritual strengths and needs (Hammer et al., 2021). This may include the support and aid of parents and carers when assessing an athlete's readiness to return to participation, especially when working with those of attention learning disorders (McKay et al., 2014).

Gender

Gender can influence injury rehabilitation in a few ways. For example, Clement et al. (2012) found that among US-based collegiate athletes, gender influenced athlete expectations of SMPs – male athletes with no prior experience of athletic training had lower expectations for athletic trainers providing a facilitative environment for rehabilitation, and female athletes with prior experience of athletic training were less likely to have realistic expectations of the athletic training. Beliefs related to gender roles may also affect help-seeking behaviors. The Sotho men of South Africa are not allowed to show their pain, whereas women are encouraged to show pain in any way possible to receive help (Nortjé & Albertyn, 2015). Among male athletes, hyper-masculinity and toughness may prevent them from seeking out mental health and/or emotional support when injured, for fear of being perceived weak (Castaldelli-Maia et al., 2019; Lim et al., 2017; Walton et al., 2021). Stigma around seeking psychological support has also been noted as a barrier for younger male athletes, and marital status (where spouses enable receptivity) as a facilitator to help-seeking behaviors (Jones, 2016).

Equally, sport support staff has not always included staff of diverse gender belonging, and until recently, female SMPs were underrepresented in professional and collegiate sport (O'Reilly et al., 2019). This may present a barrier for help-seeking behaviors for female athletes, particularly those wishing to commit to ethics of their faith. The intersection of gender and religion for Muslim women, or any other women who observe modesty, *may* necessitate a preference of a gender-concordant SMP to protect modesty, which in Islam is a religious ethic (Sajoo, 2004). This appreciation must be held with understanding that there are different ways of being a Muslim and female (Yousuf & Owens, 2023). To ensure safeguarding and respect for individual beliefs, seeking consent from the athlete to be seen by a SPP or SMP who identifies with a different gender is warranted.

For athletes who identify as transgender, sport injury and rehabilitation may also elicit multiple areas of concern that exceed those outlined previously. Risk of negative physical and mental health outcomes from anxiety and depression is high for transgendered athletes (Bretherton et al., 2021) and more pronounced for those of intersectional identity and belonging to several minoritized groups (Cicero et al., 2020). While research pertaining to gender-affirming hormone therapy (GAHT) for transgendered athletes in competitive sport is still limited and slowly growing, SPPs and SMPs must be alert to the risk of possible chronic disease implications for transgendered athletes undergoing therapy (e.g., Bretherton et al., 2021; Moore et al., 2021). The SPPs and SMPs should also be aware of possible changes to transgendered athletes' physical or mental health that could impact injury rehabilitation. To ensure safeguarding for all athletes, SPPs and SMPs, and the facilities in which they operate, must also review and establish policies and procedures that promote access and inclusivity.

Religion and Spirituality

In this chapter, *religion* is defined as a "system of beliefs in divine or superhuman power, and practices of worship or other rituals directed toward such power" (Argyle & Beit-Hallahmi, 1975, p. 1). *Spirituality*, on the other hand, is defined as an "existential aspect of their religious lives, for example, the practice of prayer throughout the day (outside a Church environment) and witness through the actions of every dimension of their lives, including sport (e.g., Romans 12:1)" (Watson & Czech, 2005, p. 27). Both have an important role in an athlete's career – to help them cope with the demands of their sport and to enhance performance (Maranise, 2013). Religious and spiritual values can also hold relevance in athletes' performance lifestyles (Balague, 1999; Howe & Parker, 2014), in how they make meaning of successes and failures (Vernacchia et al., 2000), as well as how they promote and damage mental health (Weber & Pargament, 2014).

In the sport injury context, monotheistic faith (Christianity, Judaism, and Islam) and associated values and belief practices have been found to be protective factors for both reducing susceptibility to injury and coping with injury (Koenig, 2004; Wiese-Bjornstal, 2019, 2019, November; Wiese-Bjornstal et al., 1998). Turning to faith can provide athletes with a sense of hope, help manage the stress associated with sport injury (Arvinen-Barrow et al., 2015; Najah et al., 2017), help accept the injury (Dodo et al., 2015), and encourage a sense of community social support in healing (George et al., 2002). Non-monotheistic faiths and spiritual practices may also be beneficial during sport injury. For example, when working with a coach in Zimbabwe, the author successfully facilitated thinking around the ways in which an athlete could connect daily with their traditional African spiritual healer while at a World Championship, with a goal to reduce stress responses and susceptibility to poor mental health.

Psychosocial interventions during sport injury have included mindfulness practices – a present-moment awareness with roots in Buddhism (Kabat-Zinn, 2013). Although the literature is sparse, mindfulness practice has been shown to effectively reduce injury risk (Gledhill & Ivarsson, 2020), improve rehabilitation adherence (Bennett & Lindsay, 2016), and have positive impact on mental health, well-being, mindfulness, and acceptance among injured athletes (Moesch et al., 2020; Mohammed et al., 2018). The preliminary evidence in support for using mindfulness interventions for sport injury prevention and rehabilitation makes it an appealing strategy to use with injured athletes; however, mindfulness experts have cautioned against its use without spiritual understanding (Roychowdhury et al., 2021). The SPPs and SMPs should also consider the appropriateness of using interventions rooted in Buddhism with athletes whose faith practices may conflict with Eastern philosophies or already incorporate a form of mindfulness, such as the five-times-a-day prayer – a compulsory pillar in Islam – itself a form of meditation.

Another aspect to consider with athletes who practice their faith is the possible need to adjust training and rehabilitation plans during religious observations. Christians, Jews, and Muslims practice fasting, which is a time of spiritual connection. Depending on the faith, fasting may last a day to a month-long practice, when either all, or some foods and liquid are eliminated. For Muslims, fasting during Ramadan lasts for a month, and Muslim athletes may fast from sunrise until sunset, abstaining from food and liquid intake. This can have both performance and health impacts (Burke & King, 2012; DeLang et al., 2021; Kirkendall et al., 2012; Maughan et al., 2012), including increased risk of injury, necessitating considerations for overuse and non-contact injuries (Chamari et al., 2012; DeLang et al., 2021; Eirale et al., 2013; Kirkendall et al., 2012).

While the cultural dimension of religion and spirituality has importance for athletes, those of non-white identities and Muslims do not typically disclose to teammates despite sharing other aspects of their cultural identity (Castaldelli-Maia et al., 2019). Some Muslim athletes may also turn to religious and somatic practices to support their sense of well-being, while others may seek therapy from a mental health professional. As such, understanding injured athletes' needs and preferences, and providing varied options for support, is important to ensure comprehensive care. Thus, SPPs and SMPs should (a) understand how individual athletes identify and choose to express the role of religion and spirituality in their lifestyle and injury rehabilitation, (b) be mindful of individual differences in religious and spiritual observances, (c) understand how implementing certain interventions with athletes with intersectional identities may inadvertently cause harm and/or marginalize other cultural practices, and (d) ensure the rehabilitation environment is inclusive of spaces that accommodate various religious and spiritual needs.

Race, Ethnicity, and Socioeconomic Status

When considering the interconnected and interrelated impact of race, ethnicity, and socioeconomic status on sport injury and rehabilitation, the complexity of these social structures goes beyond the scope of this chapter. As such, readers are encouraged to learn about social historical processes that have contributed to theories of racial formation, the differentiation of ethnicity from race, and the influencing experiences of socioeconomic status. What is known from society and medicine in general is that motivations and attitudes toward help-seeking behaviors of diverse racial, ethnic, and socioeconomic backgrounds may be impacted by beliefs, cultural norms, and lifestyles, given their intertwined identity. Given sport is a microcosm of society, it is reasonable to assume that the sport rehabilitation process may also depend on cultural dispositions of athlete with injuries and the professionals they work with. What follows here is a summary of how each of these social forces has been found to influence both help-seeking behaviors and sport injury rehabilitation experience.

Race and Ethnicity

Race and ethnicity have been found to influence help-seeking behaviors and rehabilitation. First, concerns around discriminatory practices by white SPPs and SMPs working with athletes from minoritized racial and ethnic backgrounds have historically been noted. Pain tolerance for Black athletes has been stereotyped and stigmatized (Druckman et al., 2018; Hollingshead et al., 2016), and racial and ethnic minoritized athletes have been underassessed or undertreated (Meghani et al., 2012). Second, environments that marginalize or are perceived to not accommodate the needs of racial and ethnic minoritized individuals may also impact perceptions of the care being provided (Johnson et al., 2004). Third, athletes who have been marginalized may choose not to seek help, as previous experiences of discriminatory practices may induce traumatic feelings and isolation. Research has also found that for some athletes, being seen by SMPs with concordant racial or ethnic backgrounds can be comforting (Zondi & Austin, 2020). It is also known that individuals of racial and ethnic backgrounds are more satisfied when being seen by healthcare providers who resemble them (Saha et al., 1999). Racial concordance has also been found to be associated with better communication (Shen et al., 2018).

Since racism is trauma, it impacts the individual across the affective, physiological, and physical channels (Carter, 2007). As such, when working with injured athletes with racial and ethnic minority backgrounds, SPPs and SMPs must consider the following: Do Black athletes of indigenous African heritage carry a possible perceived stigma on psychosocial support (Jones, 2016) and/or psychosocial care during sport injury rehabilitation, especially in interprofessional (i.e., multi-, inter-, and transdisciplinary) approaches? (For more on professional practice models, see Chapter 7.) Does implicit or explicit racial discrimination in healthcare leave certain athletes more susceptible to injury because of possible racial trauma and racial stress? Anecdotal evidence of the latter can be found in the documentary about Anton Ferdinand (Ross, 2020, November 20), highlighting that his sport performance (and injury) was undeniably impacted by overt racism.

Socioeconomic Status

For domestic and transnational (semi)professional athletes and collegiate student-athletes from low socioeconomic backgrounds who have dependence and reliance on the economic benefits of sport participation, sport injury can have serious implications. The fear of serious injury and/or losing scholarship/meal provision (Castaldelli-Maia et al., 2019) may lead to an athlete masking injury and pain and/or avoiding SMP evaluation. In the case of collegiate student-athletes, loss of scholarship may mean the athlete having to return to their domicile without academic completion due to unaffordable academic fees. This can be associated with failure in sport and academic performance and consequently has the potential to hinder social mobility. The aforementioned is also supported by Spaaij and Ryder (2022), who asserted that white middle-class males from socioeconomically privileged communities benefit more from social mobility opportunities in sport than those from underserved communities. Equally, athletes with limited financial means may lack access to SPP and SMP services. For example, sport environments that do not offer psychology services to their athletes present a barrier for low-socioeconomic-status athletes with limited resources to seek support outside their sporting environment (Brutus & Yousuf, 2019). Given the importance of addressing psychosocial aspects of sport injuries, it is imperative that SPPs, SMPs, and other service providers consider non-burdensome options for the athletes where services within sport are lacking (Brutus & Yousuf, 2019). These could include free community-based injury clinics, though this may risk/sacrifice access to specialized sport and high-performance-focused services.

Transnational Identities

Many athletes participate and compete in sport across national borders for a myriad of reasons, calling for SPPs and SMPs to be attentive to cultural differences. No two transnational athletes are the same; each has their unique intersectional identities. Because of this, SPPs and SMPs are cautioned not to make assumptions about cultural heritage but rather seek to understand if and how the athlete has acculturated and adjusted to the new home culture (D'Arcy, 2009). Despite apparent differences, there are few common factors that may or may not affect athletes' help-seeking behaviors during sport injury. Among non-dominant immigrant cultural groups, seeking mental health help may carry a stigma, resulting in an underutilization of services, dropping out of treatment, and/or waiting until symptoms have become unbearable (Dow, 2011; Sue & Sue, 1999; Tilliman, 2007). Hesitance to seek out support could also be due to fear of risking scholarship status or cultural norms where seeking out support may signify failure, and thus, there is a need to save face (Alegría et al., 2008; Breaux & Ryujin, 1999; Chang & Yoon, 2011; Sue & Sue, 1999; Tilliman, 2007). Many transnational athletes, particularly those with low socioeconomic status, may come from cultures that value collective identities, where athletic engagement and success are linked to family and community success and their ability to give back to them (Brutus & Yousuf, 2019).

Cynicism toward Western conceptualizations of medical treatment, linguistic barriers, an individual's own experiences of misdiagnosis may all influence distrust in the practitioner's ability to understand presenting needs and thus are possible reasons for avoidance of treatment (Dow, 2011). In addition, transnationals of intersectional minoritized identities may also face microaggressions in their rehabilitation environments, given biases held by multiple stakeholders (Lee & Rice, 2007). When protective factors of sport are removed due to injury, these may also compound transnational athletes' feelings of isolation (Lee & Opio, 2011), subsequently impairing both physical and mental rehabilitation during injury.

Culture of Pain

Pain, a common psychophysiological consequence of sport injury, can be heavily influenced by both the culture of sport the athlete participates in and multiple intersecting sociocultural identities of the individual. Pain includes "pain expression, pain language, the cultural meaning of suffering, traditional healers and remedies and social roles, perception and expectation" (Nortjé & Albertyn, 2015, p. 24). The meaning and experience of pain are therefore influenced by culture, and statistically significant differences in how people from different countries hold pain beliefs, appraise pain, cope with pain, and even catastrophize pain responses (Sharma et al., 2020). When injured, athletes may experience varying levels and types of pain. Some athletes, including those from Hispanic/Latino cultures (D'Arcy, 2009), may describe their pain using religious language aimed to provide meaning to the experience while seeking to understand their suffering (Bourke, 2012). Similarly, Christian biblical metaphors, use of different forms of art, spiritual rituals, and symbols have been used to support healing and to describe pain-related distress (Bourke, 2012). Some athletes may relinquish their pain to a higher power, by putting one's faith in God (e.g. in Islam).

In some African cultures, injuries and pain may be attributed to natural causes, witchcraft, and unsettled ancestral spirits, subsequently influencing the ways in which an athlete representing these cultures reacts to pain. Among the Nguni people, pain expressions are communicated through ancestral spirits, who have an active role in the living (Nortjé & Albertyn, 2015). In Sotho culture, pain is considered a form of punishment when ancestral spirits are angered (Nortjé & Albertyn, 2015). Nortjé and Albertyn (2015) also state that for some African cultures, pain experience may be influenced by historical cultural folklore, songs, and poems narrated to its members from youth, resulting in a stoical and resilient approach to dealing with pain and injury. In sub-Saharan Africa, traditional medicine continues to outweigh Western medicine, consequently making it difficult for individuals from said cultures to express and communicate pain and anxiety to Western healthcare professionals (Schlemmer & Marsh, 2006). Since there is a growing number of African athletes living and competing in other parts of the world (e.g., Okpara, 2019), SPPs and SMPs should develop awareness and understanding of how traditional cultural perceptions of pain perceptions influence the athletes they work with.

In Chinese culture, Buddhism, Taoism, and Confucianism are likely to affect an injured athlete's views on pain and injury (D'Arcy, 2009). In Chinese culture, pain is a result of blocked Qi and is resolved by removing the blockage to return to a state of harmony with the universe. Chinese athletes with injuries may also see verbalizing pain as incongruent with spiritual beliefs. Recent research with middle-aged transnational Chinese female table tennis players living in New Zealand (Liu & Pringle, 2020) explored experiences of pain and injuries and found that the athletes were willing to tolerate moderate pain for the benefit of enhancing community solidarity and collective interest. This is in contrast with research conducted in Western cultural contexts, where athletes are more likely to tolerate moderate pain to prove their own individual capability (Liu & Pringle, 2020).

Language can influence pain expressions, as the vocabulary used to describe physical and emotional pain may vary across different national cultures and gender. For example, Irish rugby players who retired from sport due to injury used profanities when discussing their emotions related to injury and rehabilitation (Arvinen-Barrow et al., 2017). In Australia, women have been found to use more words and graphic language to describe their pain and to focus on sensory aspects of pain, while men have been found to use fewer words and less-descriptive language, focusing on the pain event itself and on their emotions (Strong et al., 2009). Equally, research in Finland with patients who speak Swedish as a first and Finnish as a second language found that expressing pain in second language negatively influences communication and assessment related to affective aspects of pain (Mustajoki et al., 2018). This supports the need for SPPs and SMPs to be aware of regional differences in pain expression without assuming homogeneity. For example, assuming all individuals from the Nordic countries experience and express pain in the same way would marginalize these individuals. While cultural differences in pain expressions and pain language exist, it is critical that SPPs and SMPs do not assume that an athlete will respond to pain a certain way because of their cultural belonging. For example, *assuming* that Chinese or African American athletes are stoic with pain tolerance marginalizes their pain experience and omits other information that may be important (e.g., D'Arcy, 2009). Both SPPs and SMPs are also reminded not to impose their cultural worldviews and beliefs on the athlete and their family members and are reminded to treat the individual with best care that fits the pain complaint (D'Arcy, 2009).

Developing Multicultural Competency in Practice

When working with athletes with injuries, the aim for SPPs and SMPs is to provide support through injury rehabilitation, minimizing the risk of re-injury, and cultivating a sense of well-being and belonging. To do this effectively with athletes from diverse backgrounds, it is imperative for the SPPs and the SMPs to look inward and consider how they experience the environment as an ongoing process. Examining multicultural forces affords the SPPs and SMPs an opportunity to better understand the athletes they work with and what may hinder their recovery progression. To develop multicultural competence, SPPs and SMPs are encouraged to engage in specific self-reflective practices, with a goal to develop cultural reflexivity and sensitivity and cultural humility.

Cultural Reflexivity and Sensitivity

Cultural reflexivity and sensitivity refer to the process of self-reflection and exploration of one's own identity and worldview to develop a sense of the self, being more open and responsive to alternative worldviews, cultures, and individualized experiences of clients (Saukko, 2003). Cultural reflexivity and sensitivity are generated by exploring biases, values, social position, privileges, and power (Schinke et al., 2012). The goal of this exploration is to enable a deeper appreciation for different cultures (McGannon et al., 2014; Schinke et al., 2012) in the way individuals communicate and relate to one another. The development of cultural reflexivity and sensitivity requires an authentic willingness to learn about other cultural traditions and characteristics while adapting one's own communication and behavioral approaches in a way that demonstrates sensitivity. Numerous authors have called for SPPs to make a commitment to self-reflexivity, with a goal to dismantle systemic cultures that disempower. Indeed, the field of sport and performance psychology has also seen a revision of ethics codes (e.g., the Association for Applied Sport Psychology, AASP, and the International Society of Sport Psychology, ISSP) to include a required commitment to cultural advocacy.

Cultural Humility

Cultural humility (Tervalon & Murray-Garcıa, 1998) is a dynamic and lifelong process that focuses on self-reflection and personal critique, with a goal to acknowledge one's biases and how one shows up in the world. Gaining cultural humility is a lifelong commitment with no end point, in a constant re-evaluation and recognition of the shifting nature of intersecting and intertwined identities. Cultural humility differs from cultural competence – it is not only about attaining categorical knowledge about different groups of people that can lead to bias and stereotyping. Rather, it requires the SPPs and SMPs to lean in with curiosity to learn from those with whom they work and engage in a dynamic process of lifelong learning. Cultural humility also requires acceptance that one can never be fully competent in understanding the evolving nature of athletes' experiences.

Multicultural Competency in Sport Injury and Rehabilitation

For SPPs and SMPs to demonstrate multicultural competency in sport injury and rehabilitation, it is imperative for practitioners to "meet the athlete where they are" (Brutus & Yousuf, 2019). This means ensuring the athlete has personal agency (that may be culturally informed) in the injury and rehabilitation process and empowering the athlete as the expert in their culture, pain experience, and discomfort. The SPPs and SMPs should also be cognizant of athletes' experiences of possible negative stigmas, stereotypes, micro- and macro-aggressions, and financial, systemic, and environmental barriers that may impede thriving (Brutus & Yousuf, 2019). It is also important to ratify any possible concerns of mistrust, by practicing with cultural humility and centering the athletes' culture to learn from them (Miike, 2012). The aforementioned also aligns with the ethical responsibilities of professional organizations (e.g., AASP, ISSP).

Working from an intersectional lens of multicultural inclusion is complex and nuanced. To practice in a multiculturally competent manner, the SPPs and SMPs must first self-explore and be authentically present and cognizant of their own identity that shapes their worldview. This requires an active understanding of the self, an examination of how one's experiences may provide ease of inclusion or exclusion in certain groups, and how one shows up to others. It is only then one can critically examine disempowering forces, privilege, and power that may be present in professional relationships with injured athletes.

Multiculturally competent practice also necessitates an ability to maintain curiosity and cultural awareness in practice. It requires a concerted effort to consider one's own biases and seek to understand the experiences of the injured athletes. Within sport injury and rehabilitation, it is incumbent upon SPPs and SMPs to refrain from over-pathologizing behavioral symptoms, recognizing the dangers of misdiagnosis, particularly when in the athletes' own culture, such responses may be considered normal stress-responses (Dow, 2011). The SPPs and SMPs must also aim to create a culture and environment of belonging and acceptance and have the ability to acknowledge privilege and power in the professional relationship, with a readiness to relinquish it (Brutus & Yousuf, 2019).

Instead of exploring one's self, some researchers have suggested that SPPs and SMPs may let go of the self and be no one when working with clients. Consistent with Buddhist philosophy, such approach enables presence with the injured athlete while fostering interpersonal mindfulness (Andersen, 2020; Andersen & Ivarsson, 2016), though adopting such approach comes with its own concerns. First, it assumes a cultural philosophy that may not align with the athlete. Second, by letting go of self and becoming no one, the SPP or the SMP is not actively examining their cultural positioning and the cultural contextual forces that exist around them. Instead, SPPs and SMPs should practice multicultural competency by broaching conversations with an integrated, congruent, or infusing style that considers the intersectional and dynamic nature of the athletes' identities (Day-Vines et al., 2007) without reinforcing disempowering stereotypes and assumptions. That way, SPPs and SMPs can be active change agents and advocates, and those who commit to an infusing style of practice go beyond their professional duty, where social justice advocacy is valued personally as a way of life.

Practical Recommendations for Sport Medicine Professionals

In addition to developing multicultural competency through cultural reflexivity, sensitivity, and humility, SPPs and SMPs are also encouraged to promote multicultural acceptance using three main psychosocial strategies: creating inclusive spaces and practices, building trusting relationships, and adopting strength-based approaches with athletes with injuries.

Create Inclusive Spaces and Practices

Creating inclusive spaces and practices means that injured athletes, regardless of their intersecting sociocultural characteristics, have access to physical and psychological spaces that make them feel welcomed, accepted, safe, and comfortable. Facilitative actions for creating inclusive spaces and practices include removing or reducing financial barriers to access rehabilitation services (e.g., access to a psychologist, podiatrist) and continuing other support services (e.g., meal provisions) for low-income athletes (Brutus & Yousuf, 2019). Other facilitative actions include being mindful of possible disparities in access to virtual healthcare spaces utilized during rehabilitation (e.g., smartphone apps) due to physical, financial, or other limitations. It is also important to ensure that face-to-face provisions of care are physically accessible, welcoming to varied gender expressions, and respectful of religious and cultural preferences.

Examples of creating inclusive psychological spaces and practices include honoring athletes' feelings of collective community duty as reason for their need to heal from injury quickly without reducing or disputing their motives (Brutus & Yousuf, 2019) and validating shared experiences of feeling marginalized by practices that do not take account of their needs, without gaslighting or demonstrating fragility in the alliance. It is also beneficial to provide athletes with community resources, where athletes may share their experiences and/or difficulty, while fostering autonomy and independence in their healthcare decisions from a non-restrictive perspective.

Inclusive practices also include ensuring diversity in the sport medicine team. This may include non-medical professionals, such as pastors, religious leaders, folk healers, language teachers and/or interpreters, and those from minoritized backgrounds. Equally, ensuring all intake forms, such as a sport inventory protocol (Taylor et al., 2018), are comprehensive to account for an athlete's identity, values, and beliefs and to avoid possible confusion that may occur due to language barriers. Use of visual pain scales and measurements may also be useful, especially if an athlete comes from a culture where pain management is limited (D'Arcy, 2009).

Build Trusting Relationships

Having a trusting relationship means that athletes, regardless of their intersecting sociocultural characteristics, feel a sense of security with the SPP or SMP they are working with. They also trust that the SPP or SMP will seek to understand their cultural preferences and experiences and help guide the athletes to a resolution by fostering positive feelings of hope and self-esteem. Paramount to creating a trusting relationship is the ability to listen and empower the athlete in their rehabilitation and learn from them. This speaks to cultural humility in building trust, where SPPs and SMPs accept never fully knowing everything about another person's culture. Meeting athletes "where they are," refraining from making assumptions, ensuring they feel heard and seen for their individuality and cultural alignment, while also seeking to build relationships with culture experts to support one's cultural learning, will ultimately build trust and rapport in the relationship.

Adopt a Strength-Based Approach

A strength-based approach to care means that athletes, regardless of their intersecting sociocultural characteristics, feel like the SPP or SMP they are working with is recognizing the benefits of varied personal strengths and social and community networks that support their well-being. A strength-based approach is an individualized approach supporting athletes of intersectional identities, accepting that cultural approaches/mechanisms may not align with their treatment provider (Brutus & Yousuf, 2019). The SPPs and SMPs can and should learn from the athlete what has previously helped them to cope with adversity and challenges. This should lead to encouraging the athlete to draw on cultural capital (Yosso, 2005), as well as positive influences and strengths from their community, family, and life that has enabled a sense of well-being in the past (Brutus & Yousuf, 2019), consequently affirming cultural alliance.

Conclusion

Working from a multicultural paradigm and recognizing that athletes identify with many intersecting identities requires SPPs and SMPs to extend beyond traditional models of support during sport injury. Such an approach necessitates both understanding of the cultural experiences of the athletes and commitment to cultural reflexivity, sensitivity, and humility. The SPPs and SMPs are also encouraged to commit to being active change agents and lifelong learners in understanding biases, dismantling barriers, and providing access to all in a way that supports the athlete's sense of belonging and resilience. By adopting a multicultural paradigm to guide one's work, the relationship between SPPs/SMPs and the athlete is enriched, which can increase adherence and facilitate injury recovery.

Case Study

Assia is a 21-year-old French Algerian female soccer player with a blended family competing at a professional club in the United Kingdom (UK). Assia's mother is of Cameroonian descent, and father of Algerian descent, both based in Algeria. Assia completed her schooling in a faith-based school in Algeria, with enhanced teaching methods for children with speech impediments. Assia is bilingual, fluent in French and Arabic. She has limited command of the English language but has committed to learning with the help of a club-sponsored tutor. Her speech impediment is not apparent when conversing in French but pronounced when attempting to speak English. Assia's friends and family describe her as a warm and sociable individual. Assia moved to the UK when she was 18 on a professional football contract seven months before the COVID-19 SARS pandemic sent the country into lockdown. Assia shares a house with two teammates, both of English heritage, in a town that has only a small ethnic community. She generally gets along well with her teammates but often turns down a night out at a restaurant or club with her teammates. The club provides lunch of high nutrition after training, but the team and staff notice that Assia comes 15 minutes later to the dining area and never eats any meat, as it is not halal. Her housemates have also noticed a small mat that has images of a mosque at the side of her bed and have joked about it being her comfort blanket.

About a month before lockdown, Assia picked up a foot fracture. Her sports medicine team included a strength and conditioning coach, a medical doctor, a physiotherapist, a psychologist, and a player welfare officer. While she appeared to be recovering well, her housemates noticed that Assia was beginning to isolate herself and was sleeping less. As the pandemic brought a halt to training, Assia locked down alone as her housemates went home to their parents. Assia could not get home to hers. The club pivoted to provide all athletes with fitness equipment to support their fitness. Shortly after the beginning of lockdown, the world was left in shock as they witnessed the murder of George Floyd by a police officer. During team meetings over Zoom, Assia would hear her teammates and staff share their opinions, which she felt was dismissive of her experience as a Black Arabic woman. When she tried to speak up about her experiences, she felt ignored, which made her feel angry.

Over time, Assia became increasingly agitated and withdrawn during the Zoom calls. Her sports medicine team members struggled to ascertain her progress in healing and her general health. "I am fine, and no, I am not in pain," Assia would respond when asked about how she was doing. Her sports medicine team gave her a rehabilitation fitness program to adhere to, told her to download a mindfulness application on her phone, and implemented some self-talk interventions. A week later, when her SMP was trying to assess Assia's progress over Zoom, her default response was once again short: "I am fine, and no, I am not in pain." In a sports medicine team meeting later that evening, the SMP provided an update on Assia to the team and described her as aggressive, dismissive, and rude.

Questions

1. What intersecting identities and sociocultural factors are important to consider when working with Assia?
2. What might be some protective factors for Assia during injury rehabilitation?
3. What contextual elements might have explained Assia's stress response to her injury and rehabilitation?
4. What are some of the stereotype threats and microaggressions presented in this case?
5. What personal and sociocultural provisions might the sports medicine team have considered in her support?

References

Addo, I. Y. (2020). Double pandemic: Racial discrimination amid coronavirus disease 2019. *Social Sciences & Humanities Open*, *2*(1), 100074. https://doi.org/10.1016/j.ssaho.2020.100074

Alegría, M., Chatterji, P., Wells, K., Cao, Z., Chen, C., Takeuchi, D., . . . Meng, X. (2008). Disparity in depression treatment among racial and ethnic minority populations in the United States. *Psychiatric Services*, *59*(11), 1264–1272. https://doi.org/10.1176/ps.2008.59.11.1264

American Psychological Association. (2022). *APA dictionary of psychology*. https://dictionary.apa.org/

Andersen, M. B. (2020). Identity and the elusive self: Western and Eastern approaches to being no one. *Journal of Sport Psychology in Action*, *11*(4), 243–253. https://doi.org/10.1080/21520704.2020.1825026

Andersen, M. B., & Ivarsson, A. (2016). A methodology of loving kindness: How interpersonal neurobiology, compassion, and transference can inform researcher-participant encounters and storytelling. *Qualitative Research in Sport, Exercise and Health*, *8*(1), 1–20. https://doi.org/10.1080/2159676X.2015.1056827

Argyle, M., & Beit-Hallahmi, B. (1975). *The social psychology of religion*. Routledge & Kegan Paul.

Arvinen-Barrow, M., Clement, D., Hamson-Utley, J. J., Zakrajsek, R. A., Kamphoff, C. S., Lee, S.-M., . . . Martin, S. B. (2016). Athletes' expectations about sport injury rehabilitation: A cross-cultural study. *Journal of Sport Rehabilitation*, *25*(4), 338–347. https://doi.org/10.1123/jsr.2015-0018

Arvinen-Barrow, M., Clement, D., Hamson-Utley, J. J., Zakrajsek, R. A., Lee, S. M., Kamphoff, C., . . . Martin, S. B. (2015). Athletes' use of mental skills during sport injury rehabilitation. *Journal of Sport Rehabilitation*, *24*(2), 189–197. https://doi.org/10.1123/jsr.2013-0148

Arvinen-Barrow, M., Hurley, D., & Ruiz, M. C. (2017). Transitioning out of professional sport: The psychosocial impact of career-ending injuries among elite Irish rugby football union players. *Journal of Clinical Sport Psychology*, *10*(1). https://doi.org/10.1123/jcsp.2016-0012

Balague, G. (1999). Understanding identity, value, and meaning when working with elite athletes. *The Sport Psychologist*, *13*(1), 89–98. https://doi.org/10.1123/tsp.13.1.89

Bennett, J., & Lindsay, P. (2016). Case Study 3: An acceptance commitment and mindfulness based intervention for a female hockey player experiencing post-injury performance anxiety. *Sport and Exercise Psychology Review*, *12*(2), 36–46.

Beth, A. (2021, April 6). Altering injuries: Loss of scholarship to long-term consequences. *Inside Compliance*. http://blogs.luc.edu/compliance/?p=3873

Bohling, B. C., Luebbert, S., Borwn, A., & Haustein, D. J. (2022). *Sports medicine for special groups*. PM&R Knowledge Now®. Retrieved November 4, 2022, from https://now.aapmr.org/sports-medicine-for-special-groups/

Bourke, J. (2012). Sexual violence, bodily pain, and trauma: A history. *Theory, Culture & Society, 29*(3), 25–51. https://doi.org/10.1177/0263276412439406

Breaux, C., & Ryujin, D. H. (1999). Use of mental health services by ethnically diverse groups within the United States. *Clinical Psychologist, 52*, 4–15.

Bretherton, I., Thrower, E., Zwickl, S., Wong, A., Chetcuti, D., M, G., . . . Cheung, A. S. (2021). The health and well-being of transgender Australians: A national community survey. *LGBT Health, 8*, 42–49. https://doi.org/10.1089/lgbt.2020.0178

Brewer, B. W., & Petitpas, A. J. (2017). Athletic identity foreclosure. *Current Opinion in Psychology, 16*, 118–122. https://doi.org/10.1016/j.copsyc.2017.05.004

Brutus, A., & Yousuf, S. (2019). Meeting student-athletes where they are: Counseling and psychological services for college student-athletes of diverse racial, ethnic, and socioeconomic backgrounds. In M. J. Loughran (Ed.), *Counseling and psychological services for college student-athletes* (pp. 221–244). FIT Publishing.

Buffington, M., & Lai, A. (2011). Resistance and tension in feminist teaching. *Visual Arts Research, 37*(2), 1–13. https://doi.org/10.5406/visuartsrese.37.2.0001

Burke, L. M., & King, C. (2012). Ramadan fasting and the goals of sports nutrition around exercise. *Journal of Sports Sciences, 30*(1), 21–31. https://doi.org/10.1080/02640414.2012.680484

Butryn, T. M. (2002). Critically examining white racial identity and privilege in sport psychology consulting. *The Sport Psychologist, 16*(3), 316–336. https://doi.org/10.1123/tsp.16.3.316

Carter, R. T. (2007). Racism and psychological and emotional injury: Recognizing and assessing race-based traumatic stress. *The Counseling Psychologist, 35*(1), 13–105. https://doi.org/10.1177/0011000006292033

Castaldelli-Maia, J. M., Gallinaro, J. G. D. M., Falcão, R. S., Gouttebarge, V., Hitchcock, M. E., Hainline, B., . . . Stull, T. (2019). Mental health symptoms and disorders in elite athletes: A systematic review on cultural influencers and barriers to athletes seeking treatment. *British Journal of Sports Medicine, 53*(11), 7070–7721. https://doi.org/10.1136/bjsports-2019-100710

Chamari, K., Haddad, M., Wong, D. P., Dellal, A., & Chaouachi, A. (2012). Injury rates in professional soccer players during Ramadan. *Journal of Sports Sciences, 30*(1), 93–102. https://doi.org/10.1080/02640414.2012.696674

Chang, D. F., & Yoon, P. (2011). Ethnic minority clients' perceptions of the significance of race in cross-racial therapy relationships. *Psychotherapy Research, 21*(5), 567–582. https://doi.org/10.1080/10503307.2011.592549

Cicero, E. C., Reisner, S. L., Merwin, E. I., Humphreys, J. C., & Silva, S. G. (2020). The health status of transgender and gender nonbinary adults in the United States. *PLoS One, 15*(2), e0228765. https://doi.org/10.1371/journal.pone.0228765

Clayton, J. (2020). Multiculturalism. In A. Kobayashi (Ed.), *International encyclopedia of human geography* (2nd ed., Vol. 9, pp. 211–219). Elsevier. https://doi.org/10.1016/B978-0-08-102295-5.10296-3

Clement, D., Arvinen-Barrow, M., & LaGuerre, D. (2019). Role of religion and spirituality in sport injury rehabilitation. In B. Hemmings, N. J. Watson, & A. Parker (Eds.), *Sport, psychology and Christianity: Welfare, performance and consultancy*. Routledge.

Clement, D., Hamson-Utley, J. J., Arvinen-Barrow, M., Kamphoff, C., Zakrajsek, R. A., & Martin, S. B. (2012). College athletes' expectations about injury rehabilitation with an athletic trainer. *International Journal of Athletic Therapy & Training, 17*(4), 18–27. https://doi.org/10.1123/ijatt.17.4.18

Collins, P. H. (1998). *Fighting words: Black women and the search for Justice*. University of Minnesota Press.

Collins, P. H. (2005). *Black sexual politics: African-Americans, gender, and new racism*. Routledge.

Crenshaw, K. (1989). Demarginalizing the intersection of race and sex: A Black feminist critique of anti-discrimination doctrine, feminist theory, and antiracist politics. *University of Chicago Legal Forum, 1989*(1). http://chicagounbound.uchicago.edu/uclf/vol1989/iss1/

Cunningham, G. B. (2019). *Diversity and inclusion in sport organizations: A multilevel perspective.* Routledge.

Danylchuk, K., & Grbac, D. (2016). International student-athletes in Canadian interuniversity sport (CIS): Perceptions, motivations, and experiences. *Journal of Intercollegiate Sport, 9*(1), 50–72.

D'Arcy, Y. (2009). The effect of culture on Pain. *Nursing Made Incredibly Easy, 7*(3), 5–7. https://doi.org/10.1097/01.NME.0000350931.12036.c7

David, E. J. R., Okazaki, S., & Giroux, D. (2014). A set of guiding principles to advance multicultural psychology and its major concepts. In F. T. L. Leong, L. Comas-Díaz, G. C. Nagayama Hall, V. C. McLoyd, & J. E. Trimble (Eds.), *APA handbook of multicultural psychology* (Vol. 1, Theory and research, pp. 85–104). American Psychological Association. https://doi.org/10.1037/14189-005

Davis, R. W., & Ferrara, M. S. (1995). Sports medicine and athletes with disabilities. In K. P. DePauw & S. J. Gavron (Eds.), *Disability and sport* (pp. 133–149). Human Kinetics.

Day-Vines, N. L., Wood, S. M., Grothaus, T., Craigen, L., Holman, A., Dotson-Blake, K., & Douglass, M. J. (2007). Broaching the subjects of race, ethnicity, and culture during the counseling process. *Journal of Counseling & Development, 85*(4), 401–409. https://doi.org/10.1002/j.1556-6678.2007.tb00608.x

DeLang, M. D., Salamh, P. A., Chtourou, H., Ben, S. H., & Chamari, K. (2021). The effects of Ramadan Intermittent fasting on football players and implications for domestic football leagues over the next decade: A systematic review. *Sports Medicine (Auckland, NZ), 52*(3), 585–600. https://doi.org/10.1007/s40279-021-01586-8

Dodo, E. O., Lyoka, P. A., Chetty, I. G., & Goon, D. T. (2015). An exploration of the perceptions of spiritual rituals among elite players and coaches associated with religiosity or psychological variables. *African Journal for Physical, Health Education, Recreation and Dance, 21*(1), 103–127.

Dover Wandner, L., Devlin, A. S., & Christler, J. C. (2011). Sports-related pain: Exploring the perception of athletes' pain. *Athletic Insight: Online Journal of Sport Psychology, 3*(1), 41–57.

Dow, H. D. (2011). Migrants mental health perceptions and barriers to receiving mental health services. *Home and Health Care Management & Practice, 23*(3), 176–185. https://doi.org/10.1177/108482231039087

Druckman, J. N., Trawalter, S., Montes, I., Fredendall, A., Kanter, N., & Rubinstein, A. P. (2018). Racial bias in sport medical staff's perceptions of others' pain. *The Journal of Social Psychology, 158*(6), 721–729. https://doi.org/10.1080/00224545.2017.1409188

Eirale, C., Farooq, A., Smiley, F. A., Tol, J. L., & Chalabi, H. (2013). Epidemiology of football injuries in Asia: A prospective study in Qatar. *Journal of Science and Medicine in Sport, 16*(2), 113–117. https://doi.org/10.1016/j.jsams.2012.07.001

Eitzen, D. S., & Sage, G. H. (2009). *Sociology of North American sport* (8th ed.). Paradigm Publishers.

Eubank, M., Ronkainen, N., & Tod, D. (2020). New approaches to identity in sport. *Journal of Sport Psychology in Action, 11*(4), 215–218. https://doi.org/10.1080/21520704.2020.1835134

George, L. K., Ellison, C. G., & Larson, D. B. (2002). Explaining the relationships between religious involvement and health [Article]. *Psychological Inquiry, 13*(3), 190–200. http://search.ebscohost.com/login.aspx?direct=true&db=a9h&AN=8942223&site=ehost-live

Gledhill, A., & Ivarsson, A. (2020). Reducing sports injury risk: Making a case for psychological intervention. *The Sport and Exercise Scientist, 65*, 26–27.

Hammer, C., Podlog, L., & Gledhill, A. (2021). The upside of sports injury and disability: Personal growth following adversity. In A. Gledhill & D. Forsdyke (Eds.), *The psychology of sports injury: From risk to retirement.* Routledge.

Hollingshead, N. A., Meints, S. M., Miller, M. M., Robinson, M. E., & Hirsh, A. T. (2016). A comparison of race-related pain stereotypes held by White and Black individuals. *Journal of Applied Social Psychology, 46*(12), 718–723. https://doi.org/10.1111/jasp.12415

hooks, B. (1981). *Ain't I a woman: Black women and the search for social justice.* Routledge.

Howe, P. D., & Parker, A. (2014). Disability as a path to spiritual enlightenment: An ethnographic account of the significance of religion in Paralympic sport. *Journal of Disability and Religion, 18*(1), 8–23. https://doi.org/10.1080/15228967.2014.868988

Johnson, R., Shah, S., Arbelaez, J., Beach, M., & Cooper, L. (2004). Racial and ethnic differences in patient perceptions of bias and cultural competence in health care. *Journal of General Internal Medicine, 19*, 101–110. https://doi.org/10.1111/j.1525-1497.2004.30262.x

Jones, T.-V. (2016). Predictors of perceptions of mental illness and averseness to help: A survey of elite football players. *Journal of Mental Health*, *25*, 422–427.

Kabat-Zinn, J. (2013). *Full catastrophe living: Using the wisdom of your body and mind to face stress, pain, and illness*. Bantam Books.

Kennedy, J. T. (2021). Belonging: The secret to building engagement for employees of all backgrounds. *Leader to Leader*, *2021*(99), 45–51. https://doi.org/10.1002/ltl.20552

Kirkendall, D. T., Chaouachi, A., Aziz, A. R., & Chamari, K. (2012). Strategies for maintaining fitness and performance during Ramadan. *Journal of Sports Sciences*, *30*(1), 103–110.

Koenig, H. G. (2004). Spirituality, wellness, and quality of life. *Sex, Reproduction and Menopause*, *2*(2), 76–82.

Lee, J., & Opio, T. (2011). Coming to America: Challenges and difficulties faced by African student athletes. *Sport, Education and Society*, *16*(5), 629–644.

Lee, J. J., & Rice, C. (2007). Welcome to America? International student perceptions of discrimination. *Higher Education*, *53*, 381–409. https://doi.org/10.1007/s10734-005-4508-3

Lim, M. S. M., Bowden-Jones, H., Salinas, M., Price, J., Goodwin, G., Geddes, J., & Rogers, R. (2017). The experience of gambling problems in British professional footballers: A preliminary qualitative study. *Addiction Research and Theory*, *25*(2), 129–138. https://doi.org/10.1080/16066359.2016.121 2338

Liu, L., & Pringle, R. (2020). Mid-life Chinese women's understandings of sporting pain and injury: A non-Western cultural analysis via the Confucian concept of 'ren'. *International Review for the Sociology of Sport*. https://doi.org/10.1177/1012690220906389

Maranise, A. M. J. (2013). Superstition and religious ritual: An examination of their effects and utilization in sport. *The Sport Psychologist*, *27*(1), 83–91. https://doi.org/10.1123/tsp.27.1.83

Martin, J. J. (2005). Sport psychology consulting with athletes with disabilities. *Sport and Exercise Psychology Review*, *1*(2), 32–39.

Maughan, R. J., Zerguini, Y., Chalabi, H., & Dvorak, J. (2012). Achieving optimum sports performance during Ramadan: Some practical recommendations. *Journal of Sports Sciences*, *30*(1), 109–117. https://doi.org/10.1080/02640414.2012.696205

McFadden, T. (2022, October 26–29). *Life is like a marathon*. Association for Applied Sport Psychology 37th Annual Conference.

McGannon, K. R., Schinke, R. J., & Busanich, R. (2014). Cultural sport psychology considerations for enhancing cultural competence of practitioners. In L. S. Tashman & J. G. Cremades (Eds.), *Becoming a performance psychology professional: International perspectives on service delivery and supervision* (pp. 135–142). Routledge.

McKay, C. D., Schneider, K. J., Brooks, B. L., Mrazik, M., & Emery, C. A. (2014). Baseline evaluation in youth ice hockey players: Comparing methods for documenting prior concussions and attention or learning disorders. *Journal of Orthopedic & Sports Physical Therapy*, *44*(5), 329–335. https://doi.org/10.2519/jospt.2014.5053

Meghani, S. H., Byun, E., & Gallagher, R. M. (2012). Time to take stock: A meta-analysis and systematic review of analgesic treatment disparities for pain in the United States. *Pain Medicine*, *13*(2), 150–174. https://doi.org/10.1111/j.1526-4637.2011.01310.x

Miike, Y. (2012). "Harmony without uniformity": An Asiacentric worldview and its communicative implications. In L. A. Samovar, R. E. Porter, & E. R. McDaniel (Eds.), *Intercultural communication: A reader* (13th ed., pp. 65–80). Wadsworth Cengage Learning.

Mio, J. S., Barker, L. A., & Domenech, R. M. M. (2016). *Multicultural psychology: Understanding our diverse communities*. Oxford University Press.

Moesch, K., Ivarsson, A., & Johnson, U. (2020). "Be mindful even though it hurts": A single-case study testing the effects of a mindfulness-and-acceptance-based intervention on injured athletes' mental health. *Journal of Clinical Sport Psychology*, *14*(4), 399–421. https://doi.org/10.1123/jcsp.2019-0003

Mohammed, W. A., Pappous, A., & Sharma, D. (2018). Effect of mindfulness based stress reduction (MSBR) in increasing pain tolerance and improving the mental health of injured athletes. *Frontiers in Psychology*, *9*, 722. https://doi.org/10.3389/fpsyg.2018.00722

Moore, E., Wisniewski, A., & Dobs, A. (2021). Endocrine treatment of transsexual people: A review of treatment regimens, outcomes, and adverse effects. *The Journal of Clinical Endocrinology & Metabolism, 88*(8), 3467–3473. https://doi.org/10.1210/jc.2002-021967

Mustajoki, M., Forsén, T., & Kauppila, T. (2018). Pain assessment in native and non-native language: Difficulties in reporting the affective dimensions of pain. *Scandinavian Journal of Pain, 18*(4), 575–580. https://doi.org/10.1515/sjpain-2018-0043

Najah, A., Farooq, A., & Rejeb, R. B. (2017). Role of religious beliefs and practices on the mental health of athletes with anterior cruciate ligament injury. *Advances in Physical Education, 7*(2), 181–190. http://search.ebscohost.com/login.aspx?direct=true&db=lbh&AN=20173270420&site=ehost-live http://file.scirp.org/Html/6-1600345_76299.htm email: amiranejah@yahoo.fr

Nortjé, N., & Albertyn, R. (2015). The cultural language of pain: A South African study. *South African Family Practice, 57*(1), 24–27. https://doi.org/10.1080/20786190.2014.977034

Okpara, C. (2019, May 20). Why African players are dominating European Leagues. *The Guardian*. https://guardian.ng/sport/why-african-players-are-dominating-european-leagues/

O'Reilly, O. C., Day, M. A., Cates, W. T., Baron, J., & Westermann, R. W. (2019). The gender divide: Are female team physicians adequately represented in professional and collegiate athletics? *Orthopedic Journal of Sports Medicine, 7*(7 (Suppl. 5)). https://doi.org/10.1177/2325967119S00402

Parham, W. D. (2005). Raising the bar: Developing an understanding of athletes from racially, culturally, and ethnically diverse backgrounds. In M. B. Andersen (Ed.), *Sport psychology in practice* (pp. 201–215). Human Kinetics.

Pedersen, P. B. (1990). The multicultural perspective as a fourth force in counseling. *Journal of Mental Health Counseling, 12*(1), 93–95.

Pedersen, P. B. (1991). Multiculturism is a generic approach to counseling. *Journal of Counseling Development: Special Issue on Multiculturism as a Fourth Force, 70*(1), 6–12. https://doi.org/10.1002/j.1556-6676.1991.tb01555.x

Pedersen, P. B. (2008). Ethics, competence, and professional issues in cross-cultural counseling. In P. B. Pedersen, J. G. Draguns, & W. L. Lonne (Eds.), *Counseling across cultures* (pp. 5–20). Sage Publishing. https://doi.org/10.4135/9781483329314.n1

Popp, N., Hums, M. A., & Greenwell, T. C. (2009). Do international student-athletes view the purpose of sport differently than United States student-athletes at NCAA Division I universities? *Journal of Issues in Intercollegiate Athletics, 2*, 93–110.

Ronkainen, N. J., Kavoura, A., & Ryba, T. V. (2016). A meta-study of athletic identity research in sport psychology: Current status and future directions. *International Review of Sport and Exercise Psychology, 9*(1), 45–64. https://doi.org/10.1080/1750984X.2015.1096414

Ross, J. (2020, November 20). *Anton Ferdinand: Football, racism and me*. S. Guerra and British Broadcasting Corporation.

Roychowdhury, D., Ronkainen, N., & Guinto, M. L. (2021). The transnational migration of mindfulness: A call for reflective pause in sport and exercise psychology. *Psychology of Sport and Exercise, 56*. https://doi.org/10.1016/j.psychsport.2021.101958

Ryba, T. V. (2017). Cultural sport psychology: A critical review of empirical advances. *Current Opinion in Psychology, 15*, 123–127. https://doi.org/10.1016/j.copsyc.2017.05.003

Saha, S., Komaromy, M., Koepsell, T., & Bindman, A. (1999). Patient-physician racial concordance and perceived quality and use of health care. *Archives of Internal Medicine, 159*, 997–1004. https://doi.org/10.1001/archinte.159.9.997

Sajoo, A. B. (2004). *Muslim ethics: Emerging vistas*. I. B. Tauris.

Saukko, P. (2003). *Doing research in cultural studies*. Sage Publishing.

Schinke, R. J., & Hanrahan, S. J. (Eds.). (2009). *Cultural sport psychology*. Human Kinetics. https://doi.org/10.5040/9781492595366.ch-001.

Schinke, R. J., McGannon, K. R., Parham, W. D., & Lane, A. (2012). Toward cultural praxis: Strategies for self-reflexive sport psychology practice. *Quest, 64*(1), 34–46. https://doi.org/10.1080/00336297.2012.653264

Schlemmer, A., & Marsh, B. (2006). The effects of language barriers in a South African district hospital. *South African Medical Journal – Suid-Afrikaanse Tydskrif Vir Geneeskunde 96*(10), 1084–1087.

Sharma, S., Ferreira-Valente, A., de Williams, A. C., Haxby Abbott, J., Pais-Ribeiro, J., & Jensen, M. P. (2020). Group differences between countries and between languages in pain-related beliefs, coping, and catastrophizing in chronic pain: A systematic review. *Pain Medicine, 21*(9), 1847–1862. https://doi.org/10.1093/pm/pnz373

Shen, M. J., Peterson, E. B., Costas-Muñiz, R., Hernandez, M. H., Jewell, S. T., Matsoukas, K., & Bylund, C. L. (2018). The effects of race and racial concordance on patient-physician communication: A systematic review of the literature. *Journal of Racial and Ethnic Health Disparities, 5*(1), 117–140. https://doi.org/10.1007/s40615-017-0350-4

Spaaij, R., & Ryder, S. (2022). Sport, social mobility, and elite athletes. In W. L. A (Ed.), *The Oxford handbook of sport and society*. Oxford Academic. https://doi.org/10.1093/oxfordhb/9780197519011.013.35

Stambulova, N. B., & Ryba, T. V. (2020). Identity and cultural transition: Lessons to learn from a negative case analysis. *Journal of Sport Psychology in Action, 11*(4), 266–278. https://doi.org/10.1080/2152070 4.2020.1825025

Strong, J., Mathews, T., Sussex, R., New, F., Hoey, S., & Mitchell, G. (2009). Pain language and gender differences when describing a past pain event. *Pain, 145*(1–2), 86–95. https://doi.org/10.1016/j.pain.2009.05.018

Sue, D. W. (1978). World views and counseling. *The Personnel and Guidance Journal, 56*(8), 458–462.

Sue, D. W., Ivey, A. E., & Pedersen, P. B. (1996). *A theory of multicultural counseling and therapy*. Brooks/Cole.

Sue, D. W., & Sue, D. (1999). *Counseling the culturally different: Theory and practice* (5th ed.). John Wiley & Sons.

Taylor, J., Simpson, D., & Brutus, A. L. (2018). Interviewing: Asking the right questions. In J. Taylor (Ed.), *Assessment in applied sport psychology*. Human Kinetics.

Tervalon, M., & Murray-Garcıa, J. (1998). Cultural humility versus cultural competence: A critical distinction in defining physician training outcomes in multicultural education. *Journal of Health Care for the Poor and Underserved, 9*(2), 117–125.

Tilliman, D. G. (2007). *The utilization of counseling by the international student population on U.S. college and university campuses* (Publication Number 106). State University of New York College at Brockport. http://hdl.handle.net/20.500.12648/4582

Truong, L. K., Bekker, S., & Whittaker, J. L. (2021). Removing the training wheels: Embracing the social, contextual and psychological in sports medicine. *British Journal of Sports Medicine, 55*(9), 466–467. https://doi.org/10.1136/bjsports-2020-102679

Vernacchia, R. A., McGuire, R. T., Reardon, J. P., & Templin, D. P. (2000). Psychosocial characteristics of Olympic track and field athletes. *International Journal of Sport Psychology, 31*(1), 5–23.

Walton, C. C., Rice, S., Gao, C. X., Butterworth, M., Clements, M., & Purcell, P. (2021). Gender differences in mental health symptoms and risk factors in Australian elite athletes. *BMJ Open Sport & Exercise Medicine, 7*. https://doi.org/10.1136/bmjsem-2020-000984

Watson, N., & Czech, D. R. (2005). The use of prayer in sport: Implications for sport psychology consulting. *Athletic Insight: Online Journal of Sport Psychology, 7*(4), 26–35.

Weber, S. R., & Pargament, K. I. (2014). The role of religion and spirituality in mental health *Current Opinion in Psychiatry, 27*(5), 358–363. https://doi.org/10.1097/YCO.0000000000000080

Wiese-Bjornstal, D. M. (2019). Christian beliefs and behaviours as health protective, resilience, and intervention factors in the context of sport injuries. In B. Hemmings, N. J. Watson, & A. Parker (Eds.), *Sport psychology and Christianity: Welfare, performance and consultancy* (pp. 54–70). Routledge.

Wiese-Bjornstal, D. M. (2019, November). The integrated model of religiosity and psychological response to the sport injury and rehabilitation process: A Christian illustration. *Canadian Journal for Scholarship and the Christian Faith*. https://cjscf.org/wellness/356-2/

Wiese-Bjornstal, D. M., Smith, A. M., Shaffer, S. M., & Morrey, M. A. (1998). An integrated model of response to sport injury: Psychological and sociological dynamics. *Journal of Applied Sport Psychology, 10*(1), 46–69. https://doi.org/10.1080/10413209808406377

Yosso, T. J. (2005). Whose culture has capital? A critical race theory discussion of community cultural wealth. *Race Ethnicity and Education, 8*(1), 69–91. https://doi.org/10.1080/1361332052000341006

Yousuf, S., & Owens, R. (2023). 'Doing the work': Broaching culture and diversity in sport, exercise and performance psychology consultancy practice – An intersectional consideration for working with stakeholders of marginalised racial and ethnic identities. In V. Shanmuganathan-Felton & S. Smith (Eds.), *Developing a sport psychology consultancy practice: A toolkit for students and trainees* (pp. 176–192). Routledge.

Zondi, P. C., & Austin, A. V. (2020). A question of colour: Systemic racism in sports and exercise medicine. *British Journal of Sports Medicine*. https://doi.org/10.1136/bjsports-2020-103351

Part 3

Psychosocial Strategies in Sport Injury and Rehabilitation

12 Coping with Sport Injury and Rehabilitation

Monna Arvinen-Barrow and Peter Olusoga

Chapter Objectives

- To outline the transactional theory of stress and coping.
- To apply various coping strategies to sport injury and rehabilitation.
- To examine the potential role of religion and spirituality in sport injury rehabilitation.

Introduction

Physiologically, the human body is designed to treat any stressor – including sport injury – as a threat. Instigated by the hypothalamus and known as the "fight-or-flight response," the human body responds to threat(s) by releasing hormones such as adrenaline and cortisol, resulting in a stress response aimed to protect the body from possible harm. The surge of adrenaline will prepare the body for a fight, characterized by increased heart rate, replenished energy supplies, and elevated blood pressure. Cortisol will prepare the body to focus on what is to come by suppressing non-essential bodily systems (e.g., digestive and reproductive systems), increasing glucose in the bloodstream, and activating the brain to use more glucose. Cortisol also activates the body's "natural emergency room" by ensuring it has enough substances available for tissue repair if/when necessary. The fight-or-flight response also communicates with the brain – affecting the individual's thoughts and emotions – particularly fear and numerous other mood states (Walinga, 2014).

When faced with a stressor (a threat), we, as humans, are also likely to initiate cognitive and behavioral efforts, with a goal to *cope* with the stressor and its effects (Brewer & Redmond, 2017; Walinga, 2014). *Coping* is a process where an individual attempts to change and/or avoid the situation they encounter or their emotional responses (or both). It is defined as "constantly changing cognitive and behavioral efforts to manage specific external and/or internal demands that are appraised as taxing or exceeding the resources of the person" (Lazarus & Folkman, 1984, p. 141). This process-orientated definition of *coping* also reflects the fact that coping strategies often change during the stressful episode, and several coping strategies might be employed either individually or all at once, based on an individual's dynamic perception of their likely success. The definition also distinguishes coping as separate from psychosocial strategies – which are typically implemented and used by professionals working *with* the athlete, rather than instigated by the athlete. Cox (2012) states that psychosocial strategies can become coping skills if the athlete is able to "personalize and claim ownership" (p. 214) of the taught intervention and to "integrate them into their own repertoire of psychological skills" (p. 214).

DOI: 10.4324/9781003295709-15

Existing research with sports medicine professionals (SMPs) has identified key factors that distinguish athletes who cope successfully with their injuries from those who do not. In general, these include (a) ability to maintain positive attitude, (b) ability to manage maladaptive emotional responses, and (c) ability to comply with/adhere to the rehabilitation protocol (Arvinen-Barrow et al., 2007; Clement et al., 2013; Heaney, 2006; Larson et al., 1996). With a goal to facilitate successful coping, many athletes are using personal coping skills that may have a deep personal and/or sociocultural history or meaning for them (for multicultural understanding, see Chapter 11 for more details). For example, previously injured athletes have used profanity when expressing their emotions while transitioning out of sport due to injury (Arvinen-Barrow et al., 2017) and reported turning to religious practices when injured (Arvinen-Barrow et al., 2015; Gould et al., 1997). The purpose of this chapter is to present selected coping strategies athletes are likely to use in their efforts to manage stressors related to sport injury. More specifically, this chapter will (a) outline the transactional theory of stress and coping (Lazarus & Folkman, 1984), (b) introduce selected coping strategies (i.e., humor, profanity, metaphor, and storytelling) that can have a stress-moderating effects during sport injury, (c) discuss the potential role of religion and spirituality in sport injury rehabilitation, and (d) highlight critical factors for successful coping with sport injury.

Transactional Theory of Stress and Coping

Early research exploring stress and coping in sport was clouded by inconsistent definitions of the key concepts involved. Previously, stress has been conceptualized as an environmental demand or stimulus, a response to an environmental demand, and as an interaction between the person and the environment (Olusoga & Thelwell, 2016). To address this apparent lack of conceptual precision, a framework of stress based on Lazarus's transactional theory of stress and coping (Lazarus & Folkman, 1984) proposes that individuals experience stress as a consequence of an evaluation of the situation the person is in. The *transaction* refers to the dynamic relationship between environmental demands (*i.e., stressors*) and an individual's psychological resources for dealing with them (*i.e., coping ability*). Stress responses (i.e., strain) result from a perceived imbalance between these demands and resources. Rather than conceptualizing stress as being a specific property of either the individual or the environment, it is the *meaning* constructed by an individual about their relationship with the stressor/environment (i.e., "relational meaning") that is pivotal in their experience of stress. Put simply, *stress* is a process of weighing up our demands against our perceptions of how well we think we can cope.

According to the transactional theory of stress and coping, this evaluative process of ascribing meaning to the person-environment relationship is known as appraising, and there are two main types. *Primary appraising* represents evaluation of whether a particular encounter represents a threat (i.e., potentially damaging to goal commitments, values, or beliefs), challenge (i.e., a potential obstacle toward goal commitments, values, or beliefs), or harm/loss (i.e., a perception that damage to goal commitments, values, or beliefs has already occurred).[1] If primary appraising is concerned with evaluating what *is* happening, *secondary appraising* involves an evaluation of what can be done. Secondary appraising involves an evaluation of coping resources, how likely coping strategies are to be effective, and whether they can be applied in a given situation.[2]

Although appraising is often the cognitive underpinning for coping, Lazarus (2006) suggested that "it is not inappropriate to refer to it as coping as well" (p. 76). Cognitive appraisals result in emotional and behavioral responses, along with the selection of appropriate (or perhaps inappropriate) coping responses. If the appraisal of the transaction results in a strain – that is, an imbalance between stressors and coping resources is perceived – the resultant outcome of the strain is dependent on how successful or effective the selected coping strategies are. It is vital, therefore, to understand the importance of coping as an integral part of how an individual navigates the stress process.

Coping Strategies

Many athletes enter the rehabilitation environment with a myriad of personal, psychological, and sociocultural factors that can either facilitate or impede successful coping with sport injury. It is also common for athletes to rely on various internalized coping strategies that bear strong personal and cultural significance. What follows is an introduction of selected coping strategies (i.e., humor, profanity, metaphors, and storytelling) that can have stress-moderating effects during sport injury and rehabilitation. Please note this list is not exhaustive but rather a reflection of strategies that have a centuries-long history in healing and healthcare.

Humor

Defined as "the capacity to perceive or express the amusing aspects of a situation" (American Psychological Association, 2022), theoretical understanding of how humor works dates back to Ancient Greece to Plato's superiority theory (i.e., putting oneself above others with humiliating putdowns) and Aristotle's play theory (i.e., playing with words or objects; Kerulis, 2020, March 23). In the 18th century, humor has been conceptualized through Freud's relief theory (i.e., humor is a mechanism to release pressures that build up in the mind) and the incongruity theory (i.e., humor comes from two things that do not fit together, making it humorous; Kerulis, 2020, March 23).

It is "likely that humor is as old as healing. Hippocrates, for instance, advised his patients to 'contemplate on comic things' to facilitate recovery" (Francia et al., 2015, cited in Piemonte & Abreu, 2020, p. 608). According to Kuiper and Martin (1998), "the stress-moderating effects of humor appear to operate, at least in part, through more positive appraisals and more realistic cognitive processing of environmental information" (p. 162). This supports the conceptualizations proposed in the transactional theory of stress and coping (Lazarus & Folkman, 1984). Thus far, published research into the role of humor in sport injury contexts is non-existent. Research findings from non-sport injury settings seem to suggest that humor (and laughter) can have therapeutic effects on anxiety, reduce stress and muscle tension, help control pain and discomfort, and facilitate positive mood states and overall psychological health (Abel, 2002). Humor has also been a welcome addition to the patient–healthcare provider relationship (McCabe, 2004; Scholl & Ragan, 2003) as it can release interpersonal tensions, facilitate relationships, alleviate power imbalances, and help athletes articulate their true feelings and thoughts when discussing difficult topics (Beach & Prickett, 2017; McCabe, 2004; Scholl & Ragan, 2003). While humor is not something that is prescribed as treatment, healthcare professionals (Scholl & Ragan, 2003) and sport psychology professionals (SPPs) have reported using humor in their practice for varied reasons, such as facilitating the therapeutic alliance (Pack et al., 2019, 2020).

Profanity

A unique feature of humans is the ability to use language to convey messages and meanings to others. Dating back to ancient Sanskrit, humans have assigned meaning to different patterns of sound. According to Bergen (2016), "over the last twenty-six centuries, language scholars have focused on the sanitized and saccharine type of language" (p. 3) and willfully ignored the bad types – namely, profanity. Profanity (i.e., vulgar, blasphemous, or obscene language or behavior) is generally inspired by taboo-ridden domains, such as bodily functions, sex, religion, and derogatory terms used to describe other groups of people (Steinmetz, 2016, December 15). Use of profanity violates moral foundations of purity (Sylwester & Purver, 2015), and the use of profanity is also likely to elicit unconscious biases about individuals who use it (DeFrank & Kahlbaugh, 2019). Using profanity can also be interpreted as inappropriate, antisocial, or abusive, particularly when used with an intent to belittle, hurt, or harm another person (Ashwindren et al., 2018).

Profanity, much like language in general, is an integral part of human communication. Consistent with the transactional theory of stress and coping (Lazarus & Folkman, 1984), profanity can serve as a powerful way to ascribe meaning to the person–environment relationship. Using profanity affords the expression of our experiences, intentions, and desires to be conveyed to those around us (Bergen, 2012) in an authentic and instantaneous manner (McGreal, 2017, March 24). A single curse word can convey powerful messages on how an individual appraises and emotionally responds to their stressful situation, including the strongest human emotions of anger, fear, sadness, and passion (Bergen, 2016; Jay & Janschewitz, 2008). Using profanity can also increase heart and respiratory rate, elevate body temperature, and change attentional focus. To put it simply, "bad words are powerful – emotionally, physiologically, psychologically, and socially" (Bergen, 2016, p. 1).

A sport injury research with Irish Rugby Football Union players who had experienced a career-ending injury found the use of profanity to be common when speaking about "emotions related to the injury, rehabilitation and recovery, and the factors hindering the process" (Arvinen-Barrow et al., 2017, p. 67). Using profanity can also have a cathartic effect on stress and pain (Vingerhoets et al., 2013). Research with university students has found that swearing can increase cold pressor pain tolerance and heart rate and decrease perceived pain when compared to not swearing (Stephens et al., 2009). However, benefits of swearing on pain tolerance will be lower among individuals who swear frequently in daily life when compared to non-habitual swearing (Stephens & Umland, 2011), providing further evidence for the relationship between profanity use and emotional responses to stressors such as pain.

Metaphor

Defined as a "figure of speech in which a word or phrase is applied to an object, person, or action that it does not literally denote for the purpose of creating a forceful analogy" (American Psychological Association, 2022), *metaphor(s)* have potential to offer a way to express abstract experiences in concrete terms (Lakoff & Johnson, 1980). Consistent with the transactional theory of stress and coping (Lazarus & Folkman, 1984), metaphor(s) can help assign meaning to a stressful situation, particularly when an individual is struggling to find words to describe difficult sensations, thoughts, and feelings. Metaphors can also be more than figurative expression – a plethora of research has demonstrated the value of metaphors as a tool for facilitating deeper understanding of concepts and new perspectives, as well as a vehicle for changing attitudes. In healthcare, metaphors are used as an educational tool to (a) explain medical terminology, (b) simplify mechanisms of pathogenesis, or (c) promote behavioral change (Steen, 2008).

Using metaphor(s) in injury rehabilitation is not novel. According to Stewart (2015), "communication about a patient's pain experience is a fundamental component of rehabilitation, but often requires the use of metaphoric expressions" (p. 10). Both common and self-generated metaphors of pain can be helpful in describing the sensory experience of pain (e.g., stabbing pain), the affective experience of pain (e.g., "I feel like a truck ran over me"), and the impact of pain on daily life (e.g., pain is like a strict parent with unreasonable curfew; Munday et al.,

2020; Stewart, 2015). In sport injury rehabilitation specifically, using metaphors is also not a new concept (Smith & Sparkes, 2004). A quarter century ago, Heil et al. (1998) proposed using a "patient-athlete metaphor" as a way to identifying psychological roles for all members of the injury rehabilitation team. Using a case study with a recreational athlete with chronic pain, Heil et al. demonstrated how a "patient-athlete metaphor" would highlight the central role of the athlete as the key player in the "game of rehabilitation" (p. 25) and subsequently fosters a sense of independence and control.

Storytelling

Defined as "an interactive act of using written, oral, electronic, or visual means of communication to tell a story in an effort to enable understanding of self or a situation" (Arvinen-Barrow et al., 2020, p. 209), *telling stories* has been, and continues to be, an integral part of human history. Stories are authentic experiences (Rutledge, 2011, January 16) and can take different forms – written, oral, and visual – and serve to provide a medium for organizing thoughts in a meaningful way, making sense of an experience, and expressing ourselves to the world (Scaletti & Hocking, 2010; Ward, 2007). Storytelling is also deeply rooted in our neural pathways – stories are stored and regulated by the amygdala, "the part of the brain that plays a central role in social interaction, communication, and emotion recognition" (Arvinen-Barrow et al., 2020, p. 211). A well-constructed story, and the process of storytelling, also affords the emergence of a myriad of emotions "ranging from anger, sadness, and anxiety to feelings of joy, excitement, and relief" (Arvinen-Barrow et al., 2020, p. 211). Thus, it is no surprise that the human brain prefers a story to scientific facts (McCann et al., 2019).

Consistent with the transactional theory of stress and coping (Lazarus & Folkman, 1984), storytelling can also be a creative way for an athlete to cognitively appraise and make sense of their sport injury experience. While empirical investigations into the role of storytelling in sport injury are few, using narratives and storytelling in sport injury and illness contexts is not new (Brock & Kleiber, 1994; Hyysalo, 2016; Newman et al., 2016; Roy et al., 2015; Smith & Sparkes, 2002, 2005). Indeed, sport as a cultural domain has a long history of incorporating stories into their communities (Davis, 2012), with a goal to convey motivational messages of "triumph over obstacles" and demonstrate the value of perseverance and hard work, to name a few. For more details on storytelling in sport injury, see Arvinen-Barrow et al. (2020).

Religion and Spirituality

Given that approximately three-quarters of the world's population regard religion[3] as an important aspect of life (Maoz, 2013), along with spirituality,[4] it can be an important coping strategy when faced with stressors (Peres et al., 2007). While researchers and applied practitioners have called for culturally sensitive (see Chapter 11) and holistic approaches (see Chapter 7) to injury management (Brewer & Redmond, 2017; Roy et al., 2015), much of healthcare has failed to consider the role of religion and spirituality in the process (Ledger, 2005). Considering existing sport injury risk (see Chapter 2) and psychosocial response models (see Chapters 3–6), the role of religion and spirituality in sport injury rehabilitation is multifaceted (for integrated model of religiosity and psychological response to the sport injury and rehabilitation process, see Wiese-Bjornstal, 2019, November). First, religion and spirituality can form part of an individual's psychological core, associated with stable personality variables such as attitudes, beliefs, and values (Clement et al., 2019). Second, it is also feasible to assume that religion and spirituality will also function as a coping strategy (Wiese-Bjornstal, 2019, 2019, November;

Wiese-Bjornstal et al., 1998), thus consistent with the transactional theory of stress and coping (Lazarus & Folkman, 1984):

> Religion as a system of beliefs in divine or superhuman power, and practices of prayer during injury occurrence, rehabilitation, and return to sport can provide an injured athlete a way of emotional coping including, but not limited to: reduction in the fear of unknown, tension, anger, depression, grief, and enable feelings of hopefulness and positivity during the process.
>
> (Clement et al., 2019, p. 73)

While sport sociology has long highlighted the significant role of religion and spirituality in athletes' lives (Coakley, 2009), sport psychology has only recently gained interest in understanding its relevance to athlete performance and well-being (Hemmings et al., 2019; Roychowdhury, 2019). Existing (albeit limited) research on religion, spirituality, and coping during sport injury has found that some athletes use religion and spirituality as an injury prevention strategy (Dodo et al., 2015) as well as a coping strategy with injury-related stressors (Arvinen-Barrow et al., 2015; Najah et al., 2017). Recent research with adult athletes affiliated with diverse Christian denominations found that "religious ways of coping" were predominantly positive, and that religious coping sources were used concurrently with non-religious coping strategies (Wiese-Bjornstal et al., 2022; see also Chapter 11).

Critical Success Factors

While the aforementioned strategies can be beneficial for coping with injury, pain, and rehabilitation, it is important to recognize that each can also negatively affect the coping process. In short, not everyone is comfortable with or finds value in using humor, profanity, metaphor(s), or storytelling in rehabilitation. Equally, for some, integrating religion or spirituality into rehabilitation can feel inappropriate or uncomfortable, depending on their personal beliefs and views. Before advocating for any of the previously mentioned strategies to athletes with injuries, it is imperative for the SPP, SMP, or SP to engage in reflective practice to ensure appropriateness of the approach. In no particular order, these are (a) athlete-centered approach, (b) cultural considerations, (c) professional relationship, (d) ethical considerations, (e) practitioner self-assessment, and (f) purposeful implementation.

Athlete-Centered Approach

Existing theoretical and empirical evidence suggests that adopting an athlete-centered approach to sport injury rehabilitation is likely to result in the best physical and psychosocial recovery outcomes (see Chapter 7). Consistent with this approach, it is imperative for SPPs, SMPs, and SPs to guide and encourage the athlete toward coping strategies that create the right conditions for a facilitative rehabilitation environment that fosters athlete's physical, psychological, spiritual, and social well-being.

Cultural Considerations

All athletes with injuries enter the rehabilitation process with multiple intersecting cultural identities (see Chapter 11) that will influence and are influenced by interpersonal interactions with various stakeholders. To ensure culturally competent care, SPPs, SMPs, and SPs should look inward and engage in self-reflective practices to develop their own cultural reflectivity and sensitivity and cultural humility.

Ethical Considerations

While nuanced variation in codes of ethics exists between different professions, the principle of nonmaleficence, that is, do no harm, is a priority for all (see Chapter 8). It is imperative for SPPs, SMPs, and SPs to practice ethically competent care and reflect on the appropriateness of using and advocating various coping strategies to the athletes they work with.

Practitioner Self-Assessment

Reflective practice includes continued self-assessment of one's own strengths and areas in need of improvement as a healthcare professional. Assessing one's own attitudes, biases, and skills should be an ongoing process for SPPs, SMPs, and SPs.

Professional Relationship

At the core of successful rehabilitation is a trusting and supportive working relationship between the injured athlete and the professional(s) working with them. Depending on the athlete, some of the coping strategies discussed in this chapter may have a negative impact on the professional relationship – especially when the strategies used create an incongruence with personal attitudes, beliefs, and values, for the athlete or the professional working with the athlete. For example, use of callous humor with athletes can undermine their trust in medicine (Piemonte & Abreu, 2020), and use of profanity has been found to decrease perceptions of trustworthiness, intelligence, and likability (DeFrank & Kahlbaugh, 2019), all of which are key ingredients for a good professional relationship. Linguistic differences can also create incongruence in using metaphors (Stewart, 2015), particularly when using war metaphors (e.g., painkiller, battle with injury, defense force) to describe the injury, consequences, or rehabilitation treatments. Depending on one's cultural background, references to war can be triggering, particularly for those who have been affected by war. Storytelling can also be personally, generationally, and/or socioculturally dependent. Incongruent use of stories can result in misalignment with the intended meaning and interpretation of the meaning, subsequently affecting the professional relationship between the athlete and the professional. In a similar way, reference to religious scriptures with athletes who do not share the professional's faith can also be detrimental to the professional relationship.

Purposeful Implementation

Just like psychosocial strategies, encouraging the use of coping strategies should be purposeful and appropriately timed. Professionals such as SPPs, SMPs, and SPs should be aware of the appropriateness of selected coping strategies at different stages of rehabilitation (Kamphoff et al., 2013), taking into account numerous personal, situational, and cultural factors (Clement et al., 2019).

Conclusion

Limited research has examined the use and benefits of using humor, profanity, metaphor(s), storytelling, religion, and spirituality as coping strategies during sport injury. Consistent with the transactional theory of stress and coping (Lazarus & Folkman, 1984), all the coping strategies discussed in this chapter have the potential to facilitate positive cognitive, emotional, and behavioral coping. All the strategies have the potential to help injured athletes by (a) alleviating pain, (b) moderating the stress response, and (c) providing additional ways to construct meaning to their injury experience. The chapter also emphasizes the importance of recognizing the potential negative effects of the presented strategies by highlighting critical success factors for SPPs, SMPs, and SPs to consider.

Case Study

Uloko is a 38-year-old Cirque du Soleil trapeze artist. Originally from Benin, Uloko has been touring with the Cirque for almost 20 years. Nine months ago, Uloko requested a transfer to Las Vegas, with a plan to perform for 2 more years as part of the Michael Jackson ONE show before officially retiring. While Uloko has settled well into his new life in Las Vegas, over the past six months, he has become increasingly uneasy with the religious community he has been associating himself with: "I think I am in a middle of a personal quest to re-identify myself. It is like I am revisiting and questioning my own personal values. For so many years, I have been 'on the go' and never really stopping to think and reflect."

Two months ago, Uloko fell from the trapeze during rehearsal. What looked like a harmless fall ended up having devastating consequences. A visit to the orthopedic hospital revealed a stress fracture in his right tibia and several smaller stress fractures in his fibula and femur. Routine blood work also revealed that Uloko had an untreated diabetes, which, after the fall, had exacerbated poor circulation and neuropathy – both of which Uloko had been ignoring for years – resulting in an emergency amputation of his right leg below the knee. "I have no idea how I could be so stupid. Ignoring all signs . . . I mean, I have had a blurry vision from time to time, heart rate that never seems to go down, and let's face it, I have felt the spikes in my blood sugar. But how can I be so stupid not to get myself checked?" Uloko tells his brother, who lives in Montreal, Canada, over a videocall from the hospital after the surgery.

Last night, after he had spoken to his sister who lives in London, United Kingdom, the reality of his situation hit home, hard. "I am feeling increasingly lost. I am not sure where I belong, and what am I going to do? It's not like I can just go and live with my siblings. I cannot perform anymore either. This is not a Cirque that wants freaks like me," Uloko explains to his roommate while making dance moves with his arms, and starts singing, "Don't you wish your girlfriend was freak like me . . ."

After a moment of silence, Uloko continues, saying, "Honestly, I am not even sure if I can stay in Las Vegas either . . . my visa is based on employment. But . . . where would I go? Where is home? I honestly don't know." Tears fall down his face. "Being a one-legged nomad sucks," Uloko says with a sigh.

Questions

1. Consistent with the process-oriented definition of *coping*, how would you summarize Uloko's cognitive and behavioral efforts to manage the demands of the situation?

2. What personal and sociocultural factors are likely to influence the dynamic relationship between environmental demands (i.e., *stressors*) and an individual's psychological resources for dealing with them (i.e., *coping ability*)?
3. What coping strategies outlined in this chapter may/may not be appropriate for Uloko, and why?
4. In Uloko's case, what critical success factors are important to consider in order to facilitate successful coping?

Acknowledgment

The authors would like to thank 2022 AASP CE workshop facilitators (Dr. Erin Haugen, Dr. Angel Brutus, and Kathryn Lang) and the workshop participants for their role in inspiring and conceptualizing the fictional case study used in this chapter.

Notes

1 Lazarus and Folkman (1984) point out that these stress appraisals are not mutually exclusive and can occur simultaneously. For example, harm is fused with threat because with every loss/harm comes possible negative implications for the future. Threat and challenge appraisals are not opposite ends of the same continuum and often occur simultaneously. Challenge and threat emotions can occur at the same time in stressful encounters.
2 Primary and secondary appraising are somewhat misleading terms, as primary appraising is neither more important than nor precedes, temporally, secondary appraising.
3 Defined as a "system of beliefs in divine or superhuman power, and practices of worship or other rituals directed toward such power" (Argyle, M., & Beit-Hallahmi, B., 1975). *The social psychology of religion*. Routledge & Kegan Paul.
4 Defined as an "existential aspect of their religious lives, for example, the practice of prayer throughout the day (outside a Church environment) and witness through the actions of every dimension of their lives, including sport (e.g., Romans 12: 1)" (Watson, N., & Czech, D. R., 2005, April). The use of prayer in sport: Implications for sport psychology consulting. *Athletic Insight: The Online Journal of Sport Psychology*, *17*, 4.

References

Abel, M. H. (2002). Humor, stress, and coping strategies. *HUMOR International Journal of Humor Research*, *15*(4), 365–381. https://doi.org/10.1515/humr.15.4.365
American Psychological Association. (2022). *APA dictionary of psychology*. https://dictionary.apa.org/
Argyle, M., & Beit-Hallahmi, B. (1975). *The social psychology of religion*. Routledge & Kegan Paul.
Arvinen-Barrow, M., Clement, D., Hamson-Utley, J. J., Zakrajsek, R. A., Lee, S. M., Kamphoff, C., . . . Martin, S. B. (2015). Athletes' use of mental skills during sport injury rehabilitation. *Journal of Sport Rehabilitation*, *24*(2), 189–197. https://doi.org/10.1123/jsr.2013-0148
Arvinen-Barrow, M., Clement, D., & Hemmings, B. (2020). "This is the final jump," I respond. Why, why do I utter those words? Using storytelling in sport injury rehabilitation. In W. Ross (Ed.), *Sport injury psychology: Cultural, relational, methodological, and applied considerations* (pp. 207–216). Routledge. https://doi.org/10.4324/9780367854997
Arvinen-Barrow, M., Hemmings, B., Weigand, D. A., Becker, C. A., & Booth, L. (2007). Views of chartered physiotherapists on the psychological content of their practice: A national follow-up survey in the United Kingdom. *Journal of Sport Rehabilitation*, *16*(2), 111–121. https://doi.org/10.1123/jsr.16.2.111

Arvinen-Barrow, M., Hurley, D., & Ruiz, M. C. (2017). Transitioning out of professional sport: The psychosocial impact of career-ending injuries among elite Irish rugby football union players. *Journal of Clinical Sport Psychology*, *10*(1). https://doi.org/10.1123/jcsp.2016-0012

Ashwindren, S., Shankar, V., & Zarei, N. (2018). Selected theories on the use of profanity. *International Journal of Academic Research in Business and Social Sciences*, *8*(9), 1975–1982. https://doi.org/10.6007/IJARBSS/v8-i9/4876

Beach, W. A., & Prickett, E. (2017). Laughter, humor, and cancer: Delicate moments and poignant interactional circumstances. *Health Communication*, *32*(7), 791–802. https://doi.org/10.1080/10410236.2016.1172291

Bergen, B. K. (2012). *Louder than words: The new science of how the mind makes meaning*. Basic Books.

Bergen, B. K. (2016). *What the F: What swearing reveals about our language, our brains, and ourselves*. Basic Books.

Brewer, B. W., & Redmond, C. J. (2017). *Psychology of sport injury*. Human Kinetics.

Brock, S. C., & Kleiber, D. A. (1994). Narrative in medicine: The stories of elite college athletes' career-ending injuries. *Qualitative Health Research*, *4*, 411–430.

Clement, D., Arvinen-Barrow, M., & LaGuerre, D. (2019). Role of religion and spirituality in sport injury rehabilitation. In B. Hemmings, N. J. Watson, & A. Parker (Eds.), *Sport, psychology and Christianity: Welfare, performance and consultancy*. Routledge.

Clement, D., Granquist, M., & Arvinen-Barrow, M. (2013). Psychosocial aspects of athletic injuries as perceived by athletic trainers. *Journal of Athletic Training*, *48*(4), 512–521. https://doi.org/10.4085/1062-6050-48.3.21

Coakley, J. J. (2009). *Sport in society* (10th ed.). Irwin McGraw-Hill.

Cox, R. H. (2012). *Sport psychology: Concepts and applications* (6th ed.). McGraw-Hill.

Davis, J. A. (2012). *The Olympic Games effect: How sports marketing builds strong brands*. John Wiley & Sons.

DeFrank, M., & Kahlbaugh, P. (2019). Language choice matters: When profanity affects how people are judged. *Journal of Language and Social Psychology*, *38*(1), 126–141. https://doi.org/10.1177/0261927X18758143

Dodo, E. O., Lyoka, P. A., Chetty, I. G., & Goon, D. T. (2015). An exploration of the perceptions of spiritual rituals among elite players and coaches associated with religiosity or psychological variables. *African Journal for Physical, Health Education, Recreation and Dance*, *21*(1), 103–127.

Gould, D., Udry, E., Bridges, D., & Beck, L. (1997). Coping with season-ending injuries. *The Sport Psychologist*, *11*(4), 379–399. https://doi.org/10.1123/tsp.11.4.379

Heaney, C. (2006). Physiotherapists' perceptions of sport psychology intervention in professional soccer. *International Journal of Sport and Exercise Psychology*, *4*(1), 73–86. https://doi.org/10.1080/1612197X.2006.9671785

Heil, J., Wakefield, C., & Reed, C. (1998). Patient as athlete: A metaphor for injury rehabilitation. *The Psychotherapy Patient*, *10*(3), 21–39. https://doi.org/10.1300/J358v10n03_03

Hemmings, B., Watson, N. J., & Parker, A. (Eds.). (2019). *Sport, psychology and Christianity: Welfare, performance and consultancy*. Routledge.

Hyysalo, P. (2016). *FightBack: Toinen mahdollisuus [FightBack: Second chance)* Tammi Publishers.

Jay, T., & Janschewitz, K. (2008). The pragmatics of swearing. *Journal of Politeness Research: Language, Behaviour, Culture*, *4*(2), 267–288. https://doi.org/10.1515/JPLR.2008.013

Kamphoff, C., Thomae, J., & Hamson-Utley, J. J. (2013). Integrating the psychological and physiological aspects of sport injury rehabilitation: Rehabilitation profiling and phases of rehabilitation. In M. Arvinen-Barrow & N. Walker (Eds.), *Psychology of sport injury and rehabilitation* (pp. 134–155). Routledge.

Kerulis, M. (2020, March 23). *Why do people laugh during a crisis? The role of humor part two: Examining the role of laughter during difficult times*. www.psychologytoday.com/us/blog/sporting-moments/202003/why-do-people-laugh-during-crisis-the-role-humor#:~:text=We%20have%20established%20that%20our%20current%20health%20crisis,bonds%2C%20which%20are%20vital%20during%20these%20tough%20times.

Kuiper, N. A., & Martin, R. A. (1998). Is sense of humor a positive personality characteristic? In W. Ruch (Ed.), *The sense of Humor: Explorations of a personality characteristic*. De Gruyter.

Lakoff, G., & Johnson, M. (1980). *Metaphors we live by*. The University of Chicago Press.

Larson, G. A., Starkey, C., & Zaichkowsky, L. D. (1996). Psychological aspects of athletic injuries as perceived by athletic trainers. *The Sport Psychologist*, *10*(1), 37–47. https://doi.org/10.1123/tsp.10.1.37

Lazarus, R. S. (2006). *Stress and emotion: A new synthesis*. Springer Publishing Company.

Lazarus, R. S., & Folkman, S. (1984). *Stress, appraisal, and coping*. Springer.

Ledger, S. D. (2005). The duty of nurses to meet patients' spiritual and/or religious needs [Article]. *British Journal of Nursing*, *14*(4), 220–225. http://search.ebscohost.com/login.aspx?direct=true&db=a9h&AN=16521546&site=eds-live

Maoz. (2013). The world religion dataset, 19452010: Logic, estimates, and trends. *International Interactions*, *39*(3), 265–291.

McCabe, C. (2004). Nurse-patient communication: An exploration of patients' experiences. *Journal of Clinical Nursing*, *13*(1), 41–49. https://doi.org/10.1111/j.1365-2702.2004.00817.x

McCann, S., Barto, J., & Goldman, N. (2019). Learning through story listening. *American Journal of Health Promotion*, *33*(3), 477–481. https://doi.org/10.1177/0890117119825525e

McGreal, S. A. (2017, March 24). Is using profanity a sign of honesty? Claims that swearing is a sign of honesty are highly questionable. *Psychology Today*. www.psychologytoday.com/us/blog/unique-everybody-else/201703/is-using-profanity-sign-honesty

Munday, I., Newton-John, T., & Kneebone, I. (2020). 'Barbed wire wrapped around my feet': Metaphor use in chronic pain. *British Journal of Health Psychology*, *25*(3), 814–830. https://doi.org/10.1111/bjhp.12432

Najah, A., Farooq, A., & Rejeb, R. B. (2017). Role of religious beliefs and practices on the mental health of athletes with anterior cruciate ligament injury. *Advances in Physical Education*, *7*(2), 181–190. http://search.ebscohost.com/login.aspx?direct=true&db=lbh&AN=20173270420&site=ehost-live http://file.scirp.org/Html/6-1600345_76299.htm email: amiranejah@yahoo.fr

Newman, H. J. H., Howells, K. L., & Fletcher, D. (2016). The dark side of top level sport: An autobiographic study of depressive experiences in elite sport performers. *Frontiers in Psychology*, *7*, 868. https://doi.org/10.3389/fpsyg.2016.00868

Olusoga, P., & Thelwell, R. (2016). Coach stress and associated impacts. In R. Thelwell, C. Harwood, & I. Greenlees (Eds.), *The psychology of sports coaching: Research and practice* (pp. 128–141). Routledge.

Pack, S., Arvinen-Barrow, M., Winter, S., & Hemmings, B. (2020). Sport psychology consultants' reflections on the role of humor: "It's like having another skill in your arsenal". *The Sport Psychologist*, *34*(1), 54–61. https://doi.org/10.1123/tsp.2018-0148

Pack, S., Hemmings, B., Winter, S., & Arvinen-Barrow, M. (2019). A preliminary investigation into the use of humor in sport psychology practice. *Journal of Applied Sport Psychology*, *31*(4), 494–502. https://doi.org/10.1080/10413200.2018.1514428

Peres, J. F. P., Moreira-Almeida, A., Nasello, A. G., & Koenig, H. G. (2007). Spirituality and resilience in trauma victims [Article]. *Journal of Religion & Health*, *46*(3), 343–350. https://doi.org/10.1007/s10943-006-9103-0

Piemonte, N. M., & Abreu, S. (2020). Responding to callous humor in healthcare. *AMA Journal of Ethics*, *22*(7), E608–E614. https://journalofethics.ama-assn.org/sites/journalofethics.ama-assn.org/files/2020-06/msoc1-2007_0.pdf

Roy, J., Mokhtar, A. H., Karim, S. A., & Mohanan, S. A. (2015). Cognitive appraisals and lived experiences during injury rehabilitation: A narrative account within personal and situational backdrop. *Asian Journal of Sports Medicine*, *6*(3), 1–4. https://doi.org/10.5812/asjsm.24039

Roychowdhury, D. (2019). Spiritual well-being in sport and exercise psychology. *SAGE Open*, *9*(1). https://doi.org/10.1177/2158244019837460

Rutledge, P. B. (2011, January 16). The psychological power of storytelling: Stories leap-frog technology, taking us to authentic experience. *Psychology Today*. www.psychologytoday.com/intl/blog/positively-media/201101/the-psychological-power-storytelling

Scaletti, R., & Hocking, C. (2010). Healing through story telling: An integrated approach for children experiencing grief. *New Zealand Journal of Occupational Therapy*, *57*(2), 66–71.

Scholl, J. C., & Ragan, S. L. (2003). The use of humor in promoting positive provider-patient interactions in a hospital rehabilitation unit. *Health Communication*, *15*(3), 319–330. https://doi.org/10.1207/S15327027HC1503_4

Smith, B., & Sparkes, A. C. (2002). Men, sport, spinal cord injury, and the construction of coherence: Narrative practice in action. *Qualitative Research*, *2*(2), 143–171. https://doi.org/10.1177/146879410200200202

Smith, B., & Sparkes, A. C. (2004). Men, sport, and spinal cord injury: An analysis of metaphors and narrative types *Disability and Society*, *19*(6), 613–626. https://doi.org/10.1080/0968759042000252533

Smith, B., & Sparkes, A. C. (2005). Men, sport, spinal cord injury, and narratives of hope. *Social Science and Medicine*, *61*(5), 1095–1105. https://doi.org/10.1016/j.socscimed.2005.01.011

Steen, G. (2008). The paradox of metaphor: Why we need a three-dimensional model of metaphor. *Metaphor and Symbol*, *23*(4), 213–241. https://doi.org/10.1080/10926480802426753

Steinmetz, K. (2016, December 15). Swearing is scientifically proven to help you *%$!ing deal. *TIME*. https://time.com/4602680/profanity-research-why-we-swear/

Stephens, R., Atkins, J., & Kingston, A. (2009). Swearing as a response to pain. *Neuroreport*, *20*(12), 1056–1060. https://doi.org/10.1097/WNR.0b013e32832e64b1

Stephens, R., & Umland, C. (2011). Swearing as a response to pain-effect of daily swearing frequency. *The Journal of Pain*, *12*(12), 1274–1281. https://doi.org/10.1016/j.jpain.2011.09.004

Stewart, M. (2015). The hidden influence of metaphor within rehabilitation. *SportEX Journal*, *66*, 10–14. www.co-kinetic.com/content/the-hidden-influence-of-metaphor-within-rehabilitation

Sylwester, K., & Purver, M. (2015). Twitter language use reflects psychological differences between democrats and republicans. *PLoS One*, *10*(9), e0137422. https://doi.org/10.1371/journal.pone.0137422

Vingerhoets, A., Bylsma, L. M., & Vlam, C. D. (2013). Swearing: A biopsychosocial perspective. *Psychological topics*, *22*(2), 287–304. http://hrcak.srce.hr/file/159883

Walinga, J. (2014). Stress, health, and coping. In C. Stangor & J. Walinga (Eds.), *Introduction to psychology – 1st Canadian edition*. BCcampus.

Ward, R. S. (2007). Physical therapy: Stories that must be told. *Physical Therapy*, *87*(11), 1555–1557. https://doi.org/10.2522/ptj.2007.presidential.address

Watson, N., & Czech, D. R. (2005, April). The use of prayer in sport: Implications for sport psychology consulting. *Athletic Insight: The Online Journal of Sport Psychology*, *17*, 4.

Wiese-Bjornstal, D. M. (2019). Christian beliefs and behaviours as health protective, resilience, and intervention factors in the context of sport injuries. In B. Hemmings, N. J. Watson, & A. Parker (Eds.), *Sport psychology and Christianity: Welfare, performance and consultancy* (pp. 54–70). Routledge.

Wiese-Bjornstal, D. M. (2019, November). The integrated model of religiosity and psychological response to the sport injury and rehabilitation process: A Christian illustration. *Canadian Journal for Scholarship and the Christian Faith*. https://cjscf.org/wellness/356-2/

Wiese-Bjornstal, D. M., Smith, A. M., Shaffer, S. M., & Morrey, M. A. (1998). An integrated model of response to sport injury: Psychological and sociological dynamics. *Journal of Applied Sport Psychology*, *10*(1), 46–69. https://doi.org/10.1080/10413209808406377

Wiese-Bjornstal, D. M., Wood, K. N., Principe, F. M., & Schwartz, E. S. (2022). Religiosity and ways of coping with sport injuries among Christian athletes. *Journal of the Christian Society for Kinesiology, Leisure and Sports Studies*, *7*(1). https://trace.tennessee.edu/jcskls/vol7/iss1/6

13 Patient Education in Sport Injury and Rehabilitation

Monna Arvinen-Barrow, Amanda J. Visek, and Amie Barrow

Chapter Objectives

- To introduce the purpose and benefits of patient education.
- To describe the different types, modes, and mediums of patient education in sport injury context.
- To outline the process of integrating patient education into sport injury and rehabilitation.

Introduction

Historically, healthcare has been dominated by the medical model (Engel, 1977), which ascribes to a philosophy of "immediate enforcement of compliance with prescribed regimen" (Redman, 2004, p. 2) that leaves little to no room for patient education (Redman, 2004). In its infancy, patient education was primarily didactic in nature and focused merely on providing biomedical advice (Wittink & Oosterhaven, 2018). This formative application of patient education has not been found to be highly effective and, at times, even counterproductive to patient outcomes. However, when patient education is used as a cognitive behavioral intervention strategy within biopsychosocial patient-centered care (Hashim, 2017; O'Neill, 2022), it looks and feels very different for both the patient and the healthcare provider. The purpose of this chapter is to discuss how patient education within patient-centered care can be beneficial for sport injury and rehabilitation. More specifically, this chapter will (a) define and introduce the purpose of patient education within sport injury, (b) discuss biopsychosocial benefits of effective patient education, (c) introduce different types, modes, and mediums of patient education in the sport injury context, and (d) outline the process of integrating patient education into sport injury and rehabilitation.

Construct Definition and Purpose

According to Bartlett (1985), patient education is "a planned learning experience using a combination of methods such as teaching, counseling, and behavior modification techniques which influence patients' knowledge and health behavior" (p. 323). More recently, a shift toward patient-centered education has taken place – where the education content is *"about* the patients, *with* the patients, and *for* the patients" (Hearn et al., 2019, p. 934), with a goal to ensure medical professionals "remain sensitive to all of the needs of the people they care for" (p. 934). In the context of sport injury, effective patient education typically involves two-way communication

DOI: 10.4324/9781003295709-16

between the athlete and various individuals involved in the rehabilitation process. These individuals include sports medicine professionals (SMP), sport professionals (SP), sport psychology professionals (SPP), and other significant persons in the athlete's life (e.g., parents, teammates, other family members; Stiller-Ostrowski & Kenow, 2014).

Benefits of Effective Patient Education

Consistent with the theoretical models presented in this book (see Chapters 2–6 and 19–20), patient education is a cognitive behavioral intervention that can influence both injury risk factors and a number of psychosocial responses to injury, rehabilitation, and return to participation. Most notably, patient education increases *knowledge*, which has been found to facilitate patient perceptions of competence and autonomy. Patient education is also a *shared experience* which can facilitate perceptions of relatedness (see self-determination theory; Ryan & Deci, 2002). Satisfaction with self-determination theory's three basic psychological needs (i.e., competence, autonomy, and relatedness) has been found to be associated with motivation, which is positively related to various mental and physical health outcomes (e.g., Ng et al., 2012; Podlog & Brown, 2016). Increased *knowledge* can also influence numerous cognitive appraisals and, thus, emotional and behavioral responses associated with injury (see the integrated model of psychological response to the sport injury and rehabilitation process; Wiese-Bjornstal et al., 1998). For example, Russell and Tracey (2011) found lack of understanding of injury (cognitive appraisal) was of great concern for injured athletes and a source of apprehension (emotional response) during rehabilitation. They also found *knowledge* of various behavior-focused factors, such as (a) treatment duration, (b) return to participation timeline, (c) premature return to participation risks, and (d) importance of rehabilitation adherence, were "helpful and reduced anxiety about future sport participation" (Russell & Tracey, 2011, p. 19).

Outside of sport injury, similar anxiety-reducing effects have been found (Hoving et al., 2010; Visser et al., 2001), along with other positive benefits. For example, effective patient education has been found to positively influence experiences of immunotherapy treatment outcomes and temper exaggerated patient expectations (Ihrig et al., 2023). Patient education has also been observed to increase knowledge about and improve attitudes toward receiving vaccines (Chou et al., 2014), in addition to aiding adherence to medication (Jankowska-Polańska et al., 2016). Patient education is also understood to positively influence communication and vice versa. This is important because communication is an antecedent for trust and rapport, both of which are essential ingredients of the patient–practitioner relationship within patient-centered care (Ayers & de Visser, 2018; Katz & Hemmings, 2009; Stiller-Ostrowski & Kenow, 2014). Importantly, improved communication (Louw et al., 2011) and trust in the healthcare professional (Birkhäuer et al., 2017) have been linked to better rehabilitation outcomes, thus highlighting the value of patient education as a staple intervention during rehabilitation. In fact, an evaluation of existing systematic reviews and meta-analyses found the impact of patient education in chronic diseases and obesity health outcomes was 50–80% (Lagger et al., 2010). Further, research has shown patient education can be optimized as an intervention in the treatment of specific musculoskeletal conditions. For instance, for patients diagnosed with patellofemoral pain (PFP), a recent systematic review and meta-analysis found, when combined with other treatment modalities, patient education was most effective at three months following PFP diagnosis (Winters et al., 2021). Moreover, the positive effects of patient education on health outcomes have included decreased pain and disability (Louw et al., 2011) and increased quality of life (Lagger et al., 2010).

Consequences of Ineffective Patient Education

In contrast, Forbes et al. (2021) stated ineffective patient education has been linked to poorer rehabilitation outcomes (Barwick et al., 2012), increased hospital readmissions (Hari & Rosenzweig, 2012), misuse of medications (Cumbler et al., 2009), and decreased patient satisfaction (Montini et al., 2008). Most recently, patient education of low back pain and the use of negative language within delivery of the education was found to increase patient anxiety and illness beliefs (Linskens et al., 2023) – evidence the words used in patient education can have profound consequences on rehabilitation. To aid in more effective patient education, Stewart and Loftus (2018) discuss words to avoid and suggested alternatives when delivering patient education in the realm of musculoskeletal rehabilitation.

Patient Education in Sport Injury Rehabilitation

Research has shown patients outside of sport (e.g., Hafsteinsdottir et al., 2011), and in sport (Russell & Tracey, 2011), want education on their condition, rehabilitation, and return to participation process from their treatment providers. In sport, patient education typically takes place in four main sport injury rehabilitation contexts: (a) initial intake evaluation, including medical history interviews; (b) physical examination and diagnostic testing; (c) before, during, and after treatment; and (d) when making medical recommendations (see Brewer & Redmond, 2017). It is also common for patient education to be provided by various SMPs, SPPs, and SPs. As part of the patient education process, they may educate athletes about the numerous internal and external risk factors that could have predisposed or made the athlete susceptible to sport injury. Pertinent intrinsic injury risk factors include age, previous injury, strength, and neuromuscular control (Brewer & Redmond, 2017). Other injury risk factors include maladaptive psychosomatic stress response to stressful situation(s), insufficient coping skills, and/or lack of psychological interventions (Ivarsson et al., 2017). Typical extrinsic risk factors include the environment (e.g., weather), equipment (e.g., mouthguards), and numerous sport-related factors (e.g., rules, playing surface). Recently, the importance of adequate nutrition (e.g., Turnagöl et al., 2022), sleep (e.g., Huang & Ihm, 2021), and rest and active recovery (e.g., Children's Hospital of The King's Daughters Sports Medicine & Gilmartin, 2021) have also been highlighted as injury-protective factors, and are thus likely to be topical content for injury prevention education, and also pertinent to patient education as part of injury rehabilitation.

Types of Patient Education

The type of patient education used in sport injury settings can be formal, non-formal, or informal. Formal education is planned and structured and designed by content experts. Non-formal education is planned, but not to the extent as formal education, and is often focused on offering practical knowledge. Non-formal education is typically delivered by subject experts and can take place in a myriad of flexible ways in a number of situations. Informal education is unplanned and unstructured and can be learned from anyone (e.g., from another athlete's personal experiences with injury) and does not involve "fact-checking" of the information.

The types of patient education can be delivered directly (e.g., person-to-person), indirectly (e.g., through technology, such as mobile applications), or via a combination of directly and indirectly (Akoit & Pandin, 2021). The focus of the patient education being delivered directly, indirectly, or in combination can be general (e.g., focused on generic information about the injury or rehabilitation process) or specific (e.g., focused on the patient's individual needs) and

Table 13.1 Examples of Non-Verbal Communication

Kinesics *Non-verbal communication*	*Proxemics* *Communication through space*	*Paralanguage* *Vocal components of speech*
Physical appearance	Proximity to the patient	Pitch
Punctuality	Intimate zone	Resonance
Body posture	(0–18 in/0–50 cm)	Articulation
Gestures	Personal zone	Tempo
	(18–48 in/50–120 cm)	
Touch	Social zone	Volume
Facial expressions	(48 in – 12 ft/1.20 cm-3.7 m)	
Smells and scents	Public zone	
	(Greater than 12 feet/3.7 m)	

Source: Adapted from Brewer and Redmond (2017).

aimed to educate an individual (e.g., the athlete, caregiver, sport coach) or collective group of individuals (e.g., sport team, interprofessional practice team). Depending on the desired outcome and the target audience, patient education can be delivered in-person in real time or virtually, both synchronously and asynchronously.

Modes of Patient Education

Rooted in the basics of communication (Stiller-Ostrowski & Kenow, 2014), effective patient education generally involves and is influenced by verbal and non-verbal modes of communication. Verbal communication includes both spoken and written words, whereas non-verbal communication includes three overarching dimensions – kinesics, proxemics, and paralanguage (Brewer & Redmond, 2017; see Table 13.1).

Effective patient education also considers elements of the basic two-way communication cycle: the *sender*, who communicates the *message* to the *receiver*, who responds with *feedback message* to the *sender*. This message–feedback loop involves *encoding* (i.e., selection of words, actions, gestures, and expressions) and *decoding* (i.e., a process of observation and interpretation of the encoded message) from both the sender and the receiver (Stiller-Ostrowski & Kenow, 2014); see Figure 13.1. Encoding and decoding will also involve cognitive, affective, and behavioral processes and responses.

Mediums for Patient Education

In general, patient education can be delivered through different overlapping mediums, such as oral, written/printed, audio, audiovisual, and kinesthetic methods. Table 13.2 provides select examples of patient education materials, as identified in the wider medical patient education literature.

Patient education mediums can incorporate multiple senses, such as hearing and sound, touch, itch, pressure, and sight. In the context of sport injury education, a number of other psychophysiological sensations and perceptions can also be evoked, when applicable. These include external and internal sensory systems, such as the vestibular system, spatial orientation, nociception, proprioception, equilibrioception, thermoception, as well as sense of stretch and tension.

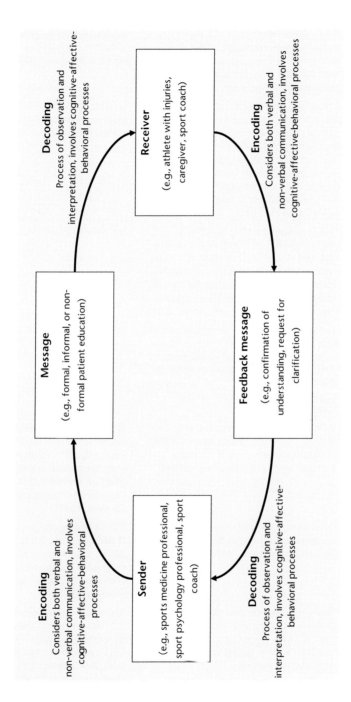

Figure 13.1 Basic communication cycle adapted to sport injury.

Table 13.2 Overview of Select Patient Education Mediums

Mediums	Description	Evidence Base
Lectures	Educational talks aimed at a particular audience, typically didactic in nature; delivered in-person and virtually, and with the help of technology, made available for asynchronous viewing.	Moderate effect on general patient outcomes compared to routine care (Theis & Johnson, 1995).
Discussions	Conversation/dialogue between two or more people; common way to deliver patient education to individuals and small groups; can take place in-person and virtually; in sport, performance-enhancement groups for athletes have been proposed to mitigate psychological distress associated with injuries (Clement et al., 2011).	Small to moderate effect size on general patient outcomes compared to routine care (Theis & Johnson, 1995).
Storytelling	Communicating a story in written, oral, electronic, or visual way to enable understanding of self or situation; helps organize thoughts, provide meaning to a lived experience, and elicit biological, emotional, and behavioral responses in the reader/listener (McCann et al., 2019).	Not yet empirically studied.
Metaphors and quotes	Metaphors are implied comparisons that help convey abstract experiences in a concrete manner (Lakoff & Johnson, 1980). Inspirational quotes combine the "art" and "science" (Cutilli, 2020) of patient education to convey key messages simply.	Not yet empirically studied.
Fact sheets and other illustrated material	Written materials, such as informational leaflets, brochures, packages or booklets, infographics, home exercise sheets, websites, and smartphone wallpapers.	Written patient education material has been found to improve patient knowledge (Friedman et al., 2011) and have a small to moderate effect on general patient outcomes compared to routine care (Theis & Johnson, 1995).
Audio materials	Educational information presented via audio recordings in the form of audiotapes, podcasts, and audiobooks.	Mixed findings for audiotapes (Friedman et al., 2011; Santo et al., 2005); however, a moderate effect on general patient outcomes compared to routine care (Theis & Johnson, 1995).
Audiovisual	Delivery of patient education through combined audio and video mediums, such as video recordings, TedTalks and YouTube videos, documentaries, and sport-related movies.	Video-based patient education intervention findings are mixed for increasing knowledge (Friedman et al., 2011), with no effect on anxiety (Trevena et al., 2006); however, videotapes have a small to moderate effect size on general patient outcomes compared to routine care (Theis & Johnson, 1995).

Mediums	Description	Evidence Base
Mobile device apps	Applications for smartphone and tablet devices designed to provide information about anatomy, conditions, and treatments; facilitate communication between different members of the rehabilitation team; aid in stress management, cognitive reframing, and tracking goal achievement and relevant rehabilitation behaviors. Note, many apps are not evidence-based; as such, always discuss with a healthcare provider in advance of use to ensure app is valid and appropriate for intended use.	Use of mobile device apps has transformed, and continues to transform, many areas of healthcare (Ventola, 2014); however, they have not yet been empirically studied in a sport rehabilitation context.
Demonstrations, stimulations, and games	Include use of 3D models, role-playing, modeling, use of simulated games, active video gaming, and so on.	No efficacy data for simulated games or role-playing has been found (Friedman et al., 2011), though demonstrations used for patient education have a large effect size on general patient outcomes compared to routine care (Theis & Johnson, 1995).

Patient Education Processes for Sport Injury and Rehabilitation

Drawing from existing literature (Agency for Healthcare Research and Quality, 2020; American Academy of Family Physicians et al., 2000; Morris, 2022), a core principle of patient education is having the requisite skills to *assess*, *plan*, *implement*, and *evaluate* (Cutilli, 2020) effective patient education interventions. What follows is a brief introduction to each in the context of sport injury and rehabilitation.

Assessment

The goal of *assessment*, within patient education, is to gain information on the educational and personal needs of the patient and determine how to best provide holistic person-centered education for the patient. In the context of injury rehabilitation, assessment typically involves the use of various objective and subjective intake forms and assessments (for a list of psychosocial assessments in sport injury, see Arvinen-Barrow et al., 2018) with the patient, as well as the use of various foundational interpersonal counseling skills (see Chapter 9). Depending on the healthcare professional's educational background and competencies, rehabilitation-focused assessment may also include the use of specific counseling approaches (e.g., motivational interviewing; Miller & Rollnick, 2013). Within the rehabilitation process, regardless of whether patient education is used for injury prevention or rehabilitation, assessment should be used to decipher patient preferences in individual learning styles, readiness to learn, and potential barriers for learning (e.g., learning disabilities, language barriers). Knowledge of these will inform the healthcare provider's planning for patient education.

Planning

The goal of *planning* is to use the knowledge gleaned from assessment(s) to inform the design of patient education materials and approaches. Well-planned patient education materials and approaches have clear purpose and outcomes, meet the patient where they are at in the rehabilitation process, and are within the scope of their abilities. Planning for effective patient education must consider pedagogical theory, patient preferences in individual learning, and scientific evidence when determining the content, types, modes, and mediums of how patient education will be delivered. Prior to implementing printable or audiovisual patient education materials, it is advisable to systematically evaluate the content developed or sourced for understandability (i.e., patient comprehension, like reading level, appropriate vocabulary) and actionability (i.e., that will aid patient rehabilitation behavior). For more on evaluating patient education materials, see Agency for Healthcare Research and Quality (2020b).

Implementation

The goal of *implementation* is to systematically incorporate the patient education plan into sport injury prevention, rehabilitation, and/or return to participation process. Implementation requires systematic commitment to the patient education process and relies on evidence-based materials and relevant knowledge from related fields (e.g., marketing, graphic design, audiovisual technology; Cutilli, 2020) while considering universal health literacy precautions (Agency for Healthcare Research and Quality, 2020a). Altogether, well-implemented patient education can aid in facilitating positive patient education outcomes.

Evaluation

The goal of *evaluation* is to appraise both strengths and challenges of the implemented patient education. Facets of patient education to consider include an assessment of the appropriateness of the educational materials and implementation processes, degree to which the intended purpose and outcomes were met, level of patient satisfaction, and extent to which patient understanding was aided and knowledge increased. Equally, it is imperative to identify patient education barriers and determine a plan for modification or revision to reduce patient education challenges.

Selected Guidelines for Effective Patient Education

In addition to having content expertise and understanding of pedagogical principles of teaching and learning, existing patient education literature (Agency for Healthcare Research and Quality, 2020a; American Academy of Family Physicians et al., 2000; Morris, 2022) highlights several interpersonal factors important for effective patient education. These include *attitudes* toward patient education, *identifying* barriers to learning, and *using strategies* to promote trust, rapport, and engagement. Table 13.3. provides selected guidelines for effective patient education as identified in the wider patient education medical literature.

Table 13.3 Selected Guidelines for Effective Patient Education

Guideline	Rationale	Selected Evidence
Communicate clearly.	Breaking educational information into small, manageable pieces can aid understanding and comprehension.	Stiller-Ostrowski and Kenow (2014)
Keep it simple; avoid medical jargon; assess, select, and create easy-to-understand patient education materials.	Injured athletes will have varying degrees of understanding of their injury, recovery, and rehabilitation. Keeping messaging simple can enhance understanding and alleviate maladaptive psychosocial responses.	Agency for Healthcare Research and Quality (2020a); Stiller-Ostrowski and Kenow (2014); van der Scheer-Horst et al. (2023)
Use structured, tailored, and interactive multi-modal patient education interventions.	Using multiple patient education mediums together can be more effective than when used in isolation.	Theis and Johnson (1995); Trevena et al. (2006)
Identify patient can'ts and can-dos.	Framing rehabilitation activities in a positive manner can facilitate sense of control and autonomy and facilitate positive rehabilitation outcomes.	Wilkoff (2022); see also Chapter 15 on self-talk
Build trust and rapport.	Trust associated with patient satisfaction, health behaviors (e.g., adherence), quality of life, and symptom severity.	Birkhäuer et al. (2017)
Check patient understanding.	Using the teach-back method and asking questions can facilitate greater patient understanding and affords quick corrections in case of misunderstanding.	Agency for Healthcare Research and Quality (2020a); Morris (2022); Trevena et al. (2006)
Consider language-related and other communication barriers.	Writing information down and in the patient's native language can be highly influential in increasing understanding and comprehension.	Morris (2022)
Consider culture, customs, and beliefs.	Cultural differences affect health beliefs and outcomes.	Mhaimeed et al. (2023); Morris (2022); see also Chapter 11
Patient education should be a continued process that includes follow-ups.	Long-term, regular patient–clinician relationship can facilitate behavior change.	Agency for Healthcare Research and Quality (2020a); American Academy of Family Physicians et al. (2000)

Conclusion

Patient education is a cognitive behavioral intervention integral to holistic injury prevention and the rehabilitation process. By combining the "art" and "science" of injury knowledge and communication, patient education can both set and temper expectations, increase personal agency, and positively affect injury outcomes. When done effectively, patient education is "simple, patient centered, and multi-modal [aimed] to meet the health literacy needs of patients/caregiver" (Cutilli, 2020, p. 267).

Case Study

Esti, a 14-year-old competitive swimmer, felt pain in her right foot while warming up at a local swim meet. "Someone kicked me, and now my toe hurts," Esti told her coach and mom. On closer inspection, all of her toes looked normal, with no signs of swelling or bruising. When palpated or flexed, Esti reported mild discomfort but no pain on her second phalange. "It is up to you whether or not you want to race," says Esti's mom. "If your toe is indeed broken, not much will be done to it. You can always take it one race at a time and see how it feels." Over the next two days, Esti swam all her races and did not think much of the toe. Two days later, she woke up with her toe swollen and bruised purple. Esti's mom made an appointment with a local orthopedic surgeon known to work with athletes. The following is a transcription of the appointment.

"Hi, Esti. I am Dr. Luu. What brings you here?"

Esti replies, "My toe hurts. Someone kicked me while warming up at a swim meet – now it's swollen and bruised. I want to know what is wrong with it and how long it will take to heal."

Dr. Luu responds, "Let me have a look."

While Esti is taking her shoes and socks off, Dr. Luu picks up one of her shoes from the floor and turns it around in his hands before placing the shoe back on the floor. While examining Esti's toe, he remarks, "Those are cool shoes. I like the thick soles. Very nice." He then says, "Do you know what a toe is made of?" Esti sits silent and shakes her head. Dr. Luu says, "A toe has three bones, and inside those bones are blood vessels. There are a couple of joints, and they move because of tendons that help the toes flex or extend. The bones are also surrounded by skin."

Esti asks, "Is my toe broken? If it is, how long will it take to heal?"

Dr. Luu answers, saying, "Well, since there are no muscles in your toe, and knowing what a toe is made of, when you see this much bruising, it's usually an indication there is a fracture of some kind. But I don't know for sure. Let us take an X-ray to confirm."

The X-ray confirms an acute fracture in the second phalange. Esti looks worried and immediately asks, "How long will it take to heal?"

Dr. Luu pauses and says, "It sounds like you are in a hurry," and then inquires, "Why are you in a rush?"

Esti says, "I have state swimming championships in two weeks, and two weeks after that, I am going to junior nationals. I need to know that I can continue to swim."

Dr. Luu responds, "I would be worried if you were an Irish dancer, and you had that broken toe. But you are not an Irish dancer, so [as a swimmer] you can train as much as your pain allows. I have seen many of these [broken] toes, and each and every one of them has eventually healed as normal."[1]

Esti looks relieved and turns to her mom and smiles a little. Dr. Luu then presents several options to Esti and says, "There are a couple of things you can do here. You can get crutches and a boot if you want to take some pressure off that toe. Or you can continue using those cool shoes you have, because they have thick, supporting soles. At swim practice, you can tape two toes together for support, but that might just feel weird."

Questions

1. What kinesics, proxemics, and paralanguage did you imagine Dr. Luu to be using as you read the case study? What effect did you imagine these to have on Esti cognitively, emotionally, and behaviorally?
2. What mediums of patient education did Dr. Luu use with Esti?
3. What additional patient education mediums could Dr. Luu have used with Esti that would likely have been beneficial, and why?
4. Considering the process of patient education, identify and justify what psychological and sociocultural factors made Dr. Luu's patient education intervention effective.

Note

1 This quote is cited from Arvinen-Barrow, M., Clement, D., & Hemmings, B. (2020). "This is the final jump," I respond. Why, why do I utter those words? Using storytelling in sport injury rehabilitation. In W. Ross (Ed.), *Sport injury psychology: Cultural, relational, methodological, and applied considerations* (pp. 207–216). Routledge. https://doi.org/10.4324/9780367854997 (p. 212).

References

Agency for Healthcare Research and Quality. (2020a). *AHRQ Health literacy universal precautions toolkit*. Agency for Healthcare Research and Quality. www.ahrq.gov/health-literacy/improve/precautions/index.html

Agency for Healthcare Research and Quality. (2020b). *The patient education materials assessment tool (PEMAT) and user's guide*. www.ahrq.gov/health-literacy/patient-education/pemat.html

Akoit, E. E., & Pandin, M. G. R. (2021). Direct, indirect, and mixed methods of health education by nurse and its impact on type 2 diabetes patients: A literature review. *medRxiv: The Reprint Server for Health Sciences*. https://doi.org/10.1101/2021.12.22.21268287

American Academy of Family Physicians, Association of Departments of Family Medicine, Association of Family Practice Residency Directors, & Society of Teachers of Family Medicine. (2000). AAFP core educational guidelines: Recommended core educational guidelines for family practice residents: Patient Education. *American Family Physician, 62*(7), 1712–1714.

Arvinen-Barrow, M., Clement, D., & Hemmings, B. (2020). "This is the final jump," I respond. Why, why do I utter those words? Using storytelling in sport injury rehabilitation. In W. Ross (Ed.), *Sport injury psychology: Cultural, relational, methodological, and applied considerations* (pp. 207–216). Routledge. https://doi.org/10.4324/9780367854997

Arvinen-Barrow, M., Hamson-Utley, J. J., & DeFreese, J. D. (2018). Sport injury, rehabilitation, and return to sport. In J. Taylor (Ed.), *Assessment in applied sport psychology* (pp. 183–198). Human Kinetics. https://doi.org/10.5040/9781492595236.ch-013

Ayers, S., & de Visser, R. (2018). *Psychology for medicine and healthcare* (2nd ed.). Sage Publishing.

Bartlett, E. (1985). At last a definition. *Patient Education and Counseling, 7*, 323–324.

Barwick, M. A., Bennett, L. M., Johnson, S. N., McGowan, J., & Moore, J. E. (2012). Training health and mental health professionals in motivational interviewing: A systematic review. *Children and Youth Services Review, 34*(9), 1786–1795. https://doi.org/10.1016/j.childyouth.2012.05.012.

Birkhäuer, J., Gaab, J., Kossowsky, J., Hasler, S., Krummenacher, P., Wernes, C., & Gerger, H. (2017). Trust in the health care professional and health outcome: A meta-analysis. *PLoS One, 12*(2), e0170988. https://doi.org/10.1371/journal.pone.0170988

Brewer, B. W., & Redmond, C. J. (2017). *Psychology of sport injury*. Human Kinetics.

Children's Hospital of The King's Daughters Sports Medicine, & Gilmartin, K. (2021). Rest and active recovery: An important step for all athletes. In *Around the blocks: A children's health resource*. www.chkd.org/Blog/Rest-and-Active-Recovery – An-Important-Step-for-All-Athletes/

Chou, T. I. F., Lash, D. B., Malcolm, B., Yousify, L., Quach, J. Y., Dong, S., & Yu, J. (2014). Effects of a student pharmacist consultation on patient knowledge and attitudes about vaccines. *Journal of the American Pharmacists Association, 54*(2), 130–137. https://doi.org/10.1331/JAPhA.2014.13114

Clement, D., Shannon, V. R., & Connole, I. J. (2011). Performance enhancement groups for injured athletes. *International Journal of Athletic Therapy & Training, 16*(3), 34–36. https://doi.org/10.1123/ijatt.16.3.34

Cumbler, E., Wald, H., & Kutner, J. (2009). Lack of patient knowledge regarding hospital medications. *Journal of Hospital Medicine, 5*(2), 83–86. https://doi.org/10.1002/jhm.566

Cutilli, C. C. (2020). Excellence in patient education: Evidence-based education that "sticks" and improves patient outcomes. *The Nursing clinics of North America, 55*(2), 267–282. https://doi.org/10.1016/j.cnur.2020.02.007

Engel, G. L. (1977). The need for a new medical model: A challenge for biomedicine. *Science, 196*(4286), 129–136. https://doi.org/10.1126/science.847460

Forbes, R., Clasper, B., Ilango, A., Kan, H., Peng, J., & Mandrusiak, A. (2021). Effectiveness of patient education training on health professional student performance: A systematic review. *Patient Education and Counseling, 104*(10), 2453–2466. https://doi.org/10.1016/j.pec.2021.02.039

Friedman, A. J., Cosby, R., Boyko, S., Hatton-Bauer, J., & Turnbull, G. (2011). Effective teaching strategies and methods of delivery for patient education: A systematic review and practice guideline recommendations. *Journal of Cancer Education, 26*(1), 12–21. https://doi.org/10.1007/s13187-010-0183-x

Hafsteinsdottir, T. B., Vergunst, M., Lindeman, E., & Schuurmans, M. (2011). Educational needs of patients with a stroke and their caregivers: A systematic review of the literature. *Patient Education and Counseling, 85*(1), 14–25. https://doi.org/10.1016/j.pec.2010.07.046

Hari, M., & Rosenzweig, M. (2012). Incidence of preventable postoperative readmissions following pancreaticoduodenectomy: Implications for patient education. *Oncology Nursing Forum, 39*(4), 408–412. https://doi.org/10.1188/12.ONF.408-412

Hashim, M. J. (2017). Patient-centered communication: Basic skills. *American Family Physician, 95*(1), 29–34. www.aafp.org/dam/brand/aafp/pubs/afp/issues/2017/0101/p29.pdf

Hearn, J., Dewji, M., Stocker, C., & Simons, G. (2019). Patient-centered medical education: A proposed definition. *Medical Teacher, 41*(8), 934–938. https://doi.org/10.1080/0142159X.2019.1597258

Hoving, C., Visser, A., Mullen, P. D., & van den Borne, B. (2010). A history of patient education by health professionals in Europe and North America: From authority to shared decision making education. *Patient Education and Counseling, 78*(3), 275–281. https://doi.org/10.1016/j.pec.2010.01.015

Huang, K., & Ihm, J. (2021). Sleep and injury risk. *Current Sports Medicine Reports, 20*(6), 286–290. https://doi.org/10.1249/JSR.0000000000000849

Ihrig, A., Richter, J., Bugaj, T. J., Friedrich, H.-C., & Maatouk, I. (2023). Between hope and reality: How oncology physicians and information providers of a cancer information service manage patients' expectations for and experiences with immunotherapies *Patient Education and Counseling, 109*, 107622. https://doi.org/10.1016/j.pec.2023.107622

Ivarsson, A., Johnson, U., Andersen, M. B., Tranaeus, U., Stenling, A., & Lindwall, M. (2017). Psychosocial factors and sport injuries: Meta-analyses for prediction and prevention *Sports Medicine, 47*(2), 353–365. https://doi.org/10.1007/s40279-016-0578-x

Jankowska-Polańska, B., Uchmanowicz, I., Dudek, K., & Mazur, G. (2016). Relationship between patients' knowledge and medication adherence among patients with hypertension. *Patient Preference and Adherence, 10*, 2437–2447. https://doi.org/doi.org/10.2147/PPA.S117269

Katz, J., & Hemmings, B. (2009). *Counselling skills handbook for the sport psychologist*. The British Psychological Society.

Lagger, G., Pataky, Z., & Golay, A. (2010). Efficacy of therapeutic patient education in chronic diseases and obesity. *Patient Education and Counseling, 79*(3), 283–286. https://doi.org/10.1016/j.pec.2010.03.015

Lakoff, G., & Johnson, M. (1980). *Metaphors we live by*. The University of Chicago Press.

Linskens, F. G., van der Scheer, E. S., Stortenbeker, I., Das, E., Staal, J. B., & van Lankveld, W. (2023). Negative language use of the physiotherapist in low back pain education impacts anxiety and illness beliefs: A randomised controlled trial in healthy respondents. *Patient Education and Counseling, 110*, 107649. https://doi.org/10.1016/j.pec.2023.107649

Louw, A., Diener, I., Butler, D. S., & Puentedura, E. J. (2011). The effect of neuroscience education on pain disability, anxiety and stress in chronic musculoskeletal pain. *Archives of Physical Medicine and Rehabilitation, 92*(12), 2041–2056. https://doi.org/10.1016/j.apmr.2011.07.198

McCann, S., Barto, J., & Goldman, N. (2019). Learning through story listening. *American Journal of Health Promotion, 33*(3), 477–481. https://doi.org/10.1177/0890117119825525e

Mhaimeed, N., Mhaimeed, N., Mhaimeed, O., Alanni, J., Burney, Z., Eshafeey, A., . . . Choi, J. (2023). Shared decision making with black patients: A scoping review. *Patient Education and Counseling, 110*, 107646. https://doi.org/10.1016/j.pec.2023.107646

Miller, W. R., & Rollnick, S. (2013). *Motivational interviewing: Helping people change* (3rd ed.). Guilford Press.

Montini, T., Noble, A. A., & Stelfox, H. T. (2008). Content analysis of patient complaints. *International Journal for Quality in Healthcare, 20*(6), 412–420. https://doi.org/10.1093/intqhc/mzn041

Morris, G. (2022). 10 ways nurses and nurse leaders can improve patient education. *NurseJournal.* https://nursejournal.org/articles/tips-to-improve-patient-education/

Ng, J. Y. Y., Ntoumanis, N., Thøgersen-Ntoumani, C., Deci, E. L., Ryan, R. M., Duda, J. L., & Williams, G. C. (2012). Self-determination theory applied to health contexts: A meta-analysis. *Perspectives on Psychological Science, 7*(4), 325–340. https://doi.org/10.1177/1745691612447309

O'Neill, N. (2022). *The eight principles of patient-centered care.* www.oneviewhealthcare.com/blog/the-eight-principles-of-patient-centered-care/

Podlog, L., & Brown, W. J. (2016). Self-determination theory: A framework for enhancing patient-centered care. *The Journal for Nurse Practitioners, 12*(6), e359–e362. https://doi.org/10.1016/j.nurpra.2016.04.022

Redman, B. K. (2004). *Advances in patient education.* Springer Publishing Company, Inc.

Russell, H. C., & Tracey, J. (2011). What do injured athletes want from their health care professionals? *International Journal of Athletic Therapy & Training, 16*(5), 18–21. https://doi.org/10.1123/ijatt.16.5.18

Ryan, R. M., & Deci, E. L. (2002). An overview of self-determination theory: An organismic dialectical perspective. In E. L. Deci & R. M. Ryan (Eds.), *Handbook of self-determination research* (pp. 3–33). University of Rochester Press.

Santo, A., Laizner, A. M., & Shohet, L. (2005). Exploring the value of audiotapes for health literacy: A systematic review *Patient Education and Counseling, 58*(3), 235–243. https://doi.org/10.1016/j.pec.2004.07.001

Stewart, M., & Loftus, S. (2018). Sticks and stones: The impact of language in musculoskeletal rehabilitation. *Journal of Orthopaedic & Sports Physical Therapy, 48*(7), 519–522. https://doi.org/10.2519/jospt.2018.0610

Stiller-Ostrowski, J., & Kenow, L. J. (2014). Communication and athlete education skills for the athletic trainer. In M. Granquist, J. J. Hamson-Utley, L. J. Kenow, & J. Stiller-Ostrowski (Eds.), *Psychosocial strategies for athletic training* (pp. 111–143). F. A. Davis.

Theis, S. L., & Johnson, J. H. (1995). Strategies for teaching patients: A meta-analysis *Clinical Nurse Specialist 9*(2), 100–105. https://doi.org/10.1097/00002800-199503000-00010

Trevena, L. J., Davey, H. M., Barratt, A., Butow, P., & Caldwell, P. (2006). A systematic review on communicating with patients about evidence. *Journal of Evaluation in Clinical Practice, 12*(1), 13–23 https://doi.org/10.1111/j.1365-2753.2005.00596.x

Turnagöl, H. H., Koşar, Ş. N., Güzel, Y., Aktitiz, S., & Atakan, M. M. (2022). Nutritional considerations for injury prevention and recovery in combat sports. *Nutrients, 14*(1), 53. https://doi.org/10.3390/nu14010053

van der Scheer-Horst, E., Rutten, G., Stortenbeker, I., Borkent, J., Swormink, W. K., Das, E., . . . van Lankveld, W. (2023). Limited health literacy in primary care physiotherapy: Does a physiotherapist use techniques to improve communication? *Patient Education and Counseling, 109,* 107624. https://doi.org/10.1016/j.pec.2023.107624

Ventola, C. L. (2014). Mobile devices and apps for health care professionals: Uses and benefits. *Pharmacy and Therapeutics: A Peer-Reviewed Journal for Managed Care and Hospital Formulary Management, 39*(5), 356–364. www.ncbi.nlm.nih.gov/pmc/articles/PMC4029126/pdf/ptj3905356.pdf

Visser, A., Deccache, A., & Bensing, J. (2001). Patient education in Europe: United differences. *Patient Education and Counseling, 44*(1), 1–5. https://doi.org/10.1016/S0738-3991(01)00111-2

Wiese-Bjornstal, D. M., Smith, A. M., Shaffer, S. M., & Morrey, M. A. (1998). An integrated model of response to sport injury: Psychological and sociological dynamics. *Journal of Applied Sport Psychology, 10*(1), 46–69. https://doi.org/10.1080/10413209808406377

Wilkoff, W. G. (2022). Give patients can'ts but also can do's. *MDedge Pediatrics*, 253388. www.mdedge.com/pediatrics/article/253388/injuries/give-patients-cants-also-can-dos?reg=1

Winters, M., Holden, S., Lura, C., Welton, N., Caldwell, D., Vicenzino, B., . . . Rathleff, M. (2021). Comparative effectiveness of treatments for patellofemoral pain: A living systematic review with network meta-analysis. *British Journal of Sports Medicine, 55*(7), 369–377. https://doi.org/10.1136/bjsports-2020-102819

Wittink, H., & Oosterhaven, J. (2018). Patient education and health literacy. *Musculoskeletal Science and Practice, 38,* 120–127. https://doi.org/10.1016/j.msksp.2018.06.004

14 Goal Setting in Sport Injury and Rehabilitation

*Monna Arvinen-Barrow, Brian Hemmings,
and Michael A. Hansen*

Chapter Objectives

- To define goal setting, types, and levels of goals in the context of sport injury and rehabilitation.
- To summarize the benefits of using different types and levels of goals during rehabilitation.
- To outline the process of setting goals during sport injury rehabilitation.

Introduction

Since the original work of Locke and Latham (1985), goal setting has become one of the most popular and widely used psychological interventions in sport (Jeong et al., 2021; Williamson et al., 2022) and is often implemented by athletes with the aim of improving performance (Weinberg & Gould, 2019). Research has identified three different types of goals, namely, outcome, performance, and process goals (e.g., Cox, 2012). Outcome goals are usually focused on the result of an event such as winning or earning a medal and involve interpersonal comparison. In contrast, performance goals often involve intrapersonal assessment, as they are typically focused on achieving a particular level of performance in comparison to one's previous performances and not to that of other competitors. Process goals are focused on the actions and required tasks in which an individual must engage in order to achieve the desired performance outcome (e.g., Cox, 2012; Weinberg & Gould, 2019). According to Cox (2012), when outcome, performance, and process goals are used in combination, athletes are more likely to experience higher levels of performance improvement and psychological development in comparison to when different goals – such as only outcome goals – are used in isolation.

The mechanistic goal-setting theory (Locke & Latham, 1990) proposes that a linear relationship exists between goals and performance. According to the original theory, difficult yet realistic, specific, and measurable goals lead to greater performance improvement when compared to vague, easy, and do-your-best goals, providing that the person who is trying to achieve the goals has accepted and taken ownership of the set goals (Locke & Latham, 1990). These theoretical principles have since been applied to the rehabilitation setting, and existing empirical research has provided support for goal setting being beneficial to athletes when injured (e.g., Beneka et al., 2007; Brewer & Redmond, 2017). This is not surprising, as athletes are naturally goal-driven and frequently use goal setting for performance enhancement. The purpose of this chapter is to discuss how goal setting can be applied within the sport injury rehabilitation context.

DOI: 10.4324/9781003295709-17

The chapter will (a) introduce the purpose of goal setting within the sport injury context, (b) discuss the ways in which injured athletes can benefit from using goal setting during rehabilitation, (c) introduce different types and levels of goals that can be beneficial during rehabilitation, and (d) outline the basic principles of goal setting during rehabilitation.

The Purpose of Rehabilitation Goal Setting

According to the integrated model of psychological response to the sport injury and rehabilitation process (Wiese-Bjornstal et al., 1998), the use of goal setting during rehabilitation is a multifaceted construct. The model proposes that when injured, athlete's use/disuse of psychological strategies (e.g., goal setting, as a behavioral response) can have an impact on their cognitive appraisal of the injury (e.g., ability to adjust their goals or rate of perceived recovery), which can have an impact on their emotional responses to the injury (e.g., feelings of frustration, anger, and attitude). The cyclical relationship between cognitions, emotions, and behaviors also functions in reverse. The use of psychological strategies such as goal setting can also have a direct impact on athletes' emotional response (e.g., facilitate emotional coping), which, in turn, can then affect cognitive appraisal of the injury (e.g., facilitate cognitive coping), which, in turn, can affect behavioral responses (e.g., facilitate behavioral coping). The model also proposes that these cognitive, emotional, and behavioral responses are mediated by a range of personal and situational factors, such as motivation, existing psychological skills, level of competition, and sports medicine team influences (for more details on the integrated model, see Chapter 3).

Given the aforementioned, it is apparent that rehabilitation goal setting can serve multiple purposes for the athlete. Since goal setting is a motivational strategy that can effectively energize athletes to become more productive and effective (Locke & Latham, 1990), its main aim should be to identify clear objectives that facilitate return back to participation both mentally and physically. At its best, a well-planned and well-structured goal-setting plan facilitates full physical and psychological recovery and affords the possibility to make substantial performance gains (Taylor & Taylor, 1997).

Benefits of Goal Setting

Research, while limited, on the use of goal setting during sport injury rehabilitation has shown multiple benefits to the athlete. Setting goals during rehabilitation has been found to have a positive effect on the athlete's physiological and psychological healing (Berengüí et al., 2021; Ievleva & Orlick, 1991). According to Beneka et al. (2007), some of the benefits include pain management when obtaining normal range of motion, muscular strengthening, and numerous sport-related skills. Goal setting can have a positive effect on the overall injury recovery process, as it has been found to enable faster physical recovery and return back to participation (DePalma & DePalma, 1989). Goal setting has also been found to impact athletes' attitude, successful appraisal/acceptance of the injury, overall confidence in the injury recovery, as well as adherence to rehabilitation (Armatas et al., 2007).

Of all the benefits, one of the main reasons goal setting appears to be useful for athletes during rehabilitation is its positive effects on adherence (e.g., Arvinen-Barrow et al., 2010; Niven, 2007). Defined as the "extent to which an individual completes behaviors as part of a treatment regimen designed to facilitate recovery from injury" (Granquist & Brewer, 2013, p. 42), *rehabilitation adherence* is an essential component for successful sport injury rehabilitation. It is therefore not surprising that (a) the relationship between rehabilitation adherence and goal setting has been well supported in the literature (Evans & Hardy, 2002), and (b) goal setting is the only psychosocial intervention that has been shown to enhance rehabilitation adherence (Brewer & Redmond, 2017). Research has found goal setting to provide the athlete with a sense of achievement and accomplishment, which can further increase adherence (Fisher et al., 1993). Goal setting has also been found to facilitate athletes' levels of motivation, effort, and persistence (for more details, see systematic review by Berengüí et al., 2021), which can also be beneficial in enhancing adherence. Over time, the use of goal setting during injury rehabilitation is also thought to increase athletes' levels of self-efficacy and self-confidence (Berengüí et al., 2021), as well as decrease athletes' feelings of 'unspiritedness' (e.g., loss of motivation and apathy; Evans & Hardy, 2002), which have been linked to increased rehabilitation adherence. Moreover, goal setting has been found to affect common rehabilitation objectives, such as communication, rehabilitation outcome assessment, as well as increasing overall rehabilitation adherence (Berengüí et al., 2021; Playford et al., 2000). As research suggests that rehabilitation adherence is a key determinant of whether or not an athlete is able to cope successfully with their rehabilitation (Arvinen-Barrow et al., 2007; Clement et al., 2013; Heaney, 2006; Lafferty et al., 2008), using goal setting during sport injury rehabilitation is highly recommended.

> Goal setting is vital . . . and very useful, very effective . . . because it is certainly for something where they (the athletes) can measure it themselves and see how they are doing Monday, Tuesday, Wednesday, Thursday and then by Friday they are getting the results that they want, so I think that's, that's certainly vital.
>
> (A Chartered Physiotherapist, cited in Arvinen-Barrow et al., 2010, used with permission of Taylor & Francis Informa UK Ltd – Books, from *Psychology of Sport Injury and Rehabilitation* by Monna Arvinen-Barrow and Natalie Walker (eds.), (1st. ed.) Copyright ©2013; permission conveyed through Copyright Clearance Center, Inc.)

Types and Levels of Goals

As sport injury can impact an athlete physically (i.e., restricts movement and use of the injured and/or the surrounding area), psychologically (i.e., changes in cognitive appraisals and mood), tangibly (i.e., restricts the accomplishment of typical daily tasks), and even financially (i.e., loss of income due to inability to work), an awareness of different types of rehabilitation goals is imperative for athletes with injuries, sports medicine professionals (SMPs), sport psychology professionals (SPPs), and any other sport professionals (SPs) working with injured athletes. According to Taylor and Taylor (1997), physical goals can provide the athlete with a clear direction for the physical aspects of recovery, whilst psychological goals can assist with issues associated with motivation, self-confidence, focus, stress, and anxiety, to name a few. Equally, performance-related goals can benefit the athlete by identifying potential areas for improvement in different areas of performance (e.g., technical and tactical development, specific physical conditioning, mental training, and return-to-form), which, during regular training, might not have received priority.

Although setting different types of goals can provide clear objectives for the rehabilitation (Flint, 1998), it is also necessary to think about how the goals can be accomplished. Typically, the ultimate aim of any rehabilitation is to heal and return to participation, which often can be a long-term process. To ensure adherence to the rehabilitation program, many athletes with injuries need daily encouragement (Hamson-Utley & Vazques, 2008). During sport injury rehabilitation, different levels of goals should also be considered (see Figure 14.1), namely, recovery, stage, daily, and lifestyle goals (Taylor & Taylor, 1997). Recovery goals are associated with the final level of recovery (long-term goals), stage goals consist of specific objectives for each of the different stages of rehabilitation (medium-term goals), and daily goals relate to everyday objectives and targets for each rehabilitation session (short-term goals). Often, daily goals can be overlooked; however, they should be set and evaluated to ensure that stage and recovery goals will be successfully attained. In addition, Taylor and Taylor (1997) recommend that goals related to the athlete's lifestyle should also be considered, as, often, existing lifestyle (i.e., sleep, diet, alcohol and drug use, relationships, work and school commitments) can either assist or hinder rehabilitation adherence and, ultimately, have an adverse

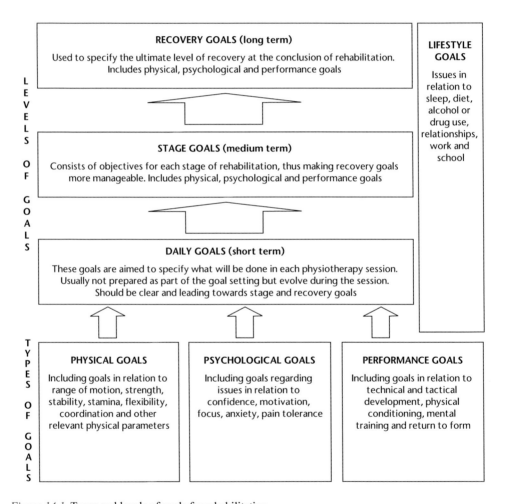

Figure 14.1 Types and levels of goals for rehabilitation.

effect on recovery outcome. White and Black (2004) also recommend identifying and setting goals for employment, social and leisure activities, and general household tasks as useful for athletes with injuries.

The Process for Using Goal Setting for Rehabilitation

Setting effective goals during injury rehabilitation should follow a systematic and organized sequence of events. These can be conceptualized in four phases: (1) assess and identify athletes' personal and physical needs for successful rehabilitation and recovery; (2) identify and set appropriate physical, psychological, and performance goals; (3) consider factors that may influence goal setting effectiveness; and (4) follow a step-by-step program to integrate goal setting into injury rehabilitation. What follows is a detailed description of the steps to provide the reader with guidance on how to improve the usefulness of goal setting in injury rehabilitation.

Phase 1: Assess and Identify Athletes' Personal and Physical Needs

One of the ways in which the assessment and identification of athletes' personal and physical needs can be facilitated is through the use of rehabilitation profiling (Taylor & Taylor, 1997). Founded in the principles of performance profiling (Butler et al., 1993), rehabilitation profiling can help SPPs and SMPs in understanding athlete perceptions of their current personal and physical factors influencing rehabilitation and recovery. Profiling provides a visual display of factors that are deemed important during rehabilitation. Once the important factors have been identified, they can provide a foundation for subsequent goal setting for the rehabilitation team (for more details, see Kamphoff et al., 2013).

Phase 2: Identifying and Setting Effective Goals: Key Characteristics

Once the athlete's important factors have been identified, it is important to ensure the planned goals are appropriate for the athlete. A number of guidelines on effective goals have been proposed in the literature (Cox, 2012; Gould, 1986; Heil, 1993b; Taylor & Taylor, 1997), all of which follow these general principles:

- Understand the importance of setting the right type of goals.
- Set goals that are specific and measurable.
- Set challenging but realistic and attainable goals.
- Set goals that are stated in a positive manner.
- Focus on the degree of, rather than on the absolute, attainment of goals.

Understand the Importance of Setting the Right Type of Goals

Flint (1998) argues that it is important to set both short- and long-term goals and, when possible, to link goals with aspects of the athlete's performance with which they are familiar (e.g., designing goals to enhance important aspects of the athlete's sport). Flint also suggests that greater emphasis should be placed on process goals since they are more likely to be within the athlete's own control and are directly linked with effort. Process goals should be linked with outcome goals and, as such, should be set for all levels of rehabilitation (short-, intermediate-, and long-term; Taylor & Taylor, 1997). The aforementioned is also supported by empirical research, as Evans et al. (2000) found support for the use of long-term, short-term, process, and performance goals during sport injury rehabilitation.

Set Goals that are Specific and Measurable

Locke and Latham (1990) proposed that vague and unmeasurable goals are not as effective as specific and measurable goals. Without the ability to measure progress, the athlete may easily feel that rehabilitation is not progressing, thus leading to decreased levels of motivation and disengagement (a behavioral response), as well as negative changes in mood (an emotional response) and irrational thoughts associated with injury, recovery, and self (a cognitive appraisal). Ensuring the goals are specific and measurable allows the athlete to evaluate progress and therefore sustain effort throughout the different phases of rehabilitation.

Set Challenging but Realistic and Attainable Goals

Existing literature appears to be in an agreement that goals that are too easy or too difficult can lead to decreased levels of motivation and thus lead to the athlete "giving up" before they even start (e.g., Cox, 2012; Gould, 1986; Heil, 1993b; Taylor & Taylor, 1997). Ensuring that goals meet the athlete's needs is of particular importance during injury rehabilitation, when their thoughts, emotions, and behaviors may already be uncharacteristic to their typical responses, owing to the injury.

Set Goals That Are Stated in a Positive Manner

Rehabilitation goals should also be set in a positive manner, with focus on what should be achieved rather than what should be avoided (Brewer & Redmond, 2017; Taylor & Taylor, 1997). Given that athletes may engage in negative self-talk during rehabilitation, using positive and functional terminology in goal setting can also assist in challenging negative and maladaptive thoughts (for more on self-talk, see Chapter 15).

Focus on the Degree, Rather Than on the Absolute Attainment, of Goals

Despite the importance of setting goals with a clear timetable for completion, it is common for a rehabilitation process to progress faster or slower than originally predicted. According to Gilbourne and Taylor (1998), "recovery is typified by an unpredictable mix of rapid progress and disappointing setbacks" (p. 135), and as such, research tends to be in favor of adopting a flexible approach to goal setting during rehabilitation (Heil, 1993a). The emphasis should be on the degree of, rather than absolute, attainment of goals to ensure desired outcomes remain reachable and meaningful for the athlete (e.g., making gradual percentage gains in range of motion). A qualitative study by Evans et al. (2000) found goal flexibility to be greatly beneficial during recovery setbacks and in dealing with unpredictable physical factors, such as swelling, soreness, and pain.

Phase 3: Identify and Consider Factors Affecting Goal Setting Effectiveness

In addition to setting effective goals, it is also important to identify and consider several other factors that can have an impact on goal setting effectiveness. These include ensuring goal setting is fully integrated into rehabilitation, considering goal setting as an individualized mutual sharing and dynamic process, understanding the importance of goal acceptance, monitoring and evaluating set goals regularly, and being aware of variability in goal setting effectiveness.

Ensure Goal Setting Is Fully Integrated into Rehabilitation

For goal setting to be successful, it is vital that athletes, SPPs, and SMPs regard goal setting as an integral part of rehabilitation. Goal setting as a psychological technique is easily paired with a behavioral outcome that can be directly linked to rehabilitation process or outcome (e.g., setting appropriate rehabilitation goals will help speed up the recovery process and improve adherence). Existing research findings indicate that many SMPs (Arvinen-Barrow, Hemmings et al., 2007; Arvinen-Barrow, Penny et al., 2010; Hamson-Utley et al., 2008) and athletes (Arvinen-Barrow et al., 2015) use goal setting during rehabilitation. Therefore, encouraging motivating athletes, SPPs, and SMPs to integrate systematic goal setting into rehabilitation and return to participation process should not be difficult if they are appropriately educated about the process and benefits of goal setting.

Consider Goal Setting as an Individualized Mutual Sharing and Dynamic Process

Flint (1998) believes that goal setting should include specific details on *how* goals are to be achieved, and this process should be educational. Sport medicine professionals involved in the process need to work together *with* the athlete to establish realistic goals for the rehabilitation program (Kolt, 2004). Through a good understanding of the goal setting process and establishing a clear desired outcome, an athlete is more likely to comply with the rehabilitation program (for more details on patient education, see Chapter 13). Evidence outside of sport injury rehabilitation has found that by using "shared decision-making" in goal setting during rehabilitation, patients have reported greater improvements in functional outcomes, an increased ownership over the decision-making process, and increases in motivation and confidence (Rose et al., 2017).

Involving the athlete in the goal setting process will also facilitate communication. When done effectively, communication can (a) increase athletes' understanding and awareness of the injury and rehabilitation process and (b) lead to better trust and rapport between the athlete and the SPPs or SMPs involved in injury rehabilitation. The systematic review by Joseph-Williams et al. (2014) found that one of the more frequently reported barriers to effective communication and collaboration between a healthcare professional and the patient is clients' cognitive appraisal of seeing the healthcare professional as an expert and perception of their own lack of knowledge to contribute meaningfully (Joseph-Williams et al., 2014). Through "shared decision-making" in goal setting, the aforementioned barrier can be addressed, and communication enhanced, thus resulting in better rehabilitation outcomes.

Goal setting during rehabilitation is also a process that evolves over time and is impacted by a number of personal (e.g., injury factors and individual differences) and situational (e.g., rehabilitation team influences) factors. Owing to this dynamic process, any goal setting during rehabilitation should be individualized and should attempt to incorporate all factors needed for successful return to participation (Jeong et al., 2021).

It appears that goal setting is often used by athletes (Arvinen-Barrow et al., 2015) and SMPs during rehabilitation, although, at times, in an unstructured way (Arvinen-Barrow et al., 2010). Setting goals during rehabilitation appears to be SMP-mandated rather than a result of a mutual dialogue between the athlete and the SMP (Arvinen-Barrow et al., 2010). Sport coaches have also highlighted the need to use goal setting during injury rehabilitation, but their role in the process has not been systematic in nature (Podlog & Dionigi, 2010). For goal setting to be effective, including the athlete, coach, and all other relevant sports medicine and sports team members in the process is vital.

Understand the Importance of Goal Acceptance

For goal setting to be successful, the athletes involved would have to accept the set goals, as without goal commitment, goal setting will be ineffective (Gilbourne et al., 1996). To increase commitment to rehabilitation goals, athletes with injuries need to feel that their opinions are valued and that their input is an integral part of the rehabilitation process as a whole (Wayda et al.,

---

I, ____(Injured athlete)____ agree to diligently fulfil my responsibilities in the rehabilitation

of my injury. These responsibilities include:

1. Taking full control of all aspects of my rehabilitation

2. Precise adherence to the rehabilitation programme designed for me

3. Attendance at all scheduled physiotherapy sessions

4. Completion of all exercises outside the rehabilitation facility

5. Full effort, focus, and intensity with all aspects of my rehabilitation regimen

6. Consistent pursuit of the goals I set in my rehabilitation goal setting programme

7. Developing psychological areas that impact my recovery and return to sport (for

    example, addressing re-injury anxieties)

8. Improving myself as an athlete during rehabilitation

9. Seeking out assistance from others when difficulties arise

I, _(Rehabilitation Professional)_ agree to diligently fulfil my responsibilities as the

rehabilitation professional in the rehabilitation of _____'s injury. These

responsibilities include:

1. Designing an individualised rehabilitation programme for the injured athlete

2. Educating the athlete about all relevant aspects of the rehabilitation process

3. Helping to establish a series of goals that will progressively lead to full recovery and

    return to sport

4. Creating a rehabilitation team with other relevant professionals

5. Being sensitive and responsive to psychological and emotional needs

6. Assisting the athlete in overcoming physical and psychological obstacles that may arise

    during rehabilitation

7. Providing the athlete with the information and skills to facilitate physical,

    psychological, and performance contributors to a successful return to sport

_____   _____

Athlete   Date

_____   _____

Rehabilitation Professional   Date

Figure 14.2 An example of a rehabilitation contract.

Copyright ©1997. Reprinted with permission from Jim Taylor, Psychological Approaches to Sports Injury Rehabilitation. Aspen Publishers Inc.

1998). These feelings of shared ownership of the goal setting process can facilitate higher levels of commitment and motivation, which, in turn, can increase rehabilitation adherence. Moreover, as goal setting is a process that should include all individuals involved in the rehabilitation, it is equally important to ensure SPPs and SMPs working with the athlete are *also* committed to the goals (Flint, 1998). A written contract to which both the athlete and the SPP or SMP are bound may be a useful tool to help promote goal commitment, adherence, motivation, and accountability in a positive way. When both parties are clear of the expectations placed upon them during rehabilitation, the recovery is likely to progress with fewer complications.

Monitor and Evaluate Set Goals Regularly

In order to maintain goal commitment, assess goal setting effectiveness, and attain goal appropriateness during the different phases of rehabilitation (for more details on different phases of rehabilitation, see Kamphoff et al., 2013), it is important to monitor, evaluate, and adjust goals during rehabilitation (Flint, 1998; Gould, 1986; Heil, 1993b; Jeong et al., 2021). Through monitoring, evaluation, and regular feedback, the athlete can better understand and appreciate their progress and subsequently increase their feelings of personal achievement, motivation, and attitude toward recovery. This can positively influence commitment, treatment compliance, and adherence, as well as overall recovery outcomes. Revisiting the written contract between the athlete and the SPP/SMP can help facilitate evaluation of previous goals and provide a guidepost for adjusting future goal-setting activities.

Be Aware of Variability in Goal Setting Effectiveness

Despite the apparent benefits of goal setting during rehabilitation, it is important to note that goal setting might not always be effective. Johnson (2000) investigated the effects of short-term psychological interventions on athletes' mood and found that when used in isolation, goal setting had no significant effects. However, when used in combination with other psychological interventions (e.g., stress management strategies, self-talk, relaxation techniques or imagery), goal setting was found to have the potential to help elevate athletes' mood during rehabilitation.

It is also important to note that not always do athletes, SPPs, and SMPs view the effectiveness of psychological interventions equally. Francis et al. (2000) found that SMPs regarded the use of short-term goals as an effective technique for treatment and believed that athletes who set goals during rehabilitation were more likely to cope better with their injuries. Conversely, the athletes in the study viewed goal setting as useful for coping with injuries but rated the importance of setting short-term goals considerably lower than the SMPs. Nevertheless, if the basic guidelines of systematic goal setting phases as outlined in this chapter are followed, these differences in opinions about the effectiveness will be highlighted, and as a result, adjustments to the goal setting program can be made to ensure it meets the needs of everyone involved.

Phase 4: A Step-by-Step Program to Integrate Goal Setting into Injury Rehabilitation

When setting goals for rehabilitation, the aforementioned principles can ensure goals are set appropriately for each athlete in a way that meets their individualized needs. The process for setting effective goals should always begin with a conversation between the SMP and the athlete in which critical physical aspects of rehabilitation will be discussed and explained (Taylor & Taylor, 1997). This should be followed by setting clear goals for each of the components of physical recovery: range of motion, strength, stability, stamina, flexibility, and any other relevant physical parameters. Psychological goals should be discussed in a similar manner, and depending on the rehabilitation setting, the athlete could discuss these with SPP or SMP or with their interprofessional rehabilitation team. Secondly, strategies for achieving goals need to be agreed upon and learned by athletes. By doing so, the athlete is more likely to feel a sense of control (Boyle, 2003; Kolt & Andersen, 2004), which has been found to have an effect on rehabilitation adherence. Thirdly, and perhaps most importantly, the set goals need to be revised and assessed on a regular basis in order for them to be effective (Gould, 1986). Monitoring, evaluation, and adjusting goals can be done through various methods, such as diaries, meetings, graphs, and rehabilitation contracts (Butler, 1997).

Process of Goal Setting during Sport Injury Rehabilitation

1. Start with a conversation between the rehabilitation professionals and the athlete.
2. Set clear goals for each of the components of physical recovery: range of motion, strength, stability, stamina, flexibility, and any other relevant physical parameters.
3. Discuss psychological goals in a similar manner. You can, if you wish, use a tool such as rehabilitation profiling (for more details, see Kamphoff et al., 2013).
4. Agree upon any strategies needed for achieving goals.
5. Remember to monitor, evaluate, and adjust goals regularly.

Source: Original text from Taylor and Taylor (1997) and the table from Arvinen-Barrow & Hemmings (2013). Copyright ©2013 from *Psychology of Sport Injury and Rehabilitation* by Monna Arvinen-Barrow and Natalie Walker (eds.). Reproduced by permission of Taylor and Francis Group, LLC, a division of Informa plc. This permission does not cover any third party copyrighted work which may appear in the material requested. User is responsible for obtaining permission for such material separately from this grant.

Conclusion

The importance of setting goals during sport injury rehabilitation has been highlighted in the past literature (Brewer & Redmond, 2017). While very little published research has been conducted in the past decade, empirical evidence in support can be found in earlier research investigating athletes representing a range of sports and various competitive levels (for more details, see systematic review by Berengüí et al., 2021). For many athletes, the hardest thing is to try to pace their recovery appropriately and not to progress too fast (Samples, 1987; cited in Wagman & Khelifa, 1996, p. 257). Through goal setting, appropriate pace of progression can be identified and monitored. Since goal setting often forms an integral part of an athlete's everyday training when not injured, it makes sense to continue similar procedures during rehabilitation. Thus, the integration of goal setting into the rehabilitation process is not only profitable but, with the right guidance and support, should also be easily transferable (Taylor & Taylor, 1997).

Case Study

Dadi is a 32-year-old military service member with aspirations to join the country's elite special operations unit. As a condition of approving their request to attend the selection process, Dadi's commanding officer has stipulated that in order to demonstrate their abilities and commitment, Dadi must first attend and pass a notoriously difficult small unit tactics and leadership course. Dadi has attempted this small unit tactics and leadership course twice before. The first attempt was cut short due to an extremely poisonous spider bite, and the second attempt ended prematurely due to grade III ankle sprain. Dadi's doctor and physical therapist have advised that full recovery could take up to six weeks, and that Dadi should use an Aircast for the first two weeks. Dadi has been ignoring their doctor and physical therapist's advice by returning to regular exercise a mere three days after the injury. When asked why Dadi was not wearing the Aircast, Dadi replied, "It is useless. It gets in the way and doesn't do anything anyway."

Six weeks later, Dadi is still not ready to return to the leadership course. The ankle continues to be sore, swells up from time to time, and Dadi is still experiencing significant localized pain. Dadi has also become increasingly agitated, losing their temper over minor hassles and with their squad-mates while on duty. Dadi has also started to do long road marches and runs alone after duty hours and, upon returning to their room, regularly consumes alcohol to dull the pain.

During a weekend barbeque with a few friends from the unit, after a couple of beers, Dadi shares their doubts about attempting the small unit tactics and leadership course for the third time. "The next leadership course is in two months. My road march and run times are slow, no matter how hard I train. The pain seems to be increasing and not decreasing. I am just not good enough to do this. It's my third attempt . . . so what is the point of even trying if I can't graduate?" Dadi confides to their friends. "I mean . . . I am trying, doing more than asked, and get nowhere. I might as well not re-enlist and quit the military when my contract expires."

Questions

1. What key elements of Dadi's experience would you want to address with goal setting?
2. With reference to the integrated model of psychological response to sport injury and rehabilitation, what factors from Dadi's experience may have affected their cognitive appraisal?
3. What types of goals could be beneficial for Dadi, and why?
4. In Dadi's case, what factors do you think are important to consider for goal setting effectiveness?

References

Armatas, V., Chondrou, E., Yiannakos, A., Galazoulas, C., & Velkopoulos, C. (2007). Psychological aspects of rehabilitation following serious athletic injuries with special reference to goal setting: A review study. *Physical Training*. http://ejmas.com/pt/ptframe.htm

Arvinen-Barrow, M., Clement, D., Hamson-Utley, J. J., Zakrajsek, R. A., Lee, S. M., Kamphoff, C., . . . Martin, S. B. (2015). Athletes' use of mental skills during sport injury rehabilitation. *Journal of Sport Rehabilitation, 24*(2), 189–197. https://doi.org/10.1123/jsr.2013-0148

Arvinen-Barrow, M., Hemmings, B., Weigand, D. A., Becker, C. A., & Booth, L. (2007). Views of chartered physiotherapists on the psychological content of their practice: A national follow-up survey in the United Kingdom. *Journal of Sport Rehabilitation, 16*(2), 111–121. https://doi.org/10.1123/jsr.16.2.111

Arvinen-Barrow, M., Penny, G., Hemmings, B., & Corr, S. (2010). UK chartered physiotherapists' personal experiences in using psychological interventions with injured athletes: An interpretative phenomenological analysis. *Psychology of Sport and Exercise, 11*(1), 58–66. https://doi.org/10.1016/j.psychsport.2009.05.004

Beneka, A., Malliou, P., Bebetsos, E., Gioftsidou, A., Pafis, G., & Godolias, G. (2007). Appropriate counselling techniques for specific components of the rehabilitation plan: A review of the literature. *Physical Training*. http://ejmas.com/pt/ptframe.htm

Berengüí, R., Castejón, M. A., & Martínez-Alvarado, J. R. (2021). Goal setting in sport injury rehabilitation: A systematic review. *Journal of Physical Education and Sport*, *21*(6), 3569–3576. https://doi.org/10.7752/jpes.2021.06482

Boyle, S. (2003). Goal setting: The injured athlete. *Swim*, *20*(1), 18–19.

Brewer, B. W., & Redmond, C. J. (2017). *Psychology of sport injury*. Human Kinetics.

Butler, R. J. (1997). Psychological principles applied to sports injuries. In S. French (Ed.), *Physiotherapy: A psychosocial approach* (2nd ed., pp. 155–168). Butterworth-Heinemann.

Butler, R. J., Smith, M., & Irwin, I. (1993). The performance profile in practice. *Journal of Applied Sport Psychology*, *5*(1), 48–63. https://doi.org/10.1080/10413209308411304

Clement, D., Granquist, M., & Arvinen-Barrow, M. (2013). Psychosocial aspects of athletic injuries as perceived by athletic trainers. *Journal of Athletic Training*, *48*(4), 512–521. https://doi.org/10.4085/1062-6050-48.3.21

Cox, R. H. (2012). *Sport psychology: Concepts and applications* (6th ed.). McGraw-Hill.

DePalma, M. T., & DePalma, B. (1989). The use of instruction and the behavioural approach to facilitate injury recovery. *Athletic Training*, *24*, 217–219.

Evans, L., & Hardy, L. (2002). Injury rehabilitation: A goal-setting intervention study. *Research Quarterly for Exercise and Sport*, *73*(3), 310–319. https://doi.org/10.1080/02701367.2002.10609025

Evans, L., Hardy, L., & Flemming, S. (2000). Intervention strategies with injured athletes: An action research study. *The Sport Psychologist*, *14*(2), 188–206. https://doi.org/10.1123/tsp.14.2.188

Fisher, A. C., Mullins, S. A., & Frye, P. A. (1993). Athletic trainers' attitudes and judgements of injured athletes' rehabilitation adherence. *Journal of Athletic Training*, *28*(1), 43–47. https://pubmed.ncbi.nlm.nih.gov/16558203/

Flint, F. A. (1998). Specialized psychological interventions. In F. A. Flint (Ed.), *Psychology of sport injury* (pp. 29–50). Human Kinetics.

Francis, S. R., Andersen, M. B., & Maley, B. (2000). Physiotherapists' and male professional athletes' views on psychological skills for rehabilitation. *Journal of Science and Medicine in Sport*, *3*(1), 17–29. https://doi.org/10.1016/S1440-2440(00)80044-4

Gilbourne, D., & Taylor, A. H. (1998). From theory to practice: The integration of goal perspective theory and life development approaches within an injury specific goal-setting program. *Journal of Applied Sport Psychology*, *10*(1), 124–139. https://doi.org/10.1080/10413209808406381

Gilbourne, D., Taylor, A. H., Downie, G., & Newton, P. (1996). Goal-setting during sports injury rehabilitation: A presentation of underlying theory, administration procedure, and an athlete case study. *Sports Exercise and Injury*, *2*, 192–201.

Gould, D. (1986). Goal setting for peak performance. In J. M. Williams (Ed.), *Applied sport psychology: Personal growth to peak performance* (pp. 133–148). Mayfield.

Granquist, M. D., & Brewer, B. W. (2013). Psychological aspects of rehabilitation adherence. In M. Arvinen-Barrow & N. Walker (Eds.), *The psychology of sport injury and rehabilitation* (pp. 40–53). Routledge.

Hamson-Utley, J. J., Martin, S., & Walters, J. (2008). Athletic trainers' and physical therapists' perceptions of the effectiveness of psychological skills within sport injury rehabilitation programs. *Journal of Athletic Training*, *43*(3), 258–264. https://doi.org/10.4085/1062-6050-43.3.258

Hamson-Utley, J. J., & Vazques, L. (2008). The comeback: Rehabilitating the psychological Injury. *Athletic Therapy Today*, *13*(5), 35–38. https://doi.org/doi.org/10.1123/att.13.5.35

Heaney, C. (2006). Physiotherapists' perceptions of sport psychology intervention in professional soccer. *International Journal of Sport and Exercise Psychology*, *4*(1), 73–86. https://doi.org/10.1080/1612197X.2006.9671785

Heil, J. (1993a). A comprehensive approach to injury management. In J. Heil (Ed.), *Psychology of sport injury* (pp. 137–149). Human Kinetics.

Heil, J. (Ed.). (1993b). *Psychology of sport injury*. Human Kinetics.

Ievleva, L., & Orlick, T. (1991). Mental links to enhanced healing: An exploratory study. *The Sport Psychologist*, *5*(1), 25–40. https://doi.org/10.1123/tsp.5.1.25

Jeong, Y. H., Healy, L. C., & McEwan, D. (2021). The application of goal setting theory to goal setting interventions in sport: A systematic review. *International Review of Sport and Exercise Psychology*. https://doi.org/10.1080/1750984X.2021.1901298

Johnson, U. (2000). Short-term psychological intervention: A study of long-term-injured athletes. *Journal of Sport Rehabilitation*, *9*(3), 207–218. https://doi.org/10.1123/jsr.9.3.207

Joseph-Williams, N., Elwyn, G., & Edwards, A. (2014). Knowledge is not power for patients: A systematic review and thematic synthesis of patient-reported barriers and facilitators to shared decision making. *Patient Education and Counseling*, *94*(3), 291–309. https://doi.org/10.1016/j.pec.2013.10.031

Kamphoff, C., Thomae, J., & Hamson-Utley, J. J. (2013). Integrating the psychological and physiological aspects of sport injury rehabilitation: Rehabilitation profiling and phases of rehabilitation. In M. Arvinen-Barrow & N. Walker (Eds.), *Psychology of sport injury and rehabilitation* (pp. 134–155). Routledge.

Kolt, G. S. (2004). Injury from sport, exercise, and physical activity. In G. S. Kolt & M. B. Andersen (Eds.), *Psychology in the physical and manual therapies* (pp. 247–267). Churchill Livingstone.

Kolt, G. S., & Andersen, M. B. (Eds.). (2004). *Psychology in the physical and manual therapies*. Churchill Livingstone Inc.

Lafferty, M. E., Kenyon, R., & Wright, C. J. (2008). Club-based and non-clubbased physiotherapists' views on the psychological content of their practice when treating sports injuries. *Research in Sports Medicine*, *16*(4), 295–306. https://doi.org/10.1080/15438620802523378

Locke, E. A., & Latham, G. P. (1985). The application of goal-setting to sports. *Journal of Sport Psychology*, *7*(3), 205–222. https://doi.org/10.1123/jsp.7.3.205

Locke, E. A., & Latham, G. P. (1990). *A theory of goal setting and task performance*. Prentice Hall.

Niven, A. (2007). Rehabilitation adherence in sport injury: Sport physiotherapists' perceptions. *Journal of Sport Rehabilitation*, *16*(2), 93–110. https://doi.org/10.1123/jsr.16.2.93

Playford, E. D., Dawson, L., Limbert, V., Smith, M., Ward, C. C., & Wells, R. (2000). Goal-setting in rehabilitation: Report of a workshop to explore professionals perceptions of goal-setting. *Clinical Rehabilitation*, *14*(5), 491–496. https://doi.org/10.1191/0269215500cr343oa

Podlog, L., & Dionigi, R. (2010). Coach strategies for addressing psychosocial challenges during the return to sport from injury. *Journal of Sports Sciences*, *28*(11), 1197–1208. https://doi.org/10.1080/02640414.2010.487873

Rose, A., Rosewilliam, S., & Soundy, A. (2017). Shared decision making within goal setting in rehabilitation settings: A systematic review. *Patient Education and Counseling*, *100*(1), 65–75. https://doi.org/10.1016/j.pec.2016.07.030

Taylor, J., & Taylor, S. (1997). *Psychological approaches to sports injury rehabilitation*. Aspen.

Wagman, D., & Khelifa, M. (1996). Psychological issues in sport injury rehabilitation: Current knowledge and practice. *Journal of Athletic Training*, *31*(3), 257–261.

Wayda, V., Armenth-Brothers, F., & Boyce, B. A. (1998). Goal setting: A key to injury rehabilitation. *Athletic Therapy Today*, *3*(1), 21–25. https://doi.org/10.1123/att.3.1.21

Weinberg, R. S., & Gould, D. (2019). *Foundations of sport and exercise psychology* (7th ed.). Human Kinetics.

White, C. A., & Black, E. K. (2004). Cognitive and behavioral interventions. In G. S. Kolt & M. B. Andersen (Eds.), *Psychology in the physical and manual therapies* (pp. 93–109). Churchill Livingstone.

Wiese-Bjornstal, D. M., Smith, A. M., Shaffer, S. M., & Morrey, M. A. (1998). An integrated model of response to sport injury: Psychological and sociological dynamics. *Journal of Applied Sport Psychology*, *10*(1), 46–69. https://doi.org/10.1080/10413209808406377

Williamson, O., Swannb, C., Bennett, K. J. M., Birda, M. D., Goddard, S. G., Schweickle, M. J., & Jackman, P. C. (2022). The performance and psychological effects of goal setting insport: A systematic review and meta-analysis. *International Review of Sport and Exercise Psychology*. https://doi.org/0.1080/1750984X.2022.2116723

15 Self-Talk in Sport Injury and Rehabilitation

Kylee J. Ault-Baker, Natalie C. Walker,
and Joanne Hudson

Chapter Objectives

- To define self-talk in the context of sport injury and rehabilitation.
- To describe different types and functions of self-talk and self-talk techniques in sport injury and rehabilitation.
- To outline the roles of sports medicine and sport psychology professionals in using self-talk during sport injury rehabilitation.

Introduction

It is commonly understood that most athletes engage in some form of self-talk. Sports medicine (SMP) and sport psychology professionals (SPP) and researchers are also aware that the thoughts of an injured athlete may have a significant influence on emotions, behaviors, and recovery outcomes (Wiese-Bjornstal et al., 1998). However, the extent, frequency, content, and type of self-talk can vary depending on the situation and the individual (Zinsser et al., 2006), and factors such as competitive level and skill type moderate self-talk use (Tod et al., 2011). The purpose of this chapter is to discuss how self-talk can be beneficial for sport injury rehabilitation. The chapter will (a) define self-talk, (b) introduce the different categories (types and functions) of self-talk, (c) discuss the use of self-talk during rehabilitation, and (d) outline the process of self-talk use during rehabilitation.

Concept Definitions

According to Theodorakis et al. (2000), self-talk is "what people say to themselves either out loud or as a small voice inside their head" (p. 254). This definition highlights two aspects of self-talk. First, self-talk is expressed either overtly or covertly, and second, self-talk is comprised of statements that are addressed to oneself and not to other people in the form of conversation. Hackford and Schwenkmezger (1993) defined self-talk as a "dialogue [through which] the individual interprets feelings and perceptions, regulates and changes evaluations and convictions, and gives him/herself instructions and reinforcement" (p. 355). This definition offers both the notion that self-talk is concerned with making self-statements but also alludes to some of the specific uses of self-talk. Rooted in the preceding definitions and existing research, in this chapter, self-talk is defined as intrapersonal conversation that (a) represents verbalizations or statements addressed to the self, (b) is multidimensional in nature (e.g., with frequency and valence

DOI: 10.4324/9781003295709-18

properties), (c) has interpretive elements associated with the content of statements employed, (d) is dynamic, and (e) serves a function for the athlete (i.e., can be instructional and/or motivational; Hardy, 2006).

Categorizing Self-Talk: Types and Functions

Existing literature has suggested that self-talk should be categorized based on its overtness, grammatical form, self-determination, valence, and function (Van Raalte et al., 2016). What follows here is a brief discussion of different categories of self-talk as they relate to sport injury rehabilitation.

Overt and Covert Self-Talk

According to Hardy (2006), self-talk can be categorized by how self-statements are verbalized. At one end of the continuum, athletes might talk to themselves in a very *overt* fashion (i.e., externally verbalized statements), allowing others to hear what is said. At the other end of the continuum, athletes may talk to themselves *covertly*, when the verbalizations are either a small voice inside one's head or an inner dialogue that cannot be heard by others. It is likely that an athlete engages in one or both types of self-talk. To date, research has yet to provide conclusive evidence related to the effectiveness of overt compared to covert self-talk in the sport domain. However, based on similar principles in goal setting, where public goals are more effective than private goals (Kyllo & Landers, 1995), it might be expected that when statements are overt, there could be some evaluation of the individual's performance related to those statements. In this case, the individual might exert more effort to achieve the desired behaviors, such as adherence to rehabilitation, that are associated with overtly expressed statements.

Grammatical Form

Categorizing self-talk based on its *grammatical form* refers to the use of tense (e.g., present, future), person pronouns (e.g., first person, third person, collective), and style (e.g., interrogative, persuasive) used when engaging in self-talk. While most of the research has been conducted outside of sport (Van Raalte et al., 2016), evidence that does exist suggests that grammatical form may influence factors that have also been found to be important for sport injury rehabilitation. This includes self-talk's influence on performance, stress appraisals, self-efficacy, and collective efficacy (see Van Raalte et al., 2016), all of which are key psychosocial factors in sport injury, rehabilitation, and return to participation process (see Brewer & Redmond, 2017).

Assigned and Self-Determined Self-Talk

The level of self-determination (i.e., if the self-talk is "assigned" or "freely chosen"; Hardy, 2006) can also have an influence on how self-talk affects sport injury rehabilitation. Assigned self-talk is where the individual has no self-determined control over the statements (i.e., the statements are given to the athlete by someone else, such as an SMP or an SPP). Freely chosen self-talk is where the individual has completely determined their self-talk (i.e., comprised of their own statements). Often, self-talk statements can be an amalgamation of the two, as if on a continuum from completely assigned to completely freely chosen. Despite limited research on whether assigned or self-determined self-talk is more effective, it is more likely that an athlete would use more self-determined self-talk in performance settings (Hardy, 2006) and during sport injury rehabilitation. It is also likely that based on the principles of cognitive evaluation theory (Deci & Ryan, 1985), self-determined self-talk will offer more motivational benefits for the athlete (Hardy, 2006). According to cognitive evaluation theory, humans have an innate desire to feel competent and self-determined, and that feelings of self-determination for actions (i.e., behavior) are related to perceptions of control and/or choice. Given that sport injury often results in perceived lack of control (Brewer & Redmond, 2017), theoretically, self-talk chosen by the athlete should have positive effects on their self-determined motivation during sport injury rehabilitation.

Positive and Negative Self-Talk (Valence)

Typically, self-talk has been conceptualized as either positive or negative (Tod et al., 2011). Self-talk as a form of praise (Moran, 1996), that is used to keep one's focus of attention in the present (e.g., "I can do it," "Be present"), has been commonly termed positive self-talk (Weinberg, 1988). In contrast, self-talk in the form of criticism (Moran, 1996), or that presents barriers to achievement by being inappropriate, anxiety-provoking, and/or irrational (e.g., "You are useless! That was awful!"), has been coined negative self-talk (Theodorakis et al., 2000). Existing literature has suggested that self-talk with positive valence is performance-facilitating, whereas self-talk with negative valence is performance-debilitating (Hardy, 2006; Zinsser et al., 2010). In a systematic review of the literature, Tod et al. (2011) confirmed the proposed relationship between positive self-talk and performance. However, the review did not find similar effects between negative self-talk and performance. Van Raalte et al. (2016) suggested that, at times, negative statements can be considered to have a positive valence if they have a facilitative effect on performance outcome and vice versa. Van Raalte et al. (2016) also stated that "self-talk is best defined by the meaning of self-talk statements, rather than confounded with outcome" (p. 142).

In sport injury rehabilitation setting, Ievleva and Orlick (1991) were the first to study the impact of psychological interventions on athletes' recovery from sport injury. In their retrospective study with rehabilitated athletes, they reported a strong positive correlation between recovery time and the use of positive self-talk; the fast-healing athletes had a tendency to be more positive than the slower healers. Positive self-talk has also been found to generate positive emotions that are associated with enhanced quality of rehabilitation (Udry et al., 1997). In support, Rock and Jones (2002b) concluded that psychosocial interventions such as positive self-talk can have a beneficial effect on athletes' psychological well-being, particularly during setbacks in the recovery process (Rock & Jones, 2002b).

Instructional and Motivational Self-Talk (Function)

Self-talk has also been conceptualized in relation to its *function*: *instructional* and/or *motivational*. *Instructional* self-talk is thought to increase attentional focus on relevant technical aspects of performance that has been found to improve the execution of precision-based tasks requiring skill, timing, and accuracy (Hatzigeorgiardis et al., 2004; Theodorakis et al., 2000). *Motivational* self-talk is used to increase effort, enhance confidence, and/or create positive moods (Tod et al., 2011). These two broad functions of self-talk have been further refined into specific functions. Instructional self-talk has been refined into *skills* and *general* functions (Hardy et al., 2001). Skill-specific instructional self-talk statements focus on the technique or a skill and might include statements such as "Keep the hands together." Instructional general self-talk includes statements about strategies that are important for performance, such as, "Stay in second until the last bend." Motivational self-talk has been further refined into three more specific motivational functions – *arousal, mastery*, and *drive* (Hardy et al., 2001). The motivational-arousal function refers to the use of self-talk for psyching up, relaxing, and controlling arousal. The motivational-mastery function relates to mental toughness, focus of attention, confidence, and mental preparation. The motivational-drive function is concerned with goal achievement and consequently is associated with maintaining or increasing drive and effort.

The systematic review by Tod et al. (2011) suggests that both instructional and motivational self-talk has a positive effect on precision-based tasks and gross motor skill performance. Tod et al. (2011) also concluded that instructional self-talk is not consistently more effective than motivational self-talk for precision-based tasks, nor is motivational self-talk more effective than instructional self-talk for gross motor skill tasks (Tod et al., 2011). For strength- and endurance-based tasks, motivational self-talk has been found to be more effective than instructional self-talk (Tod et al., 2011). Hardy et al. (2015) have further suggested that skill level may influence the decision to use instructional or motivational self-talk; their results found that more skilled athletes performed better at a dominant foot-kicking tasks when using motivational self-talk than instructional self-talk.

Goal-Directed and Undirected Self-Talk (Function)

In addition to serving instructional and motivational functions, self-talk has also been proposed as beneficial for guiding goals and goal achievement (Latinjak et al., 2014). More commonly discussed in general psychology literature, *goal-directed* thoughts are considered to be deliberate ways to solve a problem or make progress toward a task or goal. In their research with 87 athletes, Latinjak et al. (2014) found that *goal-directed* thoughts could be organized considering two dimensions: *time orientation* (i.e., past, present, or future oriented) and *activation* (i.e., activation-oriented, not oriented toward any specific activation, and deactivation-oriented). The *time orientation* of goal-directed self-talk accounts for whether or not self-talk statements address reactions to previous events or focus on an outcome to be achieved in the future. The *activation* dimension considers if self-talk statements aim to control or create affective states.

In contrast, *undirected* self-talk is considered to be involuntary, mind-wandering, and stimulus-independent statements, where a task or goal is not spurring the undirected thoughts (Latinjak et al., 2014). Latinjak et al. (2014) found that *undirected* self-talk also consisted of two dimensions: *time perspective* (i.e., anticipatory, present-related, or retrospective) and *valence* (i.e., negative or positive). These self-talk statements were nearly always spontaneous and preceded goal-directed self-talk (Latinjak et al., 2014), thus suggesting that goal-directed self-talk may be a reaction to the undirected self-talk that occurs following an event. Latinjak et al. (2020) extended their earlier research by further identifying situational determinants and functions of goal-directed self-talk. The results from qualitative research with 97 athletes revealed goal-directed self-talk was discussed by the athletes as useful during training, competition – winning or losing – and injury. Both Latinjak et al. (2014) and Latinjak et al. (2020) suggest that injury might be a situational determinant of goal-directed self-talk use. Latinjak et al. (2020) also highlight that goal-directed self-talk may be an effective strategy for helping athletes cope with pain and injury.

Other Functions of Self-Talk

Existing literature has also noted that not all self-talk statements nicely "fit" into positive/negative motivational/instructional self-talk function dichotomies (Van Raalte et al., 2016). Van Raalte et al. (2016) highlight numerous other forms of self-talk that are used by athletes – injured or not – that have received little to no research attention in the sport psychology domain.

These include *self-compassionate, calming, self-protective, task-irrelevant*, and *humorous* self-talk. Other forms of self-talk include *associative* self-talk that focuses on bodily sensations, *dissociative* self-talk (including situation-irrelevant self-talk), and self-talk related to *escape* (Van Raalte et al., 2016), all of which could be beneficial for athletes with injuries during rehabilitation. Lastly, self-talk can also be related to enjoyment/appreciation of the moment, or focused on others, as well as take the form of repeating mantras, counting, making things to do list, and even singing to oneself (Van Raalte et al., 2016).

Benefits of Self-Talk during Sport Injury and Rehabilitation

Since the inaugural research by Ievleva and Orlick (1991), a small but growing amount of empirical studies have investigated the use of self-talk in a sport injury context (see Brewer & Redmond, 2017). The literature that does exist suggests that self-talk is a useful psychological strategy for a number of injury-related clinical outcomes, such as enhancing joint restoration, muscular strengthening, and rehearsing sport-related skills whilst injured, among other functions (Beneka et al., 2007). Beneka et al. (2013) also found self-talk to be beneficial during a balance task and found that both instructional and motivational self-talk significantly improved overall rehabilitation performance of athletes with knee injuries.

The use of self-talk during sport injury and rehabilitation also has psychosocial benefits. For example, it has been found to positively affect mood (Beneka et al., 2013; Naoi & Ostrow, 2008), decrease perceptions of pain (Beneka et al., 2013; Naoi & Ostrow, 2008), and reframe athletes' cognitions during the rehabilitation process (Rock & Jones, 2002a). A series of studies exploring the use of coping strategies by injured athletes have also provided further support for the benefits of self-talk at the elite level. Of the sample of Olympic wrestlers interviewed, 80% stated that they used thought control strategies as a means of coping with their injuries (Gould, Eklund et al., 1993). Rational thinking and self-talk have also been reported as the most popular coping strategies among injured national championship–level figure skaters (Gould, Finch et al., 1993) and athletes who experienced season-ending injuries (Gould et al., 1997).

Models of Self-Talk

Hardy et al. (2009) proposed a conceptual framework with a goal to explain factors believed to mediate performance–self-talk relationship. According to the framework, *personal* factors (e.g., personality, beliefs, preferences, and cognitive processing) and *situational* factors (e.g., setting, coach characteristics) as antecedents influence both *self-talk* and its *cognitive, motivational, behavioral*, and *affectual* consequences. Following a thorough review of the recent self-talk literature, Van Raalte et al. (2016) expanded on the original framework by Hardy et al. (2009). The sport-specific model for self-talk "highlights the dynamic interrelationships" (Van Raalte et al., 2016, p. 141) between self-talk and the various antecedents, mechanisms, and behaviors. Central to the model is *self-talk*, which, as outlined earlier, can serve numerous functions and vary in *valence*, linguistic *grammatical properties*, and *overtness*. The model also assumes that numerous *personal* and *contextual* factors impact two bidirectionally interacting systems. These systems (system 1 and system 2) also influence, and are influenced by, self-talk and behavior. The model also proposed a one-directional relationship between self-talk and behavior, which in turn is proposed to affect contextual factors.

Consistent with the Hardy et al. (2009) conceptualization, the *personal* factors include personality, beliefs, preferences, and cognitive processing. The *contextual* factors consist of the situational factors outlined in the Hardy et al. (2009) framework, including the setting and coach characteristics, among others. The two systems in the sport-specific self-talk model focus on the various deliberate and autonomous mechanisms related to self-talk.

System 2 includes the various *cognitive mechanisms* that are required for information processing. These include *deliberate* mental effort, *rational* thought, and *emotional* neutrality. System 2 is governed by rules and logic, is amenable to change when presented with new information and perspectives, and functions as an unbiased "monitor" of thoughts and behaviors (Van Raalte et al., 2016). Self-talk that is processed in system 2 is categorized into *proactive* and *reactive* self-talk. Proactive self-talk focuses on a specific intention of a future outcome, and reactive self-talk operates in response to system 1–generated self-talk statements that are being processed in system 2. System 1 includes the various *affective mechanisms* that generate associations and impressions with affective valence. System 1 is predominantly automatic, difficult to modify, and possibly even below the level of awareness (Van Raalte et al., 2016). Currently, little research has explicitly investigated the applicability of the systems-based model of self-talk in sport or in sport injury rehabilitation.

Self-Talk Techniques

Since positive self-talk has generally been advocated as more useful than negative self-talk (Zinsser et al., 2010), a common goal of self-talk interventions has been to help athletes reduce negative self-talk and increase more positive self-talk. This practice is not entirely aligned with existing research evidence (Tod et al., 2011), as an inconsistent effect has been detected for the possible benefits of positive self-talk over the use of negative self-talk. Hamilton et al. (2007) describe negative self-talk as "challenging" self-talk, thus providing support for the importance of focusing on the meaning and interpretation of the self-talk's content. For example, following an unacceptable or undesired behavior (e.g., missing a rehabilitation session), an athlete might

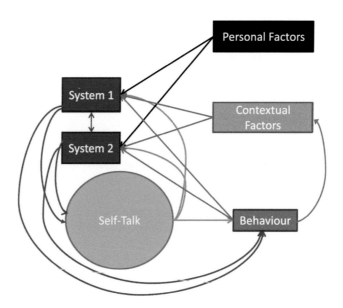

Figure 15.1 Sport-specific model of self-talk.

Source: Reprinted from Psychology of Sport and Exercise, 22, Judy L. Van Raalte, Andrew Vincent, & Britton W. Brewer, Self-talk: Review and sport-specific model, 139–148. Copyright ©(2016) with permission from Elsevier.

give themselves a "talking to" (e.g., "You idiot, this will not help you!"), which can act as a motivator not to repeat the same behavior in the future. This type of self-talk (i.e., negative statements) might only be harmful to some athletes, but for others, it might actually be facilitative (Goodhart, 1986; Van Raalte et al., 2000) and thus *functional*. The following section outlines the use of thought stopping and reframing as two potential techniques for encouraging *functional* self-talk in rehabilitation.

Thought Stopping Steps

1. Increase the athlete's awareness of the inappropriate self-talk they are using. For example, they might keep paperclips in one pocket and transfer a paperclip to the opposite pocket on each use of inappropriate self-talk in rehabilitation (Owens & Bunker, 1989). At the end of the session, the athlete can see how many paperclips they have in the "inappropriate self-talk" pocket, increasing their awareness of its use.
2. Once the athlete is aware of their use of inappropriate self-talk, the second step is to use a trigger to stop the thoughts/talk (i.e., cue word, image, or action). For example, an athlete might say "wait," visualize an image of a stop sign, or snap their fingers as a trigger to stop their inappropriate self-talk statements.
3. Finally, a more functional self-talk statement is then used to replace the previous inappropriate self-talk. This final step is important because when thought stopping techniques are used on their own without supplementary techniques, this is likely to exacerbate the problem of inappropriate self-talk.

Source: Adapted from Hardy et al. (2009). Used with permission of Taylor & Francis Informa UK Ltd – Books, from *Psychology of Sport Injury and Rehabilitation* by Monna Arvinen-Barrow and Natalie Walker (eds.), (1st. ed.) Copyright ©2013; permission conveyed through Copyright Clearance Center Inc.

Thought Stopping Technique

Thought stopping has been proposed to be useful (e.g., Bull et al., 1996) to initially stop an inappropriate thought and then allow a more functional thought to be used in its place. Thought stopping has been advocated as a deliberate self-talk technique to direct sport-related thinking (Zinsser et al., 2006).

Reframing Technique

A common response to injury is anxiety (e.g., anxieties related to pain experienced, lengthy rehabilitation anxieties, the loss of a starting place and changes to daily routines, performance outcome anxieties, pre- and/or post-operative anxiety, fitness demands and returning to peak performance anxiety, and re-injury anxiety). When faced with a potentially anxiety-provoking situation, there is a need to challenge these appraisals. This can be achieved via modifying the athlete's thoughts and self-statements associated with the situation, using reframing. Here the event or behavior stays the same, but the athlete's appraisal of the event or behavior is changed (Jones, 2003). While an abundance of research using reframing in counseling psychology exists, within sport psychology, empirical evidence is limited. There is, however, ample anecdotal evidence reporting the benefits of reframing in sport psychology (e.g., Bull et al., 1996; Porter, 2003; Syer & Connolly, 1998).

In the sport injury and rehabilitation context, an athlete's thoughts before, during, and after injury have been shown to be a critical element of the psychological response to injury

Table 15.1 Reframing Examples during Three Phases of Rehabilitation

Phase of Rehabilitation	Injury Experience	Self-Talk	Reframed Self-Talk
Phase 1	Unhelpful negative thoughts about injury severity, the significance of the injury to their future; blame themselves for injury onset; struggling to cope with the pain of the injury; concerned about the prospect of a difficult and possibly long rehabilitation process.	*"This is agony! I can't believe I went in for that tackle."*	*"I can handle this – I'm tough! I am not the only person ever to be injured. The pain prevents me from doing more damage."*
Phase 2	Loss of motivation; coping with difficult and/or lengthy rehabilitation; anxieties about becoming re-injured during rehabilitation.	*"I can't go on the board. I can't balance. I'm going to fall off and twist it again."*	*"I've balanced on an uneven surface. The board is no different. It's just the same – I can do it!"*
Phase 3	Anxieties and doubts about their return to training and competition.	*"It's not strong enough. I need more rehab before testing it in training."*	*"It has been tested throughout rehabilitation, and it has survived. It is ready."*

Note: Used with permission of Taylor & Francis Informa UK Ltd. – Books, from *Psychology of Sport Injury and Rehabilitation* by Monna Arvinen-Barrow and Natalie Walker (eds.) (1st. ed.). Copyright ©2013; permission conveyed through Copyright Clearance Center Inc.

(see Arvinen-Barrow & Granquist, 2020; Brewer & Redmond, 2017). When injured, athletes often engage in inappropriate self-talk, which is often counterproductive to rehabilitation and recovery. The SMPs and SPPs are instrumental in challenging athletes' inappropriate, self-deprecating, and maladaptive thoughts and statements. By doing so, SMPs and SPPs can reduce the detrimental impact such thoughts can have on emotional and behavioral responses during different phases of rehabilitation (see Chapter 1; Clement & Arvinen-Barrow, 2020; Kamphoff et al., 2013) to both rehabilitation and recovery outcomes (see Chapters 2–6).

Using Self-Talk in Rehabilitation

When incorporating self-talk into injury rehabilitation, SMPs and SPPs should consider several factors to maximize positive benefits. What follow are select critical success factors for SMPs and SPPs to consider.

Self-Talk Should Be Functional

The types and functions of self-talk outlined earlier in this chapter are appropriate in injury rehabilitation. It is likely that athletes will use a mixture of various self-talk statements, and at times, it is common for these to be inappropriate or self-deprecating. When struggling with injury and/or rehabilitation, an athlete might say, "I'm never going to recover from this injury." An athlete may also engage in self-talk that is self-deprecating but is also functional: "Come on, you fool, you can do this! Only four more reps!" As a reminder, negative self-talk is not always debilitative Athletes should also try to engage in more functional self-talk as it is likely to be more facilitative for rehabilitation. The SMP and the SPP can encourage an athlete to engage in many types of functional self-talk for a variety of purposes, as well as challenge the athlete when their self-talk appears to be debilitative to the rehabilitation.

Self-Talk Should Be Self-Determined

Ideally, an athlete with injuries should determine their own self-talk statements. This can be an effective way to increase feelings of autonomy, subsequently resulting in increased motivation (Ryan & Deci, 2002). When an SMP or SPP notices that an athlete's cognitive appraisals of their injury, rehabilitation, and return to sport are increasingly debilitative, the athlete is likely to need help in challenging their thoughts. It is unrealistic to expect an athlete who is engaging in debilitative self-talk to independently restructure their thoughts, so they may need assistance in doing so. While it might be tempting for the SMP or the SPP to assign new self-talk statements to the athlete, better results will be obtained through collaboration, where the athlete has ownership of the process.

Using reframing would be an effective way to help athletes change debilitative self-talk. It can also provide a framework for the athlete to record, explore, and challenge their negative thoughts in a systematic and structured way. Gaining awareness of debilitative self-talk patterns is often the most difficult part of self-talk techniques, so initial recording is a pivotal component of improving functional self-talk (Taylor & Taylor, 1997). After raising awareness, the SMP or SPP should encourage the athlete to reframe their statements into personal functional affirmations (Porter, 2003). The reframed statements should be true, or at least probable and realistic (Crossman, 2001). The athlete might also be encouraged to destroy the debilitative statements and place them in a waste bin (Porter, 2003) and to re-read the restructured functional affirmations daily, reframing any debilitating thoughts that arise. As an example, an athlete with injury might say, "I can't attack the ball anymore because it [head injury] will happen again." A challenged and reframed statement could look like, "I can attack the ball – I've done it loads before – and can make a difference to this game."

Effective Self-Talk Requires Athlete Buy-In

An athlete's belief or expectancy about intervention effectiveness is likely to be a precondition for effectiveness (e.g., Oikawa, 2004). If an athlete with injuries does not expect the self-talk statements to be useful, it would be ineffective to use self-talk techniques with them. Likewise, the SMPs' and SPPs' belief in the intervention is also likely to be a precondition for self-talk to be effective, and awareness of pre-existing beliefs and expectations is important before employing any intervention in rehabilitation. Equally, the quality of the working alliance or collaborative relationship between the SMP/SPP and the athlete can also influence the athlete's belief in, and willingness to use, self-talk (see Tod & Andersen, 2005).

Self-Talk Should Be Matched to the Level of Arousal

The process of selecting and implementing self-talk interventions with injured athletes can be challenging. Van Raalte et al. (2017) provide a helpful guidance for how to ground self-talk interventions in empirically and theoretically supported strategies rooted in the sport-specific model of self-talk (Van Raalte et al., 2016). Of the suggestions highlighted, a key aspect important for intentional self-talk interventions (system 2) is to match the self-talk to the athlete's arousal level. Instead of ignoring arousal, it is more beneficial to guide athletes with high levels of arousal to adjust their self-talk to include adaptive statements, while also acknowledging the heightened arousal. For example, when an athlete is nervous about performing a sport skill for the first time post-injury, it would be more beneficial to cue the athlete to cognitively appraise their somatic sensations as "I am excited!" than to cue them to think "I am calm" (Van Raalte et al., 2016, 2017).

Conclusion

Self-talk can have a number of functions for athletes with injuries, and its interpretation by the user is a critical determinant of the outcomes of its use. Research suggests that self-talk may be useful throughout rehabilitation for increasing injury-related clinical recovery outcomes and as a coping strategy for many biopsychosocial benefits. Future research should continue to explore the athlete's experiences of using self-talk as part of the rehabilitation process and expand the understanding of the types and functions of self-talk throughout the sport injury and rehabilitation experience.

Case Study

Justin is a 20-year-old male cheerleader who competes on a collegiate team. For the past six weeks, Justin has been engaging in rehabilitation from a grade II anterior talofibular ligament (ATFL) injury. Justin sustained an injury while training tumbling passes and landing short on his twist. He is currently in the second phase of recovery (i.e., the rehabilitative phase), and he is feeling a loss of motivation. In the training room, Sally, the SMP responsible for Justin's care, has noticed that he has been making more and more comments about his future in the sport and how the long recovery is taking. Certain exercises make Justin worried out of fear of re-injury and that he will have to take steps backward. Justin has expressed his doubts to Sally, saying, "But what if this is too much strain on my foot?" and has questioned, "Are you sure that if I fall off this balance pad, I won't hurt it more?" and "Ugh, do I really need to keep doing more of these exercises?" Sally has told Justin that these comments do not seem helpful to his rehab and that they are becoming more frequent. Justin often replies, "Yeah, well, you'd be bored too if you had to do these silly exercises instead of actually practicing." Justin has also expressed that he is uncertain that he will every fully make it through recovery, saying, "I've just got this feeling it's always going to be on my mind, and it will never be the same." Despite Justin's being a relatively pleasant person, it is clear that he is often negative about the pace that he is progressing yet has some fears about being reinjured in the rehabilitation process.

Questions

1. What specific self-talk statements would you want to modify with Justin?
2. Identify the different types and functions of the self-talk statements you are concerned about.
3. With reference to the sport-specific model of self-talk, how would you conceptualize Justin's self-talk and its impact on their rehabilitation behavior?
4. Using the quotes from the case study, reframe the statements into functional self-talk statements for Justin.

References

Arvinen-Barrow, M., & Granquist, M. D. (2020). Psychosocial considerations for rehabilitation of the injured athletic patient. In W. Prentice (Ed.), *Rehabilitation techniques for sports medicine and athletic training* (7th ed., pp. 93–116). SLACK Inc.

Beneka, A., Malliou, P., Bebetsos, E., Gioftsidou, A., Pafis, G., & Godolias, G. (2007). Appropriate counselling techniques for specific components of the rehabilitation plan: A review of the literature. *Physical Training.* http://ejmas.com/pt/ptframe.htm

Beneka, A., Malliou, P., Gioftsidou, A., Kofotolis, N., Rokka, S., Mavromoustakos, S., & Godolias, G. (2013). Effects of instructional and motivational self-talk on balance performance in knee injured. *European Journal of Physiotherapy, 56*(2), 56–63. https://doi.org/10.3109/21679169.2013.776109

Brewer, B. W., & Redmond, C. J. (2017). *Psychology of sport injury.* Human Kinetics.

Bull, S., Albinson, J. G., & Shambrook, C. J. (1996). *The mental game plan: Getting psyched for sport.* Sports Dynamics.

Clement, D., & Arvinen-Barrow, M. (2020). Psychosocial strategies for the different phases of sport injury rehabilitation. In A. Ivarsson & U. Johnson (Eds.), *Psychological bases of sport injuries* (4th ed., pp. 297–330). Fitness Information Technology.

Crossman, J. (2001). Managing thoughts, stress, and pain. In J. Crossman (Ed.), *Coping with sports injuries: Psychological strategies for rehabilitation* (pp. 128–147). Oxford University Press.

Deci, E. L., & Ryan, R. M. (1985). *Intrinsic motivation and self-determination in human behaviour.* Plenum.

Goodhart, D. E. (1986). The effects of positive and negative thinking on performance in an achievement situation. *Journal of Personality and Social Psychology, 51*(1), 117–124. https://doi.org/10.1037/0022-3514.51.1.117

Gould, D., Eklund, R. C., & Jackson, S. A. (1993). Coping strategies used by US Olympic wrestlers. *Research Quarterly for Exercise and Sport, 64*(1), 83–93. https://doi.org/10.1080/02701367.1993.10608782

Gould, D., Finch, L. M., & Jackson, S. A. (1993). Coping strategies used by national champion figure skaters. *Research Quarterly for Exercise and Sport, 64*(4), 453–468. https://doi.org/10.1080/02701367.1993.10607599

Gould, D., Udry, E., Bridges, D., & Beck, L. (1997). Coping with season-ending injuries. *The Sport Psychologist, 11*(4), 379–399. https://doi.org/10.1123/tsp.11.4.379

Hackford, D., & Schwenkmezger, P. (1993). Anxiety. In R. N. Singer, M. Murphy, & L. K. Tennant (Eds.), *Handbook of research on sport psychology* (pp. 328–364). Palgrave Macmillan.

Hamilton, R. A., Scott, D., & MacDougall, M. P. (2007). Assessing the effectiveness of self-talk interventions on endurance performance. *Journal of Applied Sport Psychology, 19*(2), 226–239. https://doi.org/10.1080/10413200701230613

Hardy, J. (2006). Speaking clearly: A critical review of the self-talk literature. *Psychology of Sport and Exercise, 7*(1), 81–97. https://doi.org/10.1016/j.psychsport.2005.04.002

Hardy, J., Begley, K., & Blanchfield, A. W. (2015). It's good but it's not right: Instructional self-talk and skilled performance. *Journal of Applied Sport Psychology, 27*(2), 132–139. https://doi.org/10.1080/10413200.2014.959624

Hardy, J., Gammage, K. L., & Hall, C. R. (2001). A descriptive study of athlete self-talk. *The Sport Psychologist, 15*(3), 306–318. https://doi.org/10.1123/tsp.15.3.306

Hardy, J., Oliver, E. J., & Tod, D. (2009). A framework for the study and application of self-talk within sport. In S. D. Mellalieu & S. Hanton (Eds.), *Advances in applied sport psychology: A review* (pp. 37–74). Routledge.

Hatzigeorgiardis, A., Theodorakis, Y., & Zourbanos, N. (2004). Self-talk in the swimming pool: The effects of self-talk on thought content and performance on water-polo tasks. *Journal of Applied Sport Psychology, 16*(2), 138–150. https://doi.org/10.1080/10413200490437886

Ievleva, L., & Orlick, T. (1991). Mental links to enhanced healing: An exploratory study. *The Sport Psychologist, 5*(1), 25–40. https://doi.org/10.1123/tsp.5.1.25

Jones, M. V. (2003). Controlling emotions in sport *The Sport Psychologist*, *17*(4), 471–486. https://doi.org/10.1123/tsp.17.4.471

Kamphoff, C., Thomae, J., & Hamson-Utley, J. J. (2013). Integrating the psychological and physiological aspects of sport injury rehabilitation: Rehabilitation profiling and phases of rehabilitation. In M. Arvinen-Barrow & N. Walker (Eds.), *Psychology of sport injury and rehabilitation* (pp. 134–155). Routledge.

Kyllo, L. B., & Landers, D. M. (1995). Goal setting in sport and exercise: A research synthesis to resolve the controversy. *Journal of Sport & Exercise Psychology*, *17*(2), 117–137. https://doi.org/10.1123/jsep.17.2.117

Latinjak, A. T., Masó, M., Calmeiro, L., & Hatzigeorgiadis, A. (2020). Athletes' use of goal-directed self-talk: Situational determinants and functions. *International Journal of Sport and Exercise Psychology*, *18*(6), 733–748. https://doi.org/10.1080/1612197x.2019.1611899

Latinjak, A. T., Zourbanos, N., López-Ros, V., & Hatzigeorgiadis, A. (2014). Goal-directed and undirected self-talk: Exploring a new perspective for the study of athletes' self-talk. *Psychology of Sport and Exercise*, *15*(5), 548–558. https://doi.org/10.1016/j.psychsport.2014.05.007

Moran, A. P. (1996). *The psychology of concentration in sport performers*. Psychology Press.

Naoi, A., & Ostrow, A. (2008). The effects of cognitive and relaxation interventions on injured athletes' mood and pain during rehabilitation. *Athletic Insight: Online Journal of Sport Psychology*, *10*(1). www.athleticinsight.com/Vol10Iss1/InterventionsInjury.htm

Oikawa, M. (2004). Does addictive distraction affect the relationship between the cognition of distraction effectiveness and depression? *Japanese Journal of Educational Psychology*, *52*(3), 287–297. https://doi.org/10.5926/jjep1953.52.3_287

Owens, D., & Bunker, L. K. (1989). *Golf: Steps to success*. Human Kinetics.

Porter, K. (2003). *The mental athlete*. Human Kinetics.

Rock, J. A., & Jones, M. V. (2002a). A preliminary investigation into the use of counseling skills in support of rehabilitation from sport injury. *Journal of Sport Rehabilitation*, *11*(4), 284–304. https://doi.org/10.1123/jsr.11.4.284

Rock, J. A., & Jones, M. V. (2002b). A preliminary investigation into the use of counseling skills in support of rehabilitation from sport injury. *Journal of Sport Rehabilitation*, *11*, 284–304.

Ryan, R. M., & Deci, E. L. (2002). An overview of self-determination theory: An organismic dialectical perspective. In E. L. Deci & R. M. Ryan (Eds.), *Handbook of self-determination research* (pp. 3–33). University of Rochester Press.

Syer, J., & Connolly, C. (1998). *Sporting body, sporting mind*. Simon & Schuster.

Taylor, J., & Taylor, S. (1997). *Psychological approaches to sports injury rehabilitation*. Aspen.

Theodorakis, Y., Weinberg, R. S., Natsis, P., Douma, I., & Kazakas, P. (2000). The effects of motivational versus instructional self-talk on improving motor performance. *The Sport Psychologist*, *14*(3), 253–271. https://doi.org/10.1123/tsp.14.3.253

Tod, D., & Andersen, M. B. (2005). Success in sport psych: Effective sport psychologists. In S. Murphy (Ed.), *The sport psych handbook* (pp. 305–314). Human Kinetics.

Tod, D., Hardy, J., & Oliver, E. (2011). Effects of self-talk: A systematic literature review. *Journal of Sport & Exercise Psychology*, *33*(4), 666–687. https://doi.org/10.1123/jsep.33.5.666

Udry, E., Gould, D., Bridges, D., & Beck, L. (1997). Down but not out: Athlete responses to season-ending injuries. *Journal of Sport & Exercise Psychology*, *19*, 229–248.

Van Raalte, J. L., Cornelius, A. E., Brewer, B. W., & Hatten, S. J. (2000). The antecedents and consequences of self-talk in competitive tennis. *Journal of Sport & Exercise Psychology*, *22*(3), 345–356. https://doi.org/10.1123/jsep.19.3.229

Van Raalte, J. L., Vincent, A., & Brewer, B. W. (2016). Self-talk: Review and sport-specific model. *Psychology of Sport and Exercise*, *22*, 139–148. https://doi.org/10.1016/j.psychsport.2015.08.004

Van Raalte, J. L., Vincent, A., & Brewer, B. W. (2017). Self-talk interventions for athletes: A theoretically grounded approach. *Journal of Sport Psychology in Action*, *8*(3), 141–151. https://doi.org/10.1080/21520704.2016.1233921

Weinberg, R. S. (1988). *The mental advantage: Developing your psychological skills in tennis*. Human Kinetics.

Wiese-Bjornstal, D. M., Smith, A. M., Shaffer, S. M., & Morrey, M. A. (1998). An integrated model of response to sport injury: Psychological and sociological dynamics. *Journal of Applied Sport Psychology*, *10*(1), 46–69. https://doi.org/10.1080/10413209808406377

Zinsser, N., Bunker, L., & Williams, J. M. (2006). Cognitive techniques for building confidence and enhancing performance. In J. M. Williams (Ed.), *Applied sport psychology: Personal growth to peak performance* (5th ed., pp. 349–381). McGraw-Hill.

Zinsser, N., Bunker, L., & Williams, J. M. (2010). Cognitive techniques for building confidence and enhancing performance. In J. M. Williams (Ed.), *Applied sport psychology: Personal growth to peak performance* (6th ed., pp. 305–335). McGraw-Hill.

16 Relaxation Techniques in Sport Injury and Rehabilitation

Caroline Heaney and Natalie C. Walker

Chapter Objectives

- To outline different types of relaxation strategies used in sport injury.
- To summarize the existing literature on using relaxation techniques during rehabilitation.
- To demonstrate the usefulness of relaxation techniques during sport injury rehabilitation.

Introduction

Several studies have explored the different stressors athletes may have to cope with when participating in sport or rehabilitating an injury. The literature suggests that aspects of competition (e.g., thinking about mistakes), interpersonal relationships (e.g., expectations from coaches or teammates), financial concerns (e.g., sponsorship), environmental conditions (e.g., the weather), and traumatic experiences (e.g., enduring a sport injury) can all test an athlete's coping resources. The key to coping with this myriad of potential stressors is for the athlete to (a) learn to become self-aware of their responses to stressors and (b) adopt appropriate psychological intervention techniques to facilitate coping. A number of psychosocial strategies have been identified as beneficial in helping athletes deal with stressors, one of which is relaxation techniques (e.g., Arvinen-Barrow et al., 2015). Research has also documented that injured athletes and sports medicine professionals (SMPs) use psychosocial strategies, including relaxation techniques, as part of rehabilitation and return to participation following an injury. In their cross-sectional research, Arvinen-Barrow et al. (2015) found relaxation was the fourth most common strategy used by injured athletes. The purpose of this chapter is to discuss how relaxation techniques can be used during sport injury rehabilitation. The chapter will (a) introduce the purpose of relaxation techniques in sport injury, (b) outline the types of relaxation techniques used in sport injury, (c) summarize existing literature on the use of relaxation techniques in sport injury, (d) discuss the ways in which relaxation techniques can be combined with other strategies during rehabilitation, and (e) provide practical suggestions on how to maximize the use of relaxation techniques during rehabilitation.

The Purpose of Relaxation Techniques in Rehabilitation

Relaxation can be defined as a temporary deliberate withdrawal from everyday activity that aims to moderate the functions of the sympathetic nervous system, which is typically activated under

DOI: 10.4324/9781003295709-19

stress (Hill, 2001). When relaxed, individuals exhibit normal blood pressure and decreases in oxygen consumption, respiratory rate, heart rate, and muscle tension (Benson & Klipper, 2000; Jacobs, 2001). Relaxation techniques therefore aim to decrease muscle tension, calm the mind, and decrease autonomic system responses (e.g., heart rate and blood pressure).

It is suggested that relaxation techniques should form an integral part of the rehabilitation process (Wiese-Bjornstal et al., 2020), and a range of relaxation techniques have been identified as beneficial for athletes with injuries. For example, Wiese-Bjornstal et al. (2020) suggest that progressive muscle relaxation (PMR), guided imagery, diaphragmatic breathing, and autogenic training are useful for athletes with injuries. Burland et al. (2019) have recommended mindfulness, guided relaxation, and breathing techniques as beneficial to increase motivation, increase self-efficacy, and decrease anxiety during sport injury. In general, relaxation techniques are considered advantageous during injury rehabilitation for two primary reasons: first, to assist athletes in coping with injury-induced pain and, second, to reduce common biopsychosocial responses to injury, such as stress and anxiety. Using relaxation techniques during rehabilitation can also help athletes focus attention, enhance confidence, and ultimately, aid healing (Brewer & Redmond, 2017). Many other psychosocial strategies that are useful during sport injury rehabilitation (e.g., imagery) also rely on a foundation of relaxation to enhance effectiveness. Although presented separately in this book, often, psychosocial strategies are integrated within a psychological skills training package. For example, using relaxation techniques to produce a relaxed state can also be conducive to generating mental images for different types of imagery (for more details on imagery in rehabilitation, see Chapter 17).

Types of Relaxation Techniques

In sport, the term "relaxation" or "relaxation techniques" has been used to describe a range of methods through which an athlete can facilitate physical and psychological well-being. These methods are commonly split into two categories: physical (somatic) and mental (cognitive) relaxation (Brewer & Redmond, 2017). The primary aim of physical relaxation techniques is to release physical tension in the body. Mental relaxation techniques focus on the mind rather than the body and are underpinned by a belief that a relaxed mind will physically relax the body. In this chapter, we will focus on four relaxation techniques that have been shown to be particularly effective for sport injury rehabilitation – PMR (physical), breath control techniques (physical), mindfulness (mental), and relaxation imagery (mental).

Progressive Muscle Relaxation (PMR)

Based on the early work of Jacobson (1938), PMR aims to teach the individual what it feels like to relax, by contrasting the feeling of tension in specific muscle groups with the feeling of relaxation in those same muscle groups. PMR consists of learning to sequentially tense and then relax groups of muscles, paying attention to the feelings of tension and relaxation to help the athlete become aware of when muscles are tense and how to relax them (Brewer & Redmond, 2017). Athletes are encouraged to observe early signals of stress and anxiety and to scan their muscles frequently for any tension experienced throughout the situation (e.g., a rehabilitation session; Hill, 2001). The scanning required to perform PMR involves having the athlete note signs of muscular tension during the day, and by scanning the body at least twice a day, they should be able to implement the relaxation response in a short time by using deep breathing (Crossman, 2001). When any tension is experienced, the athlete is instructed to tense these muscles, hold this tension for a count of seven, and then release the tension, noticing the difference in sensation between tension and relaxation (Hill, 2001).

When implementing PMR, after initial deep breaths, subsequent breaths should be steady and shallow, with inhalations coming in through the nose and exhalations going out through the mouth. The inhalation should lead smoothly into exhalation and not be forced or include a pause between the two (i.e., holding one's breath). The tension phase should last approximately 7–10 seconds, and the relaxation phase should last approximately 25–30 seconds. During the relaxation phase, the facilitator of the PMR (e.g., the SMP) should adopt a lowered tone of voice compared with the tension phase (for more details, see Crossman, 2001). The first few sessions can take up to 30 minutes, and it is recommended that athletes follow a the script for 16 muscle groups when first learning PMR (Crossman, 2001). With practice, less time is required, and the aim is for the athlete to be able to develop the ability to relax quickly. Various PMR scripts are widely available in both written and audiovisual formats that could be used in rehabilitation settings.

Öst (1988) developed an applied variant of the PMR technique with the aim of teaching an athlete to relax within 20 minutes to 30 seconds. The first phase of training involves a 15-minute PMR routine practiced twice a day. The second phase of training is a "release-only" phase that takes five to seven minutes to complete, where the muscle relaxation is initiated without deliberate prior muscle tension. The time to complete the "release-only" routines is reduced to two to three minutes, using the instructional cue word "relax." The time is further reduced until only a few seconds are required to achieve desired relaxation outcome, and then practiced for specific situations (e.g., in-between rehabilitation exercises). The goal is to initiate a fast relaxation response as and when required, which can be beneficial for athletes during the rehabilitation process and beyond.

Breath Control Techniques

Correct breathing is fundamental to achieving a relaxed state. A link exists between breathing and the system controlling our physiological arousal. Stimulation of the sympathetic nervous system (when anxious) leads to breaths that are short, shallow, and irregular, whereas stimulation of the parasympathetic nervous system (when calm and confident) is associated with smooth, deep, and rhythmic breaths (Keable, 1989). Slow breathing is therefore considered to have stress-relieving properties and is one of the easiest yet most effective ways to control stress, anxiety, and muscle tension (Weinberg & Gould, 2019). A wide range of breath control techniques exist. For the purposes of this chapter, centering, diaphragmatic, and ratio breathing are described, as they are particularly effective during sport injury rehabilitation.

Centering

Centering (also known as the "centering breath") is a relaxation technique that focuses attention on the task at hand. There are a variety of different ways to centering breath, but the most common appears to be changing the focus of attention from the athlete's head to their center of gravity, hence giving a feeling of stability and balance. This feeling of stability, balance, and control is the prompt to relax (Harwood, 1998). One key feature of centering is that, over time, and with practice, it provides a method of relaxing quickly. A deep breath is all that an athlete, who has practiced centering, needs to remove the feelings of anxiety (e.g., on a new, more challenging rehabilitation exercise producing re-injury anxiety). The athlete can then refocus their attention on what needs to be done and how they are going to do it, rather than on the possible negative consequences.

Sample Centering Exercise

- Stand with your feet shoulder-width apart and bend the knees slightly.
- Relax the neck, arms, and shoulder muscles.
- Direct your thoughts inwards to check and alter your muscle tension and breathing, by focusing on the abdominal muscles and how they expand as you breathe in. Try to feel the heaviness in your muscles.
- Take a slow, deep breath (from the diaphragm), trying to limit the movement of the chest cavity.
- Concentrate on your breathing and the heaviness of your muscles, clearing the mind of all irrelevant thoughts, and say "relax."
- Now, focus your attention on the rehabilitation activity and what you need to do to perform it.

Source: Adapted from Harwood (1998). Used with permission of Taylor & Francis Informa UK Ltd. – Books, from *Psychology of Sport Injury and Rehabilitation* by Monna Arvinen-Barrow and Natalie Walker (eds.) (1st. ed.). Copyright ©2013; permission conveyed through Copyright Clearance Center Inc.

Diaphragmatic Breathing

Diaphragmatic breathing (sometimes known as abdominal breathing) is a technique which involves taking slow deep breaths into the lower part of the lungs, strengthening the diaphragm and making breathing more efficient (Brewer & Redmond, 2017). It emphasizes the downward expansion of the chest cavity that causes the abdomen to swell. The first step in diaphragmatic breathing (as in all other breath control techniques) is to guide the athlete to become aware of their regular breathing patterns. When engaging in diaphragmatic breathing exercises, if the athlete's chest rises more than their abdomen, they should be shown how they could breathe differently. They should be explained about the benefits of changing their breathing. The aim of diaphragmatic breathing is for the athlete to try to feel their ribs expanding and moving as air is inhaled, and then the ribs recoiling as they exhale. The athlete should be aware of how the lungs and diaphragm work. For example, athletes should know that the diaphragm forms the roof of the abdomen, and at rest, it is domed in shape. When it is contracted, it flattens, making more room in the chest for air to be inhaled. When the diaphragm is relaxed, it returns to its dome shape, helping to force the air out. The movement of the diaphragm affects the position of the internal organs, and hence, when contracted, it pushes down on these organs and causes the abdomen to swell a little. Athletes might find diaphragmatic breathing useful just prior to a specific rehabilitation exercise, with a goal to relax as a preparation for the activity and to help focus on the task. Diaphragmatic breathing can also be encouraged during rehabilitation exercises to improve the intensity and effort of the work.

Ratio Breathing

Ratio breathing is a deep-breathing technique focusing on the number of inhalations compared with exhalations (e.g., a ratio of four inhalations to seven exhalations). The individual counts the ratio of breaths, providing a distraction from negative thoughts. The technique can be easily explained to an athlete using visual images, for example, asking them to imagine an open palm and to think of the counting of their breaths as the gaps between their fingers. It is also useful for the athlete practicing ratio breathing to understand the arousal mechanism that ratio breathing is aimed to affect. The athlete engaged in ratio breathing should understand that their levels of arousal are controlled by the autonomic nervous system, which is not under our conscious control. As such, when under stress, what happens in our bodies might not be what we want to

---

Diaphragmatic Breathing Exercise

- Lie on your back and take small breaths in via the nose and exhale out of the mouth, letting air just fall out of the lungs (do not force it).
- Gradually increase the size of your breaths until slow and deep (no holding of breath).
- You should be taking a maximum 12 breaths (inhale/exhale) per minute.
- Place the palm of your hands on the bottom of your ribs, with the fingertips touching.
- On exhaling, relax the abdomen, shoulders, and chest.
- Take in a big breath via the nose and notice what happens to the abdomen and ribs (for many, the chest will rise more than the abdomen).

Note: For a more visual impact of current breathing patterns, it is also possible to use paper or plastic cups instead of using the hands. Similarly, it is possible to replicate this exercise standing. For example, in front of a mirror, without upper-body clothing, place your hands flat against your stomach (palms on bottom of ribs, with fingertips touching).

Source: Adapted from McConnell (2011). Used with permission of Taylor & Francis Informa UK Ltd. – Books, from *Psychology of Sport Injury and Rehabilitation* by Monna Arvinen-Barrow and Natalie Walker (eds.) (1st. ed.). Copyright ©2013; permission conveyed through Copyright Clearance Center Inc.

---

happen (e.g., increased heart rate, increased breathing rate). When arousal levels are heightened, an individual needs to activate the parasympathetic nervous system, which is associated with a relaxed state. This can be achieved through taking slow, controlled, longer "out" breaths (hence the longer exhale ratio compared with inhalation).

Mindfulness

In recent years, mindfulness has become increasingly popular among athletes. Cottraux (2007), cited in Bernier et al. (2009, p. 320), has defined *mindfulness* as "a mental state resulting from voluntarily focusing one's attention on one's present experience in its sensorial, mental, cognitive and emotional aspects, in a non-judgmental way." Mindfulness uses a range of meditation, breathing methods, guided imagery, and other practices to relax the body and mind and help reduce stress. Mindfulness encourages individuals to engage in non-judging awareness of their internal experience occurring at each moment, such as bodily sensations, cognitions, and emotions, and to environmental stimuli, such as sights and sounds, with an attitude of curiosity, openness, and acceptance (Baer, 2003; Bagheri et al., 2021).

During injury rehabilitation, mindfulness can be seen as beneficial to help injured athletes in achieving a relaxed state of mind and body and to become more aware of their injury situation. It may be useful in drawing an athlete's focus to the private events that they are experiencing throughout their rehabilitation, as well as encouraging such events to come and go without trying to control the experiences (Mahoney & Hanrahan, 2011). Mindful attention may also be useful to draw athletes' focus to rehabilitation exercises to ensure correct execution of movements and to gain maximum benefits from physical interventions (Mahoney & Hanrahan, 2011).

Whilst research points toward a growing interest in the use of mindfulness interventions in sport injury rehabilitation, experts have cautioned against its adoption without a spiritual understanding (Roychowdhury et al., 2021). It would also be appropriate to consider the appropriateness of such an intervention for those athletes whose faith may conflict with Eastern philosophies. Equally, it would be important to establish if an athlete has already adopted another form of meditation (e.g., Islam prayer), as lack of consideration for such factors may inadvertently do more harm (see Chapters 11 and 12).

Sample Mindfulness Meditation Program

- Breathing meditation
- Body scan meditation
- Sitting meditation
- Walking meditation

Source: Bagheri et al. (2021).

Relaxation Imagery

Imagery is defined as the process of "using one's senses to re-create or create an experience in the mind" (Vealey & Forlenza, 2015, p. 240). Several types of imagery can be beneficial during sport injury rehabilitation (for more details, see Chapter 17), but here we focus on relaxation imagery, also known as guided or soothing imagery, which involves creating or recreating a scenario of being in a relaxing place in order to initiate a relaxation response. Such scenarios might include lying on a beach, walking around a woodland park, or whatever an athlete considers as relaxing.

Relaxation Imagery Script

- Sit or lie in a comfortable position. Close your eyes and imagine yourself lying on a beautiful beach on a warm, sunny day. Use all your senses to create an image of the beach and feel like you are there. Picture the beautiful golden sand around you, the crystal-clear warm seawater, and the clear bright-blue sky. See the waves gently lapping against the shore, and the palm trees swaying in the gentle breeze. You feel warm, calm, and relaxed.
- Breathe in and smell the sand and the warm, salty seawater. Slowly exhale and relax a little deeper. Notice the sound of the waves as they gently lap onto the beach. Listen to the gentle breeze as it softly rustles the leaves of the palm trees as you relax a little deeper. Feel the warmth of the sun shining on your skin. Feel the gentle breeze on your body. Touch the sand and feel its warmth as it runs through your fingers. You feel warm, calm, and relaxed.
- Continue to lie on the beach and see, hear, and feel the sensations of being here. Notice how calm and relaxed you feel and enjoy the feeling of relaxation as it spreads throughout your body. When you are ready, walk away from the beach and open your eyes, feeling calm and relaxed.

Benefits of Relaxation Techniques

A number of relaxation techniques have been found to be beneficial during injury rehabilitation. Based on the findings, the benefits of relaxation techniques can be typically grouped into three: (a) pain management, (b) alleviating stress and anxiety, and (c) other benefits (e.g., enhanced focus or self-confidence).

The Use of Relaxation for Pain Management

Pain inhibits breathing, reduces blood flow, and can cause muscle spasms and tension, which can actually serve to increase pain in the long term (Cousin & Philips, 1985). Relaxation is hypothesized to affect pain via (a) reducing the demand for oxygen in the tissue and lowering the levels of chemicals (such as lactic acid) that can trigger pain, (b) releasing tension in the skeletal muscle that can exacerbate pain, and (c) the release of endorphins, which interact with the opiate receptors in the brain to reduce perceptions of pain (McCaffery & Pasero, 1999). Another mechanism by which relaxation might reduce pain is via acting as an internal distraction. For example, if an injured athlete is engaging in ratio breathing, they might focus less on the pain itself and more on the breathing technique.

Several studies exploring the effects of pain management techniques in a wide range of settings have indicated that an individual's overall pain tolerance can be improved, and perceptions of pain reduced, by various types of relaxation training (Bagheri et al., 2021; Coronado et al., 2018; Cruze & Games, 2021; Madrigal & Gill, 2014). Use of relaxation training may therefore reduce the need for pain-relieving medication (Payne, 2004). For example, Bagheri et al. (2021) explored the impact of a mindfulness-based intervention on a group of female runners with patellofemoral pain over an eight-week period and found that it led to improved pain management, decreased pain intensity, and reduced pain catastrophizing. Other studies, such as Bennett and Lindsay (2016), have also found that mindfulness has improved pain management. Similar findings have been observed for other relaxation techniques. In their review of the literature, Gennarelli et al. (2020) concluded that relaxation/guided imagery was found to improve pain management in injured athletes. Similarly, Cupal and Brewer (2001) found that breathing techniques lowered perceptions of pain in athletes with anterior cruciate ligament injuries.

The Use of Relaxation to Alleviate Stress and Anxiety

Sport injury is a significant risk factor for mental health conditions among athletes (Haugen, 2022; Putukian, 2016) and commonly leads to feelings of depression, stress, and anxiety (Lichtenstein et al., 2019). As they reduce the stress response, relaxation techniques represent one of the most commonly used approaches to managing these feelings and conditions, both as a stand-alone treatment and included in a multimodal treatment package (Manzoni et al., 2008). Typical anxieties with which an injured athlete might have to cope are related to pain, rehabilitation length, potential loss of playing position, changes in daily routines, sport performance outcomes (e.g., team doing well or poorly whilst injured), pre- and/or post-operative stress, fitness demands, return to peak performance, and loss of athletic identity. Experiencing anxieties (or fear) related to re-injury during rehabilitation or return to participation is also commonplace (Kunnen et al., 2021; Kvist & Silbernagel, 2022). The impact of stress, anxiety, and other emotions can affect rehabilitation outcomes (Forsdyke et al., 2016). These stressors can interfere with recovery because the healing mechanisms of the body cannot work properly, and to maximize the effects of treatment, an athlete should be relaxed (Payne, 2004). When someone is anxious, one symptom experienced is excessive muscle tension, and this might prevent the SMP from treating the injured area effectively. In addition, the athlete might also brace their muscles during a rehabilitation exercise in an attempt to protect their injured limb, reducing the flow of blood, reducing range of movement, and increasing the risk of re-injury (Heil, 1993).

As detailed earlier, an athlete might experience anxieties related to their injury rehabilitation and return to training and competition following injury. The use of relaxation techniques during these circumstances is vital. Relaxation training, such as PMR, is useful, as it increases the athlete's awareness of their muscle physiology. For example, an athlete might inappropriately believe that they are relaxed, but with the use of relaxation training, they are able to gain greater awareness of their body and are hence enabled to become more in control. The use of breathing techniques and PMR is reported to be the most beneficial for coping with stress and anxiety associated with injury (Wagman & Khelifa, 1996).

Cupal and Brewer (2001) investigated the effects of breathing techniques and guided/relaxation imagery during sport injury rehabilitation and found that they led to decreases in re-injury anxiety. Relaxation paired with imagery exercises can also enable injured athletes to see themselves performing without anxieties (Flint, 2007; Green & Bonura, 2007; Williams & Andersen, 2007). In their review, Gennarelli et al. (2020) found that relaxation/guided imagery was effective in improving stress management and reducing re-injury anxiety in athletes with a range of injuries. Research has also found mindfulness to be effective, leading to positive outcomes, such as reduced symptoms of anxiety (Bennett & Lindsay, 2016; Moesch et al., 2020) and depression (Moesch et al., 2020).

Other Benefits of Relaxation in Rehabilitation

As well as improving pain management and reducing stress and anxiety, several other positive outcomes have been identified from using relaxation techniques during rehabilitation. These include, but are not limited to, enhanced recovery (Bennett & Lindsay, 2016), reduced healing time (Pelka et al., 2016), increased self-efficacy (Gennarelli et al., 2020), and increased acceptance (Moesch et al., 2020).

Relaxation techniques can be useful in increasing blood flow to the injured area, promoting healing and reducing the likelihood of re-injury (Heil, 1993; Taylor & Taylor, 1997). As relaxation techniques can have a direct impact on injury recovery, it is likely that an athlete's focus, feelings of self-confidence, and personal control will be enhanced. Relaxation techniques can help the athlete focus on the task at hand during rehabilitation, by redirecting their attention away from discomfort, pain, or anxiety, which can reduce the risk of re-injury. Being able to control discomfort, pain, or anxiety can also provide the athlete with a sense of achievement, which can enhance confidence. Moreover, the aforementioned process will give the athlete a sense of personal control, which is often desired by athletes with injuries (Walker, 2006).

Yukelson and Murphy (1993) stated that being an active participant in, and having some responsibility for, rehabilitation encourages positive involvement in the process. An additional advantage of using relaxation techniques during rehabilitation is its transferability to training and competition following an injury. Relaxation techniques can also help athletes in coping with other stressful situations and thus may be influential in minimizing future injury and/or re-injury.

Combining Relaxation Techniques with Other Psychological Techniques

Relaxation techniques are often combined with other psychological strategies. For example, an athlete might be encouraged to select a word that is synonymous with *relaxation* (e.g., *relax*, *calm*, *healing*, *harmony*) and to recite this cue word on exhaling (that is, pair relaxation with self-talk). The idea is that an association builds between the state of relaxation and the cue word, and over time, the cue word on its own can induce a relaxed state. The stronger the association between the cue word and relaxation, the greater the power of the cue word for the athlete. It has been recommended that the cue word should be paired at least 20 times a day with exhaling to build this skill over time (Payne, 2004). The use of an appropriate cue word is also often employed as part of centering exercises. It is also common to use relaxation techniques in combination with imagery, for example, at the start of an imagery session, to aid focus (Multhaupt & Beuth, 2018).

Whilst it is not the intention of this chapter to outline every psychosocial strategy pairing with relaxation techniques possible, it is hoped that the reader's attention is alerted to the many possibilities of using relaxation techniques in conjunction with other coping and psychosocial strategies presented in Chapters 12–18. Research has found positive results from multimodal sport psychology interventions and advocates a range of strategies as beneficial for injury rehabilitation. Gennarelli et al. (2020) concluded that relaxation imagery, positive self-talk, goal setting, counselling, emotional/written disclosure, and modelling videos all benefit sport injury recovery and lead to improvements in mood, pain management, exercise compliance, and rehabilitation adherence. When deciding on what psychosocial strategies to implement, the expertise and competences of the professional working with the athlete, as well as the preference of the athlete, should be taken into account (Payne, 2004). Techniques that appeal to an individual are more likely to gain their cooperation and result in better intervention and rehabilitation outcomes.

Guidance for Using Relaxation Techniques for Rehabilitation

Previous research indicates that the use of psychosocial strategies, including relaxation techniques, is not as common as it could be among athletes when injured. For example, Arvinen-Barrow et al. (2015) found that only 27% of the 1,283 athletes they surveyed had used psychosocial strategies during sport injury rehabilitation. Keilani et al. (2016) reported a figure of just 7% among the professional athletes they surveyed. Given the positive benefits of using relaxation techniques during sport injury, professionals around the athlete – including SMPs and sport coaches – are ideally placed to encourage the athletes to use relaxation techniques when injured. As some lack the education or confidence to deliver psychosocial strategies (e.g., Heaney et al., 2017), the purpose of this section is to offer practical guidance. Regardless of the relaxation technique employed, several prerequisites are necessary to facilitate effective relaxation. These include educating the injured athlete, providing a suitable environment for relaxation, ensuring an appropriate structure to the relaxation program, measuring relaxation effectiveness, and using appropriate relaxation techniques consistent with the phase of rehabilitation.

Educating the Athlete

Education is vital as a first step for any relaxation training (Rotella, 1982). The athlete should be educated about the purpose, benefits, and reasons for the use of relaxation. Some examples of how this might be achieved are presented throughout this chapter. The athlete should also be given opportunities to ask questions and share any apprehensions about the technique, and these should be resolved with the athlete's best interests in mind. The SMP might explain to the athlete that a relaxation technique may help them because it promotes blood supply to the injured site and blood has healing properties. They might also be informed that these techniques will give them a sense of being in control of their recovery. They do, however, need to be reminded when using PMR, for example, to take care on the tension phase when the injury location is being used and to only continue as long as they are pain-free.

Providing a Suitable Environment for Relaxation

Ensuring the environment is suitable for relaxation is important. A quiet, comfortable atmosphere is considered more facilitative to relaxation (Taylor & Taylor, 1997). However, this is not always practical in sport or rehabilitation setting. The athlete should be positioned comfortably (ideally lying down or seated in a chair). Particularly in the initial stages of learning, it is useful for the eyes to be closed and for the individual to concentrate on how their body feels and rid the mind of all other thoughts (Crossman, 2001).

Ensuring an Appropriate Structure to the Relaxation Program

Relaxation is also thought to be most effective when integrated into the structure of daily sessions (e.g., using ratio breathing during the times when pain is high; Taylor & Taylor, 1997). Relaxation is a skill, and like all other skills, it requires practice (Flint, 1998). It is also important that the athlete does not expect too much too soon, as the ability to use relaxation techniques is directly related to the amount of time spent practicing them.

Measuring Relaxation Effectiveness

It might also be useful to use physiological measures (e.g., heart rate, respiration rate, blood pressure) and psychological self-rating scales (e.g., perceived pain, anxiety) when using relaxation techniques. These measurements might help the SMP in determining the effectiveness of the technique and help the athlete see the benefits as well. Ending a rehabilitation session with relaxation is also perceived as being beneficial, since it can be a rejuvenating experience following a painful and possibly unpleasant experience (Taylor & Taylor, 1997).

Using Appropriate Relaxation Techniques during Different Phases of Rehabilitation

According to Kamphoff et al. (2013), psychosocial injury rehabilitation experience can be broadly classified into three main phases of rehabilitation – reaction to injury (phase 1), reaction to rehabilitation (phase 2), and reaction to return to sport (phase 3). It is likely that an athlete will respond differently to each of these phases; thus, ensuring appropriateness of relaxation techniques in each phase is of importance. For example, during phase 1, when pain is at its worst, using physical relaxation is important to help manage pain. In this phase, the SMP or sport psychology professional (SPP) might teach the athlete breathing techniques and encourage the use of cue words that induce a state of relaxation (Walsh, 2011). During phase 2, the focus might be to reduce the athlete's stress response to the injury. By integrating relaxation techniques into rehabilitation, the athlete may be better able to manage their anxieties. In this phase, the pairing of relaxation with imagery can increase effort and persistence in rehabilitation and continue to manage pain associated with rehabilitation exercises. The nature and duration of phase 2 will vary depending on the type and extent of the injury and treatment interventions, and thus the potential uses of relaxation will vary accordingly. For example, an athlete who is required to have surgery may benefit from using relaxation techniques to alleviate pre-surgery anxiety and/ or to manage post-surgery pain. In phase 3, while the athlete is likely to be eager to return to participation, it is also possible that re-injury anxiety is salient at this time (Walker & Thatcher, 2011). As such, the ability to induce a state of relaxation is an important skill and should be emphasized in response to the increase in anxiety during this phase.

Conclusion

This chapter has introduced the importance of relaxation techniques and outlined the types of relaxation techniques used in sport injury rehabilitation. The chapter then summarized the literature pertinent to the use of relaxation techniques in sport injury rehabilitation and discussed the ways in which relaxation techniques can be combined with other psychological interventions. The chapter provided practical advice to professionals (e.g., SMPs, SPPs, and coaches) on how to maximize the use of relaxation techniques with athletes during sport injury. Based on the evidence presented, a range of relaxation techniques can be of use during rehabilitation and on their return to participation. Relaxation can facilitate athletes' ability to manage and alleviate pain, to deal with stress and anxiety, and to enhance physiological recovery.

Case Study

Sangeeta is a 21-year-old female international rugby player diagnosed with a torn anterior cruciate ligament (ACL). Sangeeta is a bright prospect expected to fill in the vacancies created by the retirement of more experienced international players in the coming years. She has recently had reconstructive surgery, and while the recovery is progressing as planned, she is experiencing high levels of stress and anxiety. "The injury is weighing on me heavy. It's like . . . I have this weighted vest on my shoulders all day, every day. My pecs are tense, my shoulders are tense, and I feel like my jaw is sore," Sangeeta tells her physiotherapist during a routine treatment session.

Since sustaining her ACL injury, Sangeeta also feels under pressure to return to her previous fitness and form as soon as possible. When her surgeon informed Sangeeta that she would be on crutches for at least six weeks, followed by six to eight months of further rehabilitation, Sangeeta just sat still, silent, and clenching her jaw and fists. "I cannot believe this. This is so unfair. I was in the best shape of my life, and now this. Why?" she yells at her partner. Sangeeta gets her crutches and tries to storm off in an attempt to calm herself as she feels physically sick and her heart is pounding so hard she can hear it.

A few minutes later, Sangeeta returns and apologizes to her partner. "I am sorry, I do not mean to yell at you. It is not you. It is this ACL. I feel so angry. No, I am mad. It is so frustrating because I cannot do anything to make this better. I cannot sleep properly with this pain, and it is so hard to get around." Sangeeta's partner nods in support.

Questions

1. Based on the case description, what relaxation techniques might be beneficial for Sangeeta, and why?
2. With reference to appropriate theory, outline how and why relaxation techniques might be beneficial for Sangeeta.
3. Explain how and why combining multiple psychosocial strategies (e.g., self-talk and progressive muscle relaxation) might be useful for Sangeeta during rehabilitation.
4. Explain how and why combining multiple psychosocial strategies (e.g., relaxation imagery and self-talk) might be useful to help Sangeeta with her return to participation.

References

Arvinen-Barrow, M., Clement, D., Hamson-Utley, J. J., Zakrajsek, R. A., Lee, S. M., Kamphoff, C., . . . Martin, S. B. (2015). Athletes' use of mental skills during sport injury rehabilitation. *Journal of Sport Rehabilitation, 24*(2), 189–197. https://doi.org/10.1123/jsr.2013-0148

Baer, R. A. (2003). Mindfulness training as a clinical intervention: A conceptual and empirical review. *Clinical Psychology: Science and Practice, 10*, 125–143.

Bagheri, S., Naderi, A., Mirali, S., Calmeiro, L., & Brewer, B. W. (2021). Adding mindfulness practice to exercise therapy for female recreational runners with patellofemoral pain: A randomized controlled trial. *Journal of Athletic Training, 56*(8), 902–911. https://doi.org/10.4085/1062-6050-0214.20

Bennett, J., & Lindsay, P. (2016). Case study 3: An acceptance commitment and mindfulness based intervention for a female hockey player experiencing post-injury performance anxiety. *Sport and Exercise Psychology Review, 12*(2), 36–46.

Benson, H., & Klipper, M. Z. (2000). *The relaxation response: Updated and expanded*. Harper Collins.

Bernier, M., Thienot, E., Codron, R., & Fournier, J. F. (2009). Mindfulness and acceptance approaches in sport performance. *Journal of Clinical Sport Psychology, 3*(4), 320–333. https://doi.org/doi.org/10.1123/jcsp.3.4.320

Brewer, B. W., & Redmond, C. J. (2017). *Psychology of sport injury*. Human Kinetics.

Burland, J. P., Toonstra, J. L., & Howard, J. S. (2019). Psychosocial barriers after anterior cruciate ligament reconstruction: A clinical review of factors influencing postoperative success. *Sports Health: A Multidisciplinary Approach, 11*(6), 528–534. https://doi.org/10.1177/1941738119869333

Coronado, R. A., Bird, M. L., Van Hoy, E. E., Huston, L. J., Spindler, K. P., & Archer, K. R. (2018). Do psychosocial interventions improve rehabilitation outcomes after anterior cruciate ligament reconstruction? A systematic review. *Clinical Rehabilitation, 32*(2), 287–298. https://doi.org/10.1177/0269215517728562

Cousin, M. J., & Philips, G. D. (1985). Acute pain management. In M. J. Cousin & G. D. Philips (Eds.), *Clinics in critical care medicine*. Churchill.

Crossman, J. (2001). Managing thoughts, stress, and pain. In J. Crossman (Ed.), *Coping with sports injuries: Psychological strategies for rehabilitation* (pp. 128–147). Oxford University Press.

Cruze, E., & Games, K. E. (2021). Mindfulness training's effect of pain outcomes in musculoskeletal pain: A systematic review. *Journal of Sports Medicine & Allied Health Sciences, 7*(2), 1–12. https://doi.org/10.25035/jsmahs.07.02.01

Cupal, D. D., & Brewer, B. W. (2001). Effects of relaxation and guided imagery on knee strength, re-injury anxiety, and pain following anterior cruciate ligament reconstruction. *Rehabilitation Psychology, 46*(1), 28–43. https://doi.org/10.1037/0090-5550.46.1.28

Flint, F. A. (1998). Integrating sport psychology and sports medicine in research: The dilemmas. *Journal of Applied Sport Psychology, 10*(1), 83–102. https://doi.org/10.1080/10413209808406379

Flint, F. A. (2007). Modeling in injury rehabilitation: Seeing helps believing. In D. Pargman (Ed.), *Psychological bases of sport injuries* (3rd ed., pp. 95–108). Fitness Information Technology.

Forsdyke, D., Smith, A., Jones, M., & Gledhill, A. (2016). Psychosocial factors associated with outcomes of sports injury rehabilitation in competitive athletes: A mixed studies systematic review. *British Journal of Sports Medicine, 50*(9), 537–544. https://doi.org/10.1136/bjsports-2015-094850

Gennarelli, S. M., Brown, S. M., & Mulcahey, M. K. (2020). Psychosocial interventions help facilitate recovery following musculoskeletal sports injuries: A systematic review. *The Physician and Sportsmedicine, 48*(4), 370–377. https://doi.org/10.1080/00913847.2020.1744486

Green, L. B., & Bonura, K. B. (2007). The use of imagery in the rehabilitation of injured athletes. In D. Pargman (Ed.), *Psychological bases of sport injuries* (3rd ed., pp. 131–147). Fitness Information Technology.

Harwood, C. (1998). *Handling pressure*. The National Coaching Foundation.

Haugen, E. (2022). Athlete mental health & psychological impact of sport injury. *Operative Techniques in Sports Medicine, 30*(1), 150898. https://doi.org/10.1016/j.otsm.2022.150898

Heaney, C., Rostron, C. L., Walker, N. C., & Green, A. J. K. (2017). Is there a link between previous exposure to sport injury psychology education and UK sport injury rehabilitation professionals' attitudes and behaviour towards sport psychology? *Physical Therapy in Sport, 23*(1), 99–104. https://doi.org/10.1016/j.ptsp.2016.08.006

Heil, J. (1993). A framework of psychological assessment. In J. Heil (Ed.), *Psychology of sport injury* (pp. 73–87). Human Kinetics.

Hill, K. L. (2001). *Frameworks for sport psychologists*. Human Kinetics.

Jacobs, G. D. (2001). The physiology of mind-body interactions: The stress response and the relaxation response. *Journal of Alternative & Complementary Medicine, 7*, 583–592. https://doi.org/10.1089/107555301753393841

Jacobson, E. (1938). *Progressive relaxation*. University of Chicago Press.

Kamphoff, C. S., Thomae, J., & Hamson-Utley, J. J. (2013). Integrating the psychological and physiological aspects of sport injury rehabilitation: Rehabilitation profiling and phases of rehabilitation. In M. Arvinen-Barrow & N. Walker (Eds.), *The psychology of sport injury and rehabilitation* (pp. 134–155). Routledge.

Keable, D. (1989). *The management of anxiety: A manual for therapists*. Churchill Livingstone.

Keilani, M., Hasenöhrl, T., Gartner, I., Krall, C., Fürnhammer, J., Cenik, F., & Crevenna, R. (2016). Use of mental techniques for competition and recovery in professional athletes. *Wiener klinische Wochenschrift*, *128*(9), 315–319. https://doi.org/10.1007/s00508-016-0969-x

Kunnen, M., Dionigi, R. A., Litchfield, C., & Moreland, A. (2021). Psychological barriers negotiated by athletes returning to soccer (football) after anterior cruciate ligament reconstructive surgery. *Annals of Leisure Research*. https://doi.org/10.1080/11745398.2021.2010224

Kvist, J., & Silbernagel, K. G. (2022). Fear of movement and reinjury in sports medicine: Relevance for rehabilitation and return to sport. *Physical Therapy*, *102*(2), pzab272. https://doi.org/10.1093/ptj/pzab272

Lichtenstein, M. B., Gudex, C., Andersen, K., Bojesen, A. B., & Jørgensen, U. (2019). Do exercisers with musculoskeletal injuries report symptoms of depression and stress? *Journal of Sport Rehabilitation*, *28*(1), 46–51. https://doi.org/10.1123/jsr.2017-0103

Madrigal, L., & Gill, D. L. (2014). Psychological responses of division I female athletes through injury recovery: A case study approach. *Journal of Clinical Sport Psychology*, *8*(2), 276–298. https://doi.org/10.1123/wspaj.2014-0024

Mahoney, J., & Hanrahan, S. (2011). A brief educational intervention using acceptance and commitment therapy: Four injured athletes' experiences. *Journal of Clinical Sport Psychology*, *5*(3), 252–273. https://doi.org/10.1123/jcsp.5.3.252

Manzoni, G. M., Pagnini, F., Castelnuovo, G., & Molinari, E. (2008). Relaxation training for anxiety: A ten-years systematic review with meta-analysis. *BCM Psychiatry*, *8*, 41–52. https://doi.org/10.1186/1471-244X-8-41

McCaffery, M., & Pasero, C. (1999). Assessment: Underlying complexities, misconceptions, and practical tools. In M. McCaffery & C. Pasero (Eds.), *Pain clinical manual* (2n ed., pp. 35–102). Mosby.

McConnell, A. (2011). *Breathe strong perform better*. Human Kinetics.

Moesch, K., Ivarsson, A., & Johnson, U. (2020). "Be mindful even though it hurts": A single-case study testing the effects of a mindfulness-and acceptance-based intervention on injured athletes' mental health. *Journal of Clinical Sport Psychology*, *14*(4), 399–421. https://doi.org/10.1123/jcsp.2019-0003

Multhaupt, G., & Beuth, J. (2018). The use of imagery in athletic injury rehabilitation: A systematic review. *German Journal of Sports Medicine*, *69*(3), 57–63. https://doi.org/10.5960/dzsm.2018.316

Ost, L. G. (1988). Applied relaxation: Description of an effective coping technique. *Scandinavian Journal of Behavior Therapy*, *17*, 83–96.

Payne, S. (2004). Relaxation techniques. In G. S. Kolt & M. B. Andersen (Eds.), *Psychology in the physical and manual therapies* (pp. 111–124). Churchill Livingstone.

Pelka, M., Heidari, J., Ferrauti, A., Meyer, T., Pfeiffer, M., & Kellmann, M. (2016). Relaxation techniques in sports: A systematic review on acute effects on performance. *Performance Enhancement & Health*, *5*(2), 47–59.

Putukian, M. (2016). The psychological response to injury in student athletes: A narrative review with a focus on mental health. *British Journal of Sports Medicine*, *50*(3), 145–149.

Rotella, R. J. (1982). Psychological care of the injured athlete. In D. N. Kulund (Ed.), *The injured athlete* (pp. 213–224). Lippincott.

Roychowdhury, D., Ronkainen, N., & Guinto, M. L. (2021). The transnational migration of mindfulness: A call for reflective pause in sport and exercise psychology. *Psychology of Sport and Exercise*, *56*. https://doi.org/10.1016/j.psychsport.2021.101958

Taylor, J., & Taylor, S. (1997). *Psychological approaches to sports injury rehabilitation*. Aspen.

Vealey, R. S., & Forlenza, S. T. (2015). Understanding and using imagery in sport. In J. M. Williams & V. Krane (Eds.), *Applied sport psychology: Personal growth to peak performance* (7th ed., pp. 240–273). McGraw Hill.

Wagman, D., & Khelifa, M. (1996). Psychological issues in sport injury rehabilitation: Current knowledge and practice. *Journal of Athletic Training*, *31*(3), 257–261.

Walker, N. (2006). *The meaning of sports injury and re-injury anxiety assessment and intervention* University of Wales.

Walker, N., & Thatcher, J. (2011). The emotional response to athletic injury: Re-injury anxiety. In J. Thatcher, M. V. Jones, & D. Lavallee (Eds.), *Coping and emotion in sport* (2nd ed., pp. 235–259). Routledge.

Walsh, A. E. (2011). The relaxation response: A strategy to address stress. *International Journal of Athletic Therapy & Training, 16*(2), 20–23. https://doi.org/10.1123/ijatt.16.2.20

Weinberg, R. S., & Gould, D. (2019). *Foundations of sport and exercise psychology* (7th ed.). Human Kinetics.

Wiese-Bjornstal, D. M., Wood, K. N., & Kronzer, J. R. (2020). Sport injuries and psychological sequelae. In G. Tenenbaum & R. C. Eklund (Eds.), *Handbook of sport psychology* (4th ed., pp. 751–772). John Wiley & Sons, Inc.

Williams, J. M., & Andersen, M. B. (2007). Psychosocial antecedents of sport injury and interventions for risk reduction. In G. Tenenbaum & R. C. Eklund (Eds.), *Handbook of sport psychology* (3rd ed., pp. 379–403). Wiley.

Yukelson, D., & Murphy, S. (1993). Psychological considerations in injury prevention. In P. A. F. H. Renstrom (Ed.), *Sports injuries: Basic principles of prevention and care* (pp. 321–333). Blackwell Scientific Publications.

17 Imagery in Sport Injury and Rehabilitation

*Monna Arvinen-Barrow, Damien Clement,
Brian Hemmings, and Jessica L. Ford*

Chapter Objectives

- To define imagery in the context of sport injury and rehabilitation.
- To describe the different functions, types, and benefits of imagery in sport injury and rehabilitation.
- To outline the process of using imagery during sport injury rehabilitation.

Introduction

Many athletes, sport coaches, and sport psychology professionals (SPPs) appreciate the usefulness of mental imagery in enhancing sport performance (Simonsmeier et al., 2020). A wealth of research evidence exists in support of imagery being one of the most popular performance-enhancement techniques in sport (e.g., DeFrancesco & Burke, 1997; Hall & Rodgers, 1989; Miller & Munroe-Chandler, 2019; Pain et al., 2011; Simonsmeier et al., 2020). It appears that athletes of all levels frequently use imagery (Arvinen-Barrow et al., 2008; Arvinen-Barrow et al., 2007), and that elite, high-level, and successful athletes use significantly more imagery than their novice, lower-level, and less-successful counterparts (e.g., Arvinen-Barrow et al., 2008; Callow & Hardy, 2001; Cumming & Hall, 2002a, 2002b; Munroe-Chandler & Guerrero, 2017).

Athletes also use imagery at different times of the season (e.g., Arvinen-Barrow et al., 2008; Cumming & Hall, 2002a; Munroe et al., 1998). Imagery use goes beyond sport type classification (e.g., team vs. individual, open vs. closed, and fine vs. gross motor skill). For example, athletes in alpine skiing, basketball, Brazilian jujitsu, dance, fencing, field hockey, figure skating, floorball, football, grappling, gymnastics, handball, ice hockey, judo, martial arts, motocross, mountain biking, power lifting, rugby, soccer, squash, synchronized skating, tennis, track-and-field, triathlon, volleyball, wheelchair basketball, and wheelchair rugby have reported using imagery (e.g., Arvinen-Barrow et al., 2007, 2008; Budnik-Przybylska et al., 2020; Cederström et al., 2020; Faull & Jones, 2018; Hall et al., 1990; Martin & Malone, 2013; Munroe et al., 1998; Wesch et al., 2016).

Despite the documented use of imagery by athletes of different levels in a variety of sports, and a decade on since the publication of the first edition of this chapter (Arvinen-Barrow et al., 2013), using imagery during sport injury rehabilitation continues to be largely underutilized (Arvinen-Barrow et al., 2015; Krawiec & Budnik-Przybylska, 2021; Walsh, 2005). This could be due to (a) a lack of understanding of how imagery works in a rehabilitation setting

DOI: 10.4324/9781003295709-20

(Arvinen-Barrow et al., 2015; Arvinen-Barrow et al., 2010; Walsh, 2005), (b) a lack of robust intervention studies examining the effectiveness of imagery when implemented with sport injuries (Brewer & Arvinen-Barrow, 2021; Evans & Brewer, 2022; Wesch et al., 2016), or simply (c) an indication of athletes' inability to transfer skills that they normally use for performance enhancement into injury rehabilitation. The purpose of this chapter is to discuss how imagery could be applied to sport injury rehabilitation. The chapter will (a) define imagery, (b) introduce different functions and types of imagery that can be beneficial during rehabilitation, (c) discuss the ways in which athletes can benefit from using imagery during rehabilitation, and (d) outline the process of using imagery during rehabilitation.

Concept Definitions

In the context of sport, Morris et al. (2005) and Denis (1985) have defined *imagery* as a cognitive process that involves creating or re-creating an object, scene, sensation, event, or activity experience as though it were occurring in overt, physical reality. The visualization process is generated from memorial information that stems from the past or may take place in the future. The process involves "quasi-sensorial, quasi-perceptual, and quasi-affective characteristics, that is under the volitional control of the imager, and which may occur in the absence of the real stimulus antecedents normally associated with the actual experience" (Morris et al., 2005, p. 19).

In "lay terms," imagery can be described as an activity which involves creating a clear mental picture of the sporting situations, which can mean the venue, the performance, the conditions, the people, the emotions, and the feelings. Imagery is underpinned by the assumption that the mind does not differentiate between real and actual scenarios; when an athlete is imagining an activity, the brain reacts as if the activity were actually being executed (Krawiec & Budnik-Przybylska, 2021). When applied to sport injury rehabilitation, *imagery* refers to an activity in which the athlete can create images related to the injury, rehabilitation, and the return to participation. These include, but are not limited to, the healing process, the injured body part fully healed and restored to normal levels of functioning, the rehabilitation setting, successfully completing rehabilitation exercises, and dealing with pain and any emotions associated with the injury and recovery process.

Functions of Imagery

Typically, the sport psychology literature has identified five intersecting imagery types as useful to athletes (Hall et al., 1998). According to Hall et al. (1998), these include *cognitive-specific imagery* (CS; imagining specific sport skills), *cognitive-general imagery* (CG; imagining executing entire plays/routines and sections of a performance), *motivational-specific imagery* (MS; imagining winning a medal), *motivational-general arousal imagery* (MG; imagining controlling stress, anxiety, and arousal), and *motivational-general mastery imagery* (MGM; imagining feeling confident). Rarely have these been described in an injury rehabilitation setting (Monsma et al., 2009), as the focus of rehabilitation imagery has been on the usefulness (and effectiveness) of healing, pain management, the rehabilitation process, and performance imagery during sport injury rehabilitation (Miller & Munroe-Chandler, 2019).

Sordoni et al. (2000) were the first to explore the functions (i.e., the *why*) of imagery use during rehabilitation. Their findings indicated that rehabilitation imagery serves both a cognitive and motivational function. In a subsequent study, Sordoni et al. (2002) extended their earlier work by stating that athletes with injuries used imagery for cognitive, motivational, and healing purposes. Milne et al. (2005) support the three functions of imagery outlined previously, their results suggesting that athletes use significantly more imagery for motivational and cognitive purposes than for healing purposes. Milne et al. (2005) also found a relationship between cognitive imagery and task self-efficacy. They did not find motivational imagery to be a predictor for coping self-efficacy, thus implying that in sport injury rehabilitation, motivational imagery is not as important a source of self-efficacy as it is in a sport performance context.

Driediger et al. (2006) provided important information about how to build a foundation for imagery use during rehabilitation. The results revealed that athletes used imagery for motivational purposes, mainly in the form of reinforcing recovery goals (i.e., imagining being fully recovered). The findings also suggested that the actual imagery content also varied, as the athletes reported using healing, pain management, and performance imagery. Evans et al. (2006) extend the aforementioned, as they found that imagery functions and imagery use vary depending on the rehabilitation stage of the athlete. Based on Evans et al. (2006), athletes appear to use healing, pain management, and performance imagery during the early and mid-phases of rehabilitation. Performance imagery (cognitive-specific imagery) is typically used for performance enhancement and not for rehabilitation. The use of cognitive-specific imagery (e.g., imagining successful execution of technical skills) was found to have a positive effect on athletes' motivation, attitude, and self-confidence. During the latter phases, however, athletes appeared to use cognitive-specific, cognitive-general, and motivational-general mastery imagery. Imagery was also used to maintain a positive attitude and to increase self-confidence. Miller and Munroe-Chandler (2019) have provided similar guidance for imagery type and different phases of rehabilitation. They recommend motivational-general mastery, cognitive-general, and pain-management imagery type immediately following an injury. During rehabilitation, cognitive-specific, cognitive-general, motivational-specific, pain management, and healing imagery have been proposed as beneficial, depending on the phase of rehabilitation (see Miller & Munroe-Chandler, 2019).

Based on the literature reviewed, it is clear that imagery during rehabilitation can serve motivational, cognitive, healing, pain management, and sport performance/skill-related functions. Matching the function of imagery with the rehabilitation phase (see Kamphoff et al., 2013) and the imagery type appears to be beneficial for recovery. It is important to understand the meaning behind the imagery use, as it can have an impact on the effectiveness of the chosen imagery function and type for achieving the desired outcome.

Types of Imagery

Rooted in existing literature (Flint, 1998; Morris et al., 2005; Rotella, 1982, 1985; Rotella & Heyman, 1993), Walsh (2005) synthesized that there are four main types (i.e., the *what*) of imagery beneficial to sport injury rehabilitation. These include *healing imagery* (i.e., visualizing and feeling the injured body part healing), *pain management imagery* (i.e., assisting the athlete to cope with the pain associated with the injury), *rehabilitation process imagery* (i.e., assisting the athlete in dealing with possible challenges during the rehabilitation program), and *performance imagery* (i.e., practicing physical skills and imagining themselves performing successfully and injury-free). Recently, two additional types of imagery have been used in an injury rehabilitation context: *compassion-focused imagery* (i.e., showing affection toward the self and others; Campbell et al., 2019) and *dynamic motor imagery* (i.e., physically executing the intended movement while simultaneously imagining it occurring; Cederström et al., 2020). What follows is an introduction to each type of imagery.

Healing Imagery

Healing imagery refers to images in which the athlete will see the injured body part healing (e.g., imagining seeing ruptured muscle tissue getting better). Healing imagery can be used to envision the internal processes and anatomical healing that take place during rehabilitation (Walsh, 2005). For effective healing imagery, an athlete must possess a full understanding of their injury, have the ability to recreate a realistic picture of the injured area, and have an awareness of the anatomical healing process (Taylor & Taylor, 1997). They should also have knowledge of the treatment modalities employed during rehabilitation and know what the injured body part should look like once healed. Given the aforementioned, engagement in successful healing imagery requires a fair amount of knowledge and training, which unsurprisingly requires some time and effort from the individual athlete and those involved.

Only a few studies have examined the possible benefits and effects of healing imagery on sport injury rehabilitation, recovery, and the return to participation process (Cressman, 2010; Cupal & Brewer, 2001; Handegard et al., 2006; Ievleva & Orlick, 1991; Miller, 2017; Sordoni et al., 2002). Some of the main physical benefits of healing imagery include faster healing process (Ievleva & Orlick, 1991), enhanced physiological recovery (Sordoni et al., 2002), increased knee strength (Cupal & Brewer, 2001), and decreased pain (Cupal & Brewer, 2001). Research has also found healing imagery to have psychological benefits, including taking personal responsibility of the healing process (Ievleva & Orlick, 1991), decreased re-injury anxiety (Cupal & Brewer, 2001), and a greater sense of control and empowerment from injured athletes (Sordoni et al., 2002).

Pain Management Imagery

Pain management imagery requires the athlete to create images of themselves free of pain. Of the six pain management techniques identified by Fernandez and Turk (1986), three are seen as most appropriate for sport injury rehabilitation (Walsh, 2005). *Pleasant imagining* consists of visualizing yourself in a comfortable and relaxed setting, such as lying on a beach pain-free. *Pain acknowledgment* focuses on assigning pain physical properties, such as color, size, shape, sounds, and feelings. *Dramatized coping* visualizes pain as part of a challenge and reframing it as a motivational tool. These pain management imagery techniques can facilitate coping with pain, reduce pain, and subsequently assist in dealing with emotional and behavioral responses associated with injury.

Little research has examined the effectiveness of pain management imagery in sport injury rehabilitation. This is understandable, as earlier versions of the Athletic Injury Imagery Questionnaire (AIIQ and AIIQ-2; see Sordoni et al., 2000; Sordoni et al., 2002) did not include a subscale on pain management imagery. A pain management subscale was added to the AIIQ-3 (Wesch et al., 2016), but this has yet to be used in published research beyond the initial validation of the measure. Miller and Munroe-Chandler (2019) have also suggested that pain management imagery is only used in an injury rehabilitation setting. Rather than using pain management imagery, research has used different types of imagery as a strategy to alleviate pain. For example, when using a combination of relaxation techniques and guided imagery as an adjunct to physical therapy, Cupal and Brewer (2001) found reduction in pain as one of the main outcomes of the intervention. In contrast, a study investigating the effects of an intervention that combined relaxation techniques, pain management, and rehabilitation process imagery on pain found no demonstrable effects (Christakou & Zervas, 2007). Despite the lack of empirical findings to support the use of pain management imagery for rehabilitation, leading authors in the field advocate the use of imagery (be it healing, pain management, or other) as a means of alleviating pain during injury recovery and rehabilitation (Brewer & Redmond, 2017; Crossman, 2001; Walsh, 2005).

Rehabilitation Process Imagery

Rehabilitation process imagery allows the athletes with injuries to create images of the many different aspects of the process they could potentially experience, such as completing exercises, adhering to the program, overcoming setbacks and obstacles, maintaining a positive attitude, and staying focused (Heil, 1993; Ievleva & Orlick, 1991; Wiese et al., 1991). Rehabilitation process imagery can also assist athletes in dealing with the challenges that they may encounter during the process (Walsh, 2005). One of the ways in which rehabilitation process imagery is proposed to facilitate recovery is through self-efficacy. If an athlete believes and is able to visualize their ability to successfully complete an assigned rehabilitation task and/or exercise, they are more likely to be able to perform well and succeed. Green and Bonura (2007) state that rehabilitation process imagery is central to sport injury recovery, as it can enhance athletes' motivation and has a positive effect on adherence.

Research into rehabilitation process imagery is limited. One of the few studies investigating the effects of rehabilitation process imagery was a longitudinal intervention study with a male rugby player with a severely dislocated shoulder injury (Vergeer, 2006). The results supported the use of rehabilitation process imagery, as the participant reported visualizing himself making full(er) use of his shoulder. The participant also reported seeing himself performing at his pre-injury level of performance and imagining his injured arm copying the movements of his healthy arm during and after gym training. During the early stages of his rehabilitation, the participant often experienced involuntary replay images of the accident, but over the course of the rehabilitation, they had virtually disappeared. He explained how some of the images were associated with physical sensations, such as visualizing the movement of his "bone ripping." Such images were also helping him understand what had happened to his body, which he felt was facilitating his recovery. Interestingly, over the course of the physiotherapy, these images diminished as the healing progressed. Despite being able to see the head of his humerus and bone ripping, the participant reported no use of healing imagery. The participant was also not interested in trying healing imagery, as he felt that his injury was too complex, and he was not physiologically knowledgeable enough to envisage the healing process appropriately.

Performance Imagery

Performance imagery, through the mental rehearsal of sport-specific skills during rehabilitation, can have multiple benefits to athletes with injuries. As athletes often view injury as a hindering setback and as an obligatory and sometimes unnecessary time away from their sport (Taylor & Taylor, 1997), performance imagery can help maintain sport-specific skills, recognize performance gains, increase motivation, and improve the rehabilitation process (Richardson & Latuda, 1995). Performance imagery can also facilitate performance gains in areas that may not receive priority during regular training, reduce stress and anxiety, and increase confidence to return to participation (Walsh, 2005). Caution in the use of arousal-provoking images during rehabilitation is warranted, as that can result in heightened levels of somatic anxiety before returning back to sport (Monsma et al., 2009).

While research examining performance imagery in sport injury is limited (Monsma et al., 2009), what is available has typically been in support of its usefulness for athletes with injuries.

Performance imagery has been found to facilitate successful recovery (Weiss & Troxel, 1986), the speed of recovery (Ievleva & Orlick, 1991), and athletes' mood during rehabilitation and readiness to return to participation (Johnson, 2000). Performance imagery has also been linked to higher functional performance gains for muscular endurance, but not for improvements in dynamic balance and functional stability (Christakou et al., 2007). Imagery and relaxation techniques have also been found to be beneficial for the process of gaining a normal range of movement and during the joint restoration process (Beneka et al., 2007). Monsma et al. (2009) also found that imagining sport-specific images was more common among males than females and before returning to participation than at the earlier stages of rehabilitation.

Compassion-Focused Imagery

Originating from research on severe head injuries and their impact on empathy (O'Neill & McMillan, 2012), compassion-focused imagery (CFI) encourages visualizing what it is like to feel affection and warmth toward the self and others (Campbell et al., 2019). The goal of CFI is to simulate the feelings of someone who can give and experience compassion (Campbell et al., 2019; Depue & Morrone-Strupinsky, 2005) so that those impacted by head injuries can improve their quality of life, decrease critical self-talk, and improve self-reflection (Campbell et al., 2019). Not all CFI is specific to sport injuries. However, given the increasing prevalence and awareness of sport-related head injuries (Theadom et al., 2020), this emerging imagery type may be of continued importance in the sport injury rehabilitation process.

Research evidence demonstrating the effectiveness of CFI has been conflicting. CFI has been found to increase social connectedness in healthy participants (Hutcherson et al., 2008; Rockliff et al., 2008). In an injury context, use of CFI did not improve self-reported levels of empathy or self-compassion (Campbell et al., 2019), but the authors concluded that this could be due to methodological limitations (e.g., small sample size and participants' pre-existing fears of compassion). Use of CFI has also been found to decrease the physiological stress response to an experimenter-induced pain but had no impact on participant's pain tolerance (Maratos & Sheffield, 2020). While Maratos and Sheffield's (2020) research was not explicitly conducted with athletes with injuries, it provides evidence of potential utility in CFI's ability to curtail the physiological stress response in the body, particularly as it relates to pain.

Dynamic Motor Imagery

Dynamic motor imagery (DMI) combines the execution of motor imagery (visualizing tactical and kinaesthetic aspects of movement; Guillot & Collet, 2008) with actual physical practice (Cederström et al., 2020; Guillot et al., 2013). DMI was used as an intervention in a randomized controlled clinical trial that focused on traumatic knee injury (ACL, meniscus, patella) rehabilitation and should be implemented under the care of a trained sports medicine professional (SMP; Cederström et al., 2021). Cederström et al. (2020) suggested that using DMI gives individualized meaning and relevance to the rehabilitation process. This can influence motor learning (e.g., increase central nervous system involvement), increase rehabilitation adherence and intrinsic motivation, and may be associated with improved psychological readiness to return to participation. Due to physical limitations often associated with injury, it is important to note that the practice associated with DMI involves a gradual progression of movement that is monitored safely by a physical therapist (see Cederström et al., 2020).

Motor imagery (the visualization of movement) itself has been associated with the promotion of healing after an injury, as well as reduced anxiety, pain, and tension (see Dickstein & Deutsch,

2007; Guillot et al., 2013; Pastora-Bernal et al., 2021). Coupling actual movement with motor imagery (also known as DMI) has shown greater improvement in motor performance when compared to motor imagery use alone (Guillot et al., 2013). DMI has also been associated with increased enjoyment in knee injury prevention training (Cederström et al., 2020). An ongoing clinical trial investigating the impact of a 12-week motor imagery intervention program on athlete treatment following a knee injury (Cederström et al., 2021) hopes to better determine how dynamic motor imagery can be best implemented in a rehabilitation context to promote psychological readiness to return to participation.

Benefits of Imagery during Sport Injury and Rehabilitation

Existing limited research has found that athletes with injuries use imagery either spontaneously on their own (Driediger et al., 2006) or as an intervention guided by SPPs or SMPs (Arvinen-Barrow et al., 2013). What follows is a brief synthesis of the benefits of imagery during sport injury and rehabilitation, irrespective of the different imagery types outlined earlier.

Injury-Related Clinical Outcomes

Using imagery during the rehabilitation process can improve patient outcomes. For example, imagery contributed to greater improvements in knee flexion and less pain for adults that underwent knee joint arthroscopy in comparison to those who received treatment as usual (Wilczyńska et al., 2015). When compared to no-imagery control group, participants who used motor imagery before shoulder surgery were found to have greater improvements in extension, flexion, and lateral rotation and greater decrease in pain during the rehabilitation of stage II shoulder impingement syndrome (Hoyek et al., 2014).

Injury-Related Psychosocial Coping

Use of imagery has also been found to facilitate athletes' ability to better cope with their injuries (Gould et al., 1997; Rotella, 1982), the pain associated with injuries (Hamson-Utley & Vazques, 2008), and increase their perceived physical exertion during rehabilitation (Cederström et al., 2020). Some of the most notable cognitive benefits include assisting athletes in eliminating counterproductive thoughts and aiding in the development of a "positive self" (Driediger et al., 2006), improving the self-efficacy of athletes about to begin sport injury rehabilitation (Wesch et al., 2016), and helping athletes assign meaning to injury recovery (Cederström et al., 2020). Emotionally, imagery use has been found to increase overall enjoyment in the rehabilitation process (Cederström et al., 2020), increase rehabilitation motivation and subsequent rehabilitation adherence and compliance (Hamson-Utley & Vazques, 2008), and help athletes manage the emotions, anxiety, worry, and stressors typically associated with their injuries and the rehabilitation process (Hamson-Utley & Vazques, 2008; Miller, 2017; Monsma et al., 2009). Among athletes undergoing anterior cruciate ligament (ACL) reconstructive surgery for the first time, imagery training also reduced fear of re-injury and fostered confidence (Rodriguez et al., 2019). In addition to facilitating closure to injury experience (Green & Bonura, 2007), use of imagery can also help in preparing for successful return back to pre-injury level of performance physically (i.e., maintain sport-specific skills through the use of performance imagery) and psychologically (e.g., assist in increasing levels of confidence and decreasing levels of re-injury anxiety).

The Process for Using Imagery for Rehabilitation

The incorporation of imagery into injury rehabilitation should follow a systematic and organized sequence of events to increase its effectiveness within the rehabilitation context. These events can be conceptualized in terms of two phases: (a) utilizing a theoretical approach to determine the type of imagery to be used and (b) following a step-by-step program to integrate imagery into injury rehabilitation. It is advised that the aforementioned phases should be followed to increase the chances of injured athletes being able to maximize the benefits of imagery during injury rehabilitation. What follows is a description of the introductory steps as well as a brief discussion of guidelines to improve the usefulness of imagery in injury rehabilitation.

Using a Theoretical Approach to Determine the Appropriate Type of Imagery

For the chosen imagery to meet athletes' needs and to ensure the effectiveness of the implemented imagery type, understanding how imagery works is essential. Adapted from the original applied model of imagery use in sport (AMIUS; Martin et al., 1999), the first edition of this book presented an applied model of imagery use in sport injury rehabilitation (AMIUS-IR; Arvinen-Barrow et al., 2013). What follows is a revised version of the AMIUS-IR to incorporate the advances made in the theoretical applied imagery use literature (Cumming & Williams, 2012). Cumming and Williams (2012) proposed that the revised AMIUS (and, subsequently, the AMIUS-IR-Revised) can be used in a sport injury rehabilitation setting as a framework for (a) explaining the imagery phenomenon and (b) how to select the appropriate imagery type.

The revised applied model of imagery use in sport injury rehabilitation (AMIUS-IR-Revised) is centered on the *why*, *what* (type), and *how* of imagery use in sport injury rehabilitation, which acts as a determinant to the possible cognitive, affective, and behavioral outcomes of the imagery use. Grounded in existing research, the function (i.e., the *why*) of imagery use influences the types (i.e., *what*) of imagery the athletes use to achieve the desired *outcome*. The relationship between the *why* and *what* is determined by the personal meaning the individual assigns to the imagery. The model also assumes a close relationship between the *what* and the *how*; thus, these are presented concomitantly. The *why*, *what* (type), and *how* and *outcome* relationship is influenced by two pertinent antecedents: the *who* (i.e., the person using the imagery) and the *where* and *when* (i.e., the rehabilitation situation). The *what* (type) and the *how* and the *outcomes* are influenced by *imagery ability* (i.e., easiness of generating imagery content).

To determine which imagery type is most suited for the athlete with injuries, the AMIUS-IR-Revised provides a framework for factors that should be considered. First, it is imperative to determine the desired imagery function (e.g., regulate stress and anxiety). Influenced by personal meaning, the type of imagery, and its content (e.g., healing imagery, motivational-general arousal imagery) will be determined to reflect the desired imagery function. This process should consider the rehabilitation situation to ensure the desired function and outcomes are realistic and purposeful for the phase of recovery. Once the correct imagery type has been identified, those involved in the imagery process can move on to the second phase of the implementation by using a step-by-step program to integrate imagery into the injury rehabilitation.

A Step-by-Step Program to Integrate Imagery into Injury Rehabilitation

Richardson and Latuda (1995) proposed a four-step program showing how imagery could be integrated into injury rehabilitation. While this program is very useful, the authors of this chapter have modified it to include an additional step to ease any associated fears and concerns SPPs

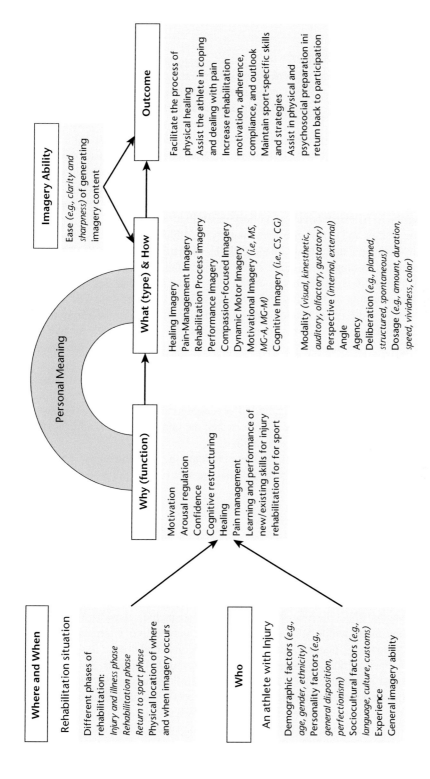

Figure 17.1 The revised applied model of imagery use in sport injury rehabilitation.

Source: Adapted from Martin et al. (1999), Cummings and Williams (2012), and Arvinen-Barrow et al. (2013).

and SMPs may have about the incorporation of imagery into injury rehabilitation. The five steps are as follows:

1. Imagery should be introduced with the intention to educate the athlete with injuries about the practical application and potential benefits of incorporating imagery into injury rehabilitation. Richardson and Latuda (1995) emphasized the importance of this step as they believe that "imagery works the best when the athlete believes it will be beneficial to the healing process" (p. 11).
2. The athlete's imagery ability needs to be informally assessed. This can be achieved by asking some, if not all, of the following questions: (a) What is your current use of imagery? (b) Describe your previous history with imagery. (c) How often have you used imagery, and in what context? (d) How effective has your past use of imagery been? and (e) How do you feel about using imagery? The information obtained can be used in the development of an imagery program to be incorporated into injury rehabilitation.
3. Depending on history and experience with imagery, an athlete with injuries may need assistance with the development of basic imagery skills. Richardson and Latuda (1995) propose 15-minute training sessions twice daily. These sessions should focus on imagery vividness and controllability, that is, the ability to create images that are vivid, clear, and realistic, in addition to incorporating all the senses (Taylor & Taylor, 1997), for a total of five minutes. Next, the focus should be switched to imagery controllability, that is, the ability to manipulate the image, making it do what they want it to (Taylor & Taylor, 1997), for five minutes. Finally, the athlete with injuries should be exposed to self-perception of the image (e.g., imagining their best ever performance, if relevant) for five minutes.
4. Once the athlete has a basic understanding of the skills introduced in step 3, they should commit to practicing until it becomes automatic. Practice should be encouraged in a variety of settings, such as before, during, and after rehabilitation-related activities and in personal time. Imagery tends to be more effective when the imagery script is athlete-created, or athlete-influenced, and/or narrated by the athlete.
5. Once the athlete has put in the necessary time practicing the use of imagery, it can be incorporated into the injury rehabilitation program, making sure to keep the process as simple and concise as possible.

Critical Success Factors

Existing research also suggests that when integrating imagery into sport injury rehabilitation, SPPs and SMPs should be mindful of the following guidelines that offer specific tips on how to maximize the usefulness of rehabilitation imagery usefulness.

1. Consider factors that affect the *how* of imagery use. These include consideration for modality (e.g., visual, kinesthetic, auditory, olfactory, gustatory), perspective (internal/external), angle, agency, deliberation (e.g., planned, structured, spontaneous), and dosage (e.g., amount, duration, speed, vividness, color), to name a few (see Cumming & Williams, 2012).
2. Consider personal and sociocultural factors that may influence imagery use. For example, when working with athletes who speak English as a second language, some of the imagery content may lose its personal and emotional meaning when scripted in non-native language.
3. Reproduce total performances. This means using all physical and psychological aspects of the injury rehabilitation experience.

4. Combine imagery with relaxation (see Chapter 16). The most important part of imagery should be to feel it physically and emotionally, and such can only be achieved if your body is relaxed, and your mind is calm.
5. Use imagery to facilitate physical and emotional well-being and feeling good.
6. Any SPPs and SMPs designing and implementing imagery interventions with injured athletes should be appropriately trained in doing so.

Conclusion

Despite existing research being limited and, on occasions, lacking empirical rigor, imagery continues to be a practical psychological intervention strategy during sport injury rehabilitation. It appears that imagery seems to positively influence injury-related clinical outcomes and psychosocial coping. This chapter provided the reader with definitions of imagery, introduced the different functions and types of injury, highlighted the benefits of rehabilitation imagery, and outlined the process of using imagery during rehabilitation.

Case Study

Rami is a 20-year-old NCAA Division III lacrosse player and honors student. During the first game of the sophomore season, Rami suffered a torn ACL (anterior cruciate ligament) in the right knee. Rami opted for ACL reconstruction surgery to increase the likelihood of returning to sport next season. The surgery required a few days off from classes, which resulted in Rami now being behind on coursework and having increased stress.

It has now been about three weeks since the initial ACL reconstruction surgery, and Rami is still in a lot of pain. Rami is adhering to the weekly physical therapy to regain strength and mobility but feels apathetic about lack of progress. Rami expressed, "I just do the same exercises every time, and I feel like nothing is improving. I know I am very difficult now, but I just cannot help it. The pain is affecting everything. The painkillers are not helping, and I hate that I cannot drive a car. Relying on friends and teammates is not fun. I feel like a burden. I wish this pain would just stop."

The head coach has tried to keep Rami involved with the lacrosse team as much as possible during recovery. It's now been eight weeks since the surgery, and the coach has noticed that Rami is becoming more withdrawn, disillusioned with the process of physical therapy, and seems to lack focus. When the coach asks Rami about physical therapy, Rami lashes out. "Come on, Coach, with all due respect, please don't ask me about it. The physio sessions are a waste of time, I am not making any progress, and I am still in pain. I might as well call it quits with lacrosse. What is the point of continuing if I never become the athlete I used to be? Besides, I am so behind on my schoolwork, too, that I don't even know where to start."

The head coach listened to Rami's outburst and remembered an athlete with ACL tear from a few years prior that found success using imagery with a certified mental performance consultant (CMPC®). The head coach passed along the CMPC®'s information to Rami. Rami has no previous experience using psychological skills but indicated willingness to try something different. That same evening, Rami scheduled an appointment and is looking forward to starting work with the CMPC® soon.

Questions

1. What key elements of Rami's experience would you want to address with imagery?
2. With reference to the integrated model of psychological response to sport injury and the rehabilitation process, what factors from Rami's experience may have affected their cognitive appraisal?
3. What type(s) of imagery might be beneficial for Rami, and why?
4. Considering the revised applied model of imagery use in sport injury rehabilitation presented in this chapter, map out Rami's case to the framework.

References

Arvinen-Barrow, M., Clement, D., Hamson-Utley, J. J., Zakrajsek, R. A., Lee, S. M., Kamphoff, C., . . . Martin, S. B. (2015). Athletes' use of mental skills during sport injury rehabilitation. *Journal of Sport Rehabilitation, 24*(2), 189–197. https://doi.org/10.1123/jsr.2013-0148

Arvinen-Barrow, M., Clement, D., & Hemmings, B. (2013). Imagery in sport injury rehabilitation. In M. Arvinen-Barrow & N. Walker (Eds.), *The psychology of sport injury and rehabilitation* (pp. 71–85). Routledge.

Arvinen-Barrow, M., Penny, G., Hemmings, B., & Corr, S. (2010). UK chartered physiotherapists' personal experiences in using psychological interventions with injured athletes: An interpretative phenomenological analysis. *Psychology of Sport and Exercise, 11*(1), 58–66. https://doi.org/10.1016/j.psychsport.2009.05.004

Arvinen-Barrow, M., Weigand, D. A., Hemmings, B., & Walley, M. (2008). The use of imagery across competitive levels and time of season: A cross-sectional study amongst synchronized skaters in Finland [Refereed]. *European Journal of Sport Sciences, 8*(3), 135–142. https://doi.org/10.1080/17461390801987968

Arvinen-Barrow, M., Weigand, D. A., Thomas, S., Hemmings, B., & Walley, M. (2007). Elite/novice athlete's imagery use in open/closed sports [Refereed]. *Journal of Applied Sport Psychology, 19*(1), 93–104. https://doi.org/10.1080/10413200601102912

Beneka, A., Malliou, P., Bebetsos, E., Gioftsidou, A., Pafis, G., & Godolias, G. (2007). Appropriate counselling techniques for specific components of the rehabilitation plan: A review of the literature. *Physical Training, 8*, 3–14. www.ejmas.com/pt/2007pt/ptart_beneka_0707.html

Brewer, B. W., & Arvinen-Barrow, M. (2021). Psychology of injury and rehabilitation. In Association for Applied Sport Psychology (AASP). In S. C. Sackett, N. Durand-Bush, & L. Tashman (Eds.), *The essential guide for mental performance consultants*. Human Kinetics Custom Content.

Brewer, B. W., & Redmond, C. J. (2017). *Psychology of sport injury*. Human Kinetics.

Budnik-Przybylska, D., Karasiewicz, K., & Kukiełko, T. (2020). Imagery, personality and injury perception in sport – mediating the effect of injury perception and imagery. *ACTA Neuropsychologica, 8*(4), 477–491. https://doi.org/10.5604/01.3001.0014.5286

Callow, N., & Hardy, L. (2001). Types of imagery associated with sport confidence in netball players of varying skills. *Journal of Applied Sport Psychology, 13*(1), 1–17. https://doi.org/10.1080/10413200109339001

Campbell, I. N., Gallagher, M., McLeod, H. J., O'Neill, B., & McMillan, T. M. (2019). Brief compassion focused imagery for treatment of severe head injury. *Neuropsychological Rehabilitation, 29*(6), 917–927. https://doi.org/10.1080/09602011.2017.1342663

Cederström, N., Granér, S., Nilsson, G., & Ageberg, E. (2020). Effect of motor imagery on enjoyment in knee-injury prevention and rehabilitation training: A randomized crossover study. *Journal of Science and Medicine in Sport, 24*(3), 258–263. https://doi.org/10.1016/j.jsams.2020.09.004

Cederström, N., Granér, S., Nilsson, G., Dahan, R., & Ageberg, E. (2021). Motor imagery to facilitate sensorimotor re-learning (MOTIFS) after traumatic knee injury: Study protocol for an adaptive randomized controlled trial. *Trials, 22*(1), 729. https://doi.org/10.1186/s13063-021-05713-8

Christakou, A., & Zervas, Y. (2007). The effectiveness of imagery on pain, edema, and range of motion in athletes with grade II ankle sprain. *Physical Therapy in Sport, 8*(3), 130–141. https://doi.org/10.1016/j.ptsp.2007.03.005

Christakou, A., Zervas, Y., & Lavallee, D. (2007). The adjunctive role of imagery on the functional rehabilitation of a grade II ankle sprain. *Human Movement Science, 26*(1), 141–154. https://doi.org/10.1016/j.humov.2006.07.010

Cressman, J. (2010). *Evaluation of the use of healing imagery in athletic injury rehabilitation* (Master's Thesis). Wilfrid Laurier University. https://scholars.wlu.ca/cgi/viewcontent.cgi?article=1995&context=etd

Crossman, J. (2001). Managing thoughts, stress, and pain. In J. Crossman (Ed.), *Coping with sports injuries: Psychological strategies for rehabilitation* (pp. 128–147). Oxford University Press.

Cumming, J., & Hall, C. (2002a). Athletes' use of imagery in the off-season. *The Sport Psychologist, 16*(2), 160–172. https://doi.org/10.1123/tsp.16.2.160

Cumming, J., & Hall, C. (2002b). Deliberate imagery practice: The development of imagery skills in competitive athletes. *Journal of Sports Sciences, 20*(2), 137–145. https://doi.org/10.1080/026404102317200846

Cumming, J., & Williams, S. E. (2012). The role of imagery in performance. In S. M. Murphy (Ed.), *Handbook of sport and performance psychology* (pp. 213–232). Oxford University Press.

Cupal, D. D., & Brewer, B. W. (2001). Effects of relaxation and guided imagery on knee strength, re-injury anxiety, and pain following anterior cruciate ligament reconstruction. *Rehabilitation Psychology, 46*(1), 28–43. https://doi.org/10.1037/0090-5550.46.1.28

DeFrancesco, C., & Burke, K. L. (1997). Performance enhancement strategies used in a professional tennis tournament. *International Journal of Sport Psychology, 28*, 185–195.

Denis, M. (1985). Visual imagery and the use of mental practice in the development of motor skills. *Canadian Journal of Applied Sport Sciences, 10*, 4S–16S.

Depue, R. A., & Morrone-Strupinsky, J. V. (2005). A neurobehavioral model of affiliative bonding: Implications for conceptualizing a human trait of affiliation. *Behavioral and Brain Sciences, 28*(3), 313–349. https://doi.org/10.1017/S0140525X05000063

Dickstein, R., & Deutsch, J. E. (2007). Motor imagery in physical therapist practice. *Physical Therapy, 87*(7), 942–953. https://doi.org/10.2522/ptj.20060331

Driediger, M., Hall, C., & Callow, N. (2006). Imagery use by injured athletes: A qualitative analysis. *Journal of Sports Sciences, 24*(3), 261–271. https://doi.org/10.1080/02640410500128221

Evans, L., & Brewer, B. W. (2022). Applied psychology of sport injury: Getting to – and moving across – The Valley of death. *Journal of Applied Sport Psychology, 34*(5), 1011–1028. https://doi.org/10.1080/10413200.2021.2015480

Evans, L., Hare, R., & Mullen, R. (2006). Imagery use during rehabilitation from injury. *Journal of Imagery Research in Sport and Physical Activity, 1*(1), 1. www.bepress.com/jirspa/vol1/iss1/art1/

Faull, A. L., & Jones, E. S. (2018). Development and validation of the Wheelchair Imagery Ability Questionnaire (WIAQ) for use in wheelchair sports. *Psychology of Sport and Exercise, 37*, 196–204. https://doi.org/10.1016/j.psychsport.2017.11.015

Fernandez, E., & Turk, D. C. (1986). *Overall and relative efficacy of cognitive strategies in attenuating pain* [Paper presentation]. The 94th Annual Convention of the American Psychological Association.

Flint, F. A. (1998). Specialized psychological interventions. In F. A. Flint (Ed.), *Psychology of sport injury* (pp. 29–50). Human Kinetics.

Gould, D., Udry, E., Bridges, D., & Beck, L. (1997). Coping with season-ending injuries. *The Sport Psychologist, 11*(4), 379–399. https://doi.org/10.1123/tsp.11.4.379

Green, L. B., & Bonura, K. B. (2007). The use of imagery in the rehabilitation of injured athletes. In D. Pargman (Ed.), *Psychological bases of sport injuries* (3rd ed., pp. 131–147). Fitness Information Technology.

Guillot, A., & Collct, C. (2008). Construction of the motor imagery integrative model in sport: A review and theoretical investigation of motor imagery use. *International Review of Sport and Exercise Psychology, 1*(1), 31–44. https://doi.org/10.1080/17509840701823139

Guillot, A., Moschberger, K., & Collet, C. (2013). Coupling movement with imagery as a new perspective for motor imagery practice. *Behavioral and Brain Functions, 9*, 1–8. https://doi.org/10.1186/1744-9081-9-8

Hall, C. R., Mack, D. E., Paivio, A., & Hausenblas, H. A. (1998). Imagery use by athletes: Development of the sport imagery questionnaire. *International Journal of Sport Psychology, 29*, 73–89.

Hall, C. R., & Rodgers, W. M. (1989). Enhancing coaching effectiveness in figure skating through a mental skills training program. *The Sport Psychologist, 4*, 1–10. https://doi.org/10.1123/tsp.3.2.142

Hall, C. R., Rodgers, W. M., & Barr, K. A. (1990). The use of imagery by athletes in selected sports. *The Sport Psychologist, 4*(1), 1–10. https://doi.org/10.1123/tsp.4.1.1

Hamson-Utley, J. J., & Vazques, L. (2008). The comeback: Rehabilitating the psychological Injury. *Athletic Therapy Today, 13*(5), 35–38. https://doi.org/doi.org/10.1123/att.13.5.35

Handegard, L. A., Joyner, A. B., Burke, K. L., & Reimann, B. (2006). Relaxation and guided imagery in the sport rehabilitation context. *Journal of Excellence, 11*, 146–164. www.zoneofexcellence.ca/Journal/Issue11/RelaxationGuidedImagery.pdf

Heil, J. (1993). Mental training in injury management. In J. Heil (Ed.), *Psychology of sport injury* (pp. 151–174). Human Kinetics.

Hoyek, N., Di Rienzo, F., Collet, C., Hoyek, F., & Guillot, A. (2014). The therapeutic role of motor imagery on the functional rehabilitation of a stage II shoulder impingement syndrome. *Disability and Rehabilitation, 36*(13), 1113–1119. https://doi.org/10.3109/09638288.2013.833309

Hutcherson, C. A., Seppala, E. M., & Gross, J. J. (2008). Loving-kindness meditation increases social connectedness. *Emotion, 8*(5), 720–724. https://doi.org/10.1037/a0013237

Ievleva, L., & Orlick, T. (1991). Mental links to enhanced healing: An exploratory study. *The Sport Psychologist, 5*(1), 25–40. https://doi.org/10.1123/tsp.5.1.25

Johnson, U. (2000). Short-term psychological intervention: A study of long-term-injured athletes. *Journal of Sport Rehabilitation, 9*(3), 207–218. https://doi.org/10.1123/jsr.9.3.207

Kamphoff, C., Thomae, J., & Hamson-Utley, J. J. (2013). Integrating the psychological and physiological aspects of sport injury rehabilitation: Rehabilitation profiling and phases of rehabilitation. In M. Arvinen-Barrow & N. Walker (Eds.), *Psychology of sport injury and rehabilitation* (pp. 134–155). Routledge.

Krawiec, J., & Budnik-Przybylska, D. (2021). Models of injury and practical tips for using imagery in rehabilitation. *Studies in Sport Humanities, 29*, 57–66. https://doi.org/10.5604/01.3001.0015.4469

Maratos, F. A., & Sheffield, D. (2020). Brief compassion-focused imagery dampens physiological pain responses. *Mindfulness, 11*, 2730–2740. https://doi.org/10.1007/s12671-020-01485-5

Martin, J. J., & Malone, L. (2013). Elite wheelchair rugby players' mental skills and sport engagement. *Journal of Clinical Sport Psychology, 7*(4), 253–263. https://doi.org/10.1123/jcsp.7.4.253

Martin, K. A., Moritz, S. E., & Hall, C. R. (1999). Imagery use in sport: A literature review and applied model. *The Sport Psychologist, 13*(3), 245–268. https://doi.org/10.1123/tsp.13.3.245

Miller, M. (2017). *A retrospective analysis: Injured youth athletes' imagery use during rehabilitation* (Master's Thesis). University of Windsor. https://scholar.uwindsor.ca/etd/6000

Miller, M., & Munroe-Chandler, K. (2019). Imagery use for injured adolescent athletes: Applied recommendations. *Journal of Sport Psychology in Action, 10*(1), 38–46. https://doi.org/10.1080/21520704.2018.1505677

Milne, M., Hall, C., & Forwell, L. (2005). Self-efficacy, imagery use, and adherence to rehabilitation by injured athletes. *Journal of Sport Rehabilitation, 14*(2), 150–167. https://doi.org/10.1123/jsr.14.2.150

Monsma, E., Mensch, J., & Farroll, J. (2009). Keeping your head in the game: Sport-specific imagery and anxiety among injured athletes. *Journal of Athletic Training, 44*(4), 410–417. https://doi.org/10.4085/1062-6050-44.4.410

Morris, T., Spittle, M., & Watt, A. P. (2005). *Imagery in sport*. Human Kinetics.

Munroe, K., Hall, C., Simms, S., & Weinberg, R. (1998). The influence of type of sport and time of season on athlete's use of imagery. *The Sport Psychologist, 12*(4), 440–449. https://doi.org/10.1123/tsp.12.4.440

Munroe-Chandler, K. J., & Guerrero, M. D. (2017). Psychological imagery in sport and performance. *Oxford Research Encyclopedia of Psychology*. https://doi.org/10.1093/acrefore/9780190236557.013.228

O'Neill, M., & McMillan, T. M. (2012). Can deficits in empathy after head injury be improved by compassionate imagery? *Neuropsychological Rehabilitation, 22*(6), 836–851. https://doi.org/10.1080/09602011.2012.691886

Pain, M., Harwood, C., & Anderson, R. (2011). Pre-competition imagery and music: The impact on flow and performance in competitive soccer. *The Sport Psychologist*, *25*(2), 212–233. https://doi.org/10.1123/tsp.25.2.212

Pastora-Bernal, J. M., Estebanez-Pérez, M. J., Lucena-Anton, D., García-López, F. J., Bort-Carballo, A., & Martín-Valero, R. (2021). The effectiveness and recommendation of motor imagery techniques for rehabilitation after anterior cruciate ligament reconstruction: A systematic review. *Journal of Clinical Medicine*, *10*(3), 428. https://doi.org/10.3390/jcm10030428

Richardson, P. A., & Latuda, L. M. (1995). Therapeutic imagery and athletic injuries. *Journal of Athletic Training*, *30*(1), 10–12. www.ncbi.nlm.nih.gov/pmc/articles/PMC1317822/pdf/jathtrain00021-0012.pdf

Rockliff, H., Gilbert, P., McEwan, K., Lightman, S., & Glover, D. (2008). A pilot exploration of heart rate variability and salivary cortisol responses to compassion-focused imagery. *Journal of Clinical Neuropsychiatry*, *5*, 132–139.

Rodriguez, R. M., Marroquin, A., & Cosby, N. (2019). Reducing fear of reinjury and pain perception in athletes with first-time anterior cruciate ligament reconstructions by implementing imagery training. *Journal of Sport Rehabilitation*, *28*(4), 385–389. https://doi.org/10.1123/jsr.2017-0056

Rotella, R. J. (1982). Psychological care of the injured athlete. In D. N. Kulund (Ed.), *The injured athlete* (pp. 213–224). Lippincott.

Rotella, R. J. (1985). The psychological care of the injured athlete. In L. K. Bunker, R. J. Rotella, & A. S. Reilly (Eds.), *Sport psychology: Psychological considerations in maximizing sport performance* (pp. 273–287). McNaughton and Gunn.

Rotella, R. J., & Heyman, S. R. (1993). Stress, injury, and the psychological rehabilitation of athletes. In J. M. Williams (Ed.), *Applied sport psychology: Personal growth to peak performance* (2nd ed., pp. 338–355). Mayfield.

Simonsmeier, B. A., Andronie, M., Buecker, S., & Frank, C. (2020). The effects of imagery interventions in sports: A meta-analysis. *International Review of Sport and Exercise Psychology*, *14*(1), 186–207. https://doi.org/10.1080/1750984X.2020.1780627

Sordoni, C., Hall, C., & Forwell, L. (2000). The use of imagery by athletes during injury rehabilitation. *Journal of Sport Rehabilitation*, *9*(4), 329–338. https://doi.org/10.1123/jsr.9.4.329

Sordoni, C., Hall, C., & Forwell, L. (2002). The use of imagery in athletic injury rehabilitation and its relationship to self-efficacy. *Physiotherapy Canada, Summer*, 177–185.

Taylor, J., & Taylor, S. (1997). *Psychological approaches to sports injury rehabilitation*. Aspen.

Theadom, A., Mahon, S., Hume, P., Starkey, N., Barker-Collo, S., Jones, K., . . . Feigin, V. L. (2020). Incidence of sports-related traumatic brain injury of all severities: A systematic review. *Neuroepidemiology*, *54*(2), 192–199. https://doi.org/10.1159/000505424

Vergeer, I. (2006). Exploring the mental representation of athletic injury: A longitudinal case study. *Psychology of Sport and Exercise*, *7*(1), 99–114. https://doi.org/10.1016/j.psychsport.2005.07.003

Walsh, M. (2005). Injury rehabilitation and imagery. In T. Morris, M. Spittle, & A. P. Watt (Eds.), *Imagery in sport* (pp. 267–284). Human Kinetics.

Weiss, M. R., & Troxel, R. K. (1986). Psychology of the injured athlete. *Athletic Training*, *21*, 104–110.

Wesch, N., Callow, N., Hall, C., & Pope, J. P. (2016). Imagery and self-efficacy in the injury context. *Psychology of Sport and Exercise*, *24*, 72–81. https://doi.org/10.1016/j.psychsport.2015.12.007

Wiese, D. M., Weiss, M. R., & Yukelson, D. P. (1991). Sport psychology in the training room: A survey of athletic trainers. *The Sport Psychologist*, *5*(1), 15–24. https://doi.org/10.1123/tsp.5.1.15

Wilczyńska, D., Łysak, A., & Podczarska-Głowacka, M. (2015). Imagery use in rehabilitation after the knee joint arthroscopy. *Baltic Journal of Health and Physical Activity*, *7*(4), 93–101. https://doi.org/10.29359/BJHPA.07.4.09

18   Social Support in Sport Injury and Rehabilitation

Monna Arvinen-Barrow, Stephen Pack,
and Travis R. Scheadler

Chapter Objectives

- To define social support and its purpose in sport injury and rehabilitation.
- To describe different mechanisms, types, and sources of social support in the context of sport injury and rehabilitation.
- To outline the process of using social support for sport injury rehabilitation.

Introduction

Social support has been one of the most rigorously and frequently researched psychosocial resources (Thoits, 1995). The notion that people feel the need to be associated with others who provide love, warmth, social ties, and a sense of belonging has long been considered as an emotionally satisfying aspect of life. Many philosophers have discussed the social needs of people, and psychologists have postulated needs for social caring and nurture (Fromm, 1955; Litwak & Szelenyi, 1969; Maslow, 1954, 1968). Social support has also been found to mediate the stress–health link, enabling individuals to better cope with stressful events, thereby reducing the likelihood stress will lead to poor health outcomes (Sarason et al., 1997). A great deal of evidence exists regarding the availability of social support and the reduced risks of mental and physical health problems (e.g., Berkman, 1984; Cohen & Wills, 1985; Thoits, 1995).

Social support has been identified as a useful coping resource when dealing with a variety of stressors in sport, such as performance pressures, relationship problems, unexpected disruption to performance routines, and depression arising from unfulfilled expectations (Gould, Eklund et al., 1993; Gould, Finch et al., 1993). High levels of particular types of social support have been linked to the maintenance of flow states (Rees & Hardy, 2004), as well as direct and indirect reductions in the effects of stress, consequently enhancing self-confidence (Rees & Freeman, 2007). Research has also demonstrated social support as beneficial to athletes when dealing with sport-related burnout (Rees, 2007). Sarason et al. (1990) also proposed social support as having a direct influence on performance, a notion which has since received empirical support (Freeman & Rees, 2009; Rees & Freeman, 2010; Rees & Hardy, 2004; Rees et al., 2007).

Despite many athletes preferring to "go it alone" (Hardy et al., 1996, p. 234), research seems to support the importance of social support provision, particularly during "times of need" (Rees, 2007, p. 224), such as when an athlete becomes injured. Indeed, the literature on sport-related injuries has proposed social support is an integral component of the coping process and thus a beneficial adjunct within the rehabilitation process (Arvinen-Barrow et al., 2017; Bianco, 2001;

DOI: 10.4324/9781003295709-21

Burland et al., 2018; Podlog & Eklund, 2007; Rotella & Heyman, 1993; Weiss & Troxel, 1986). The purpose of this chapter is to discuss how social support can be applied within the sport injury and rehabilitation context. The chapter will (a) introduce existing concept definitions and purposes of social support within the sport injury context, (b) describe the mechanisms of social support, (c) introduce different types of social support that can be beneficial during rehabilitation, (d) discuss potential sources of social support during rehabilitation, (e) outline the process of providing social support during rehabilitation, and (f) highlight critical success factors when providing social support to athletes with injuries.

Concept Definitions and Purpose of Social Support

Within the sport context, social support has received a high level of research attention, yet there is currently little consensus with regard to defining it as a concept. Proposed definitions have included "knowing that one is loved and that others will do all they can when a problem arises" (Sarason et al., 1990, p. 119). Specifically relating to the injury context, *social support* has been defined as a "form of interpersonal connectedness which encourages the constructive expression of feelings, provides reassurance in times of doubt, and leads to improved communication and understanding" (Heil, 1993, p. 145). Rees (2007) also described social support as a multifaceted process in which an athlete is aided by the existence of a caring and supportive network, as well as by their perception of other people's availability to provide help in times of need, and by the actual receipt of support. These definitions appear to capture a common theme with regard to people acting as a provider of resources when needed. In succinct terms, social support might be considered a coping resource or a social "fund" from which people may draw when dealing with stressors (Thoits, 1995). Scholars have argued that the primary purpose of social support during injury rehabilitation is to afford an athlete a sense of belonging and assurance, which might help convey that they are not isolated in their experience of injury and instead have a support network readily available to assist them in the rehabilitation process (Taylor & Taylor, 1997).

Mechanisms of Social Support

Social support influences injury rehabilitation by affecting an athlete's response to the injury process. According to the integrated model of psychological response to sport injury and rehabilitation process (Wiese-Bjornstal et al., 1998), social support is a situational factor affecting an athlete's cognitive appraisal of their injury, which in turn may influence their emotional and/or behavioral responses to the injury. Engagement (or lack of engagement) with social support has also been identified as a behavioral response to injury, which in turn can influence an athlete's cognitive appraisal and/or emotional response to the injury (Wiese-Bjornstal et al., 1998; for more details on the model, see Chapter 3).

Social support facilitates injury rehabilitation through two known mechanisms: by "buffering" athletes from harmful effects of injury-related stressors and by directly influencing the rehabilitation process without any association with stress (Mitchell et al., 2007; Rees, 2007). The stress-buffering model proposes that high levels of social support can provide a "shield," an indirect support mechanism against potential negative effects of injury. These include unrealistic or/negative cognitive appraisals (e.g., unrealistic rate of recovery expectations or decreased self-perception), undesired emotional responses (e.g., feelings of depression or frustration and poor emotional coping skills), and undesired behavioral responses (e.g., lack of rehabilitation adherence, substance abuse, and malingering), each having been found to have a negative effect on overall recovery outcomes of injury. The stress-buffering model also assumes that social support is not relevant to those who do not perceive their situation (that is, the injury) as stressful.

The main effects model proposes that social support can directly influence an individual's response to the injury and rehabilitation process (i.e., how an individual appraises the injury situation cognitively, emotionally, and behaviorally). Having a supportive network offers the potential to increase positive affect, therefore increasing the likelihood of an athlete being more realistic about the rate of perceived recovery (cognitive appraisal). This can subsequently cause decreased levels of frustration and a more positive attitude toward rehabilitation (emotional response), leading to the potential for enhanced treatment compliance and rehabilitation adherence (behavioral response).

Although each model describes different causal explanations of how social support works, the two are complementary (Bianco & Eklund, 2001). An athlete may view injury as stress-inducing, and based upon the number and quality of personal (e.g., confidence) and situational factors (e.g., type/severity of injury and the rehabilitation environment), social support might help both directly and indirectly. Having assistance with everyday life chores (e.g., food preparation) might have a direct impact on athletes' responses to the injury and rehabilitation process by reducing daily hassles. Such support can also enable athletes to avoid unnecessary (and potentially harmful) physical movement, consequently directly affecting the rate of physical recovery and recovery outcomes. Having a supportive sports medicine professional to work with can help athletes approach the rehabilitation process with a positive outlook, thus reducing perceived levels of stress. In contrast, a lack of tangible day-to-day support might increase the stress experienced by athletes. It is important to understand not only how social support works during injury and rehabilitation but also what types of social support can be beneficial to athletes during the rehabilitation and recovery process.

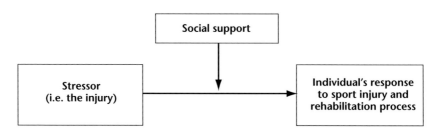

Figure 18.1 The stress-buffering effect model of social support adapted to sport injury.

Source: Adapted from Rees (2007). Copyright ©2013 from *Psychology of Sport Injury and Rehabilitation* by Monna Arvinen-Barrow and Natalie Walker (eds.). Reproduced by permission of Taylor and Francis Group, LLC, a division of Informa plc. This permission does not cover any third party copyrighted work which may appear in the material requested. User is responsible for obtaining permission for such material separately from this grant.

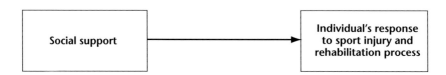

Figure 18.2 The main effects model of social support adapted to sport injury.

Source: Adapted from Rees (2007). Copyright ©2013 from *Psychology of Sport Injury and Rehabilitation* by Monna Arvinen-Barrow and Natalie Walker (eds.). Reproduced by permission of Taylor and Francis Group, LLC, a division of Informa plc. This permission does not cover any third party copyrighted work which may appear in the material requested. User is responsible for obtaining permission for such material separately from this grant.

Types of Social Support in Sport Injury Rehabilitation

Existing literature generally considers social support as a multidimensional construct (Rees & Hardy, 2000), and there is an ongoing disagreement regarding how many dimensions (or types of support) social support might comprise (Cutrona & Russell, 1990). Based on existing research (Hardy & Grace, 1991, 1993; Pines et al., 1981; Udry, 2002), five distinct types of social support are considered beneficial during sport injury rehabilitation: (1) emotional support, (2) technical support, (3) informational support, (4) tangible support, and (5) motivational support. These can be subdivided into esteem support, listening support, emotional support, emotional challenge support, shared social reality support, technical appreciation support, technical challenge support, personal assistance support, and material assistance support (see Table 18.1).

Table 18.1 Different Types of Social Support during Sport Injury Rehabilitation

Type of Support	Description of Support
Esteem support	Enacting behaviors that bolster an athlete's self-confidence, sense of competence, or self-esteem perhaps through provision of positive feedback or by demonstrating belief in the athlete's ability to cope with injury (Freeman & Rees, 2009; Rees, 2007).
Listening support	Actively listening to the athlete whilst refraining from giving advice or making judgment. This should involve sharing both positive (e.g., joys of rehabilitation success) and negative (e.g., setback frustrations) thoughts and feelings associated with rehabilitation (Taylor & Taylor, 1997).
Emotional support	Providing an athlete with impartial assistance during emotionally difficult times and demonstrating acceptance, empathy, and encouragement should they experience setbacks, thus facilitating a sense of comfort and security (Freeman & Rees, 2009; Rees & Hardy 2000)
Emotional challenge support	Challenging the athlete to do their utmost to overcome obstacles to goal achievement, and structuring support so as to facilitate motivation toward rehabilitation (Taylor & Taylor, 1997).
Shared social reality support	Acting as a "reality touchstone" by verifying an athlete's perception of the current situation and social context, thus potentially providing a sense of "normalization" (Taylor & Taylor, 1997).
Technical appreciation support	Demonstrating an acknowledgment of an athlete's achievements or reinforcing effort and intensity during a rehabilitation session (Taylor & Taylor, 1997).
Technical challenge support	Encouraging athletes to achieve more, to be excited about their work and progress, and to seek new ways in which they might rehabilitate (Taylor & Taylor, 1997).
Personal assistance support	Providing advice, guidance, and assistance in the form of time, skill, knowledge, and expertise targeted directly at problem-solving or feedback relating to rehabilitation (Rees & Hardy, 2000).
Material assistance	Providing tangible assistance, such as the provision of transport to rehabilitation, assistance with general household duties, and financial support, thus directly facilitating an athlete's chances of goal achievement (Rees, 2007; Rees & Hardy, 2000).
Motivational support	Encouraging athletes to overcome, or give into, various barriers during the rehabilitation process (Udry, 2001, 2002).

Depending on the athlete and their situation, different types of social support may be appropriate for different phases of rehabilitation (for more on rehabilitation phases, see Clement & Arvinen-Barrow, 2020b; Kamphoff et al., 2013, and Chapter 1). For example, an athlete in phase I (reaction to injury) is often mostly concerned about the pain they are experiencing. The provision of listening and emotional support, and material assistance, might be most appropriate to help athletes feel comforted and cope better with injury. During phase II (reaction to rehabilitation), an athlete is more likely to benefit from emotional challenge, technical appreciation, challenge, and motivational support, with a goal to sustain or increase motivation, rehabilitation adherence, and/or treatment compliance. During phase III (reaction to return to play), esteem support and different forms of technical and informational support can help an athlete feel more confident in their ability to return to participation and address anxiety-related concerns.

Sources of Social Support in Sport Injury Rehabilitation

Depending on personal and situational factors, the type of social support an athlete needs and prefers may vary greatly. While it is important to understand the various types of support that might be beneficial to meet the needs of an athlete with injuries, it is also important to consider potential sources of social support. During sport injury rehabilitation, athletes often interact with many individuals who might become a source of social support. These could be immediate family members, significant others, friends, sport team members (e.g., coaches, teammates), sports medicine professionals (SMPs), sport psychology professionals (SPPs), and other community members (Arvinen-Barrow et al., 2019; Caron et al., 2021; Clement & Arvinen-Barrow, 2020a; Essery et al., 2017; Iñigo et al., 2015; Ruddock-Hudson et al., 2014; Tjong et al., 2015; Yang et al., 2014). Depending on the role each has during rehabilitation, together they will form the foundation for the interprofessional care team for the athlete during rehabilitation (for more details, see Chapter 7) in the hope of ensuring a fast yet appropriate return to pre-injury (or higher) levels of fitness and performance.

Family, Friends, and Significant Others

According to Taylor and Taylor (1997), family and friends are best suited to provide emotional and listening support, as well as support in the form of emotional challenge and shared social reality (cf. Clement & Arvinen-Barrow, 2020a). Clement et al. (2015) and Ruddock-Hudson et al. (2014) noted that family and significant others comfort athletes with social support throughout each stage of the rehabilitation process. Among professional rugby players, parents were also found to provide listening support and emotional challenge support to help players regain emotional control during difficult periods (Carson & Polman, 2008). Similarly, Arvinen-Barrow et al. (2014) found that, among professional football and rugby players, families were seen as essential sources of emotional and motivational support. When an injury results in major physical limitations, the role of family as a form of tangible support (e.g., transportation to rehabilitation appointments) has also been found to be prominent (Arvinen-Barrow et al., 2014, 2017, 2019; Podlog et al., 2013). At times, family and friends have been found to pressure athletes to return to participation, sometimes too soon (Podlog et al., 2013). Family and friends should therefore be encouraged to provide social support but cautioned from pressuring athletes to return to participation too quickly.

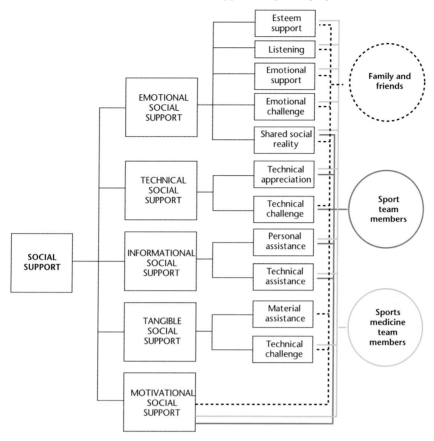

Figure 18.3 Types and sources of social support in sport injury rehabilitation.

Source: Collated from the works of Pines et al. (1981) and Udry (1997, 2002). Copyright ©2013 From *Psychology of Sport Injury and Rehabilitation* by Monna Arvinen-Barrow and Natalie Walker (eds.). Reproduced by permission of Taylor and Francis Group, LLC, a division of Informa plc. This permission does not cover any third party copyrighted work which may appear in the material requested. User is responsible for obtaining permission for such material separately from this grant.

Sport Team Members

Some scholars have suggested teammates and coaches as being well positioned to provide athletes with support in the form of technical appreciation, technical challenge, and shared social reality (Clement & Arvinen-Barrow, 2020a; Taylor & Taylor, 1997). Research has demonstrated teammates are also a source of inspiration (Carson & Polman, 2008) and motivational support (Arvinen-Barrow et al., 2014). Coaches can encourage athletes to adhere to their prescribed rehabilitation exercises (Podlog et al., 2013) and offer various other forms of emotional support (Caron et al., 2021; Ruddock-Hudson et al., 2014). Professional coaches themselves also view the provision of social support as an important part of their role by providing emotional, material, and informational support (Podlog & Eklund, 2007).

Some athletes report not receiving appropriate social support from sport team members. Arvinen-Barrow et al. (2019), for example, found some coaches questioned the severity of the professional male cricket players' injuries. Tjong et al. (2015) found lack of support from team-mates and coaches discouraged some athletes who had undergone arthroscopic shoulder stabi-lization from returning to sport. Others also have suggested how social support from coaches sometimes diminishes throughout the rehabilitation process (Ruddock-Hudson et al., 2014). Research has also highlighted disparities in how social support provision is perceived to be provided and received. Caron et al. (2021) found that coaches and teammates believed they provided the appropriate amount of social support, but athletes with injuries may have perceived a lack of emotional and esteem support from sport team members. Therefore, there is a need for sport team members to be intentional when providing social support throughout the injury rehabilitation process to ensure positive rehabilitation outcomes.

Sports Medicine Team Members

Much research suggests SMPs are well positioned to provide all types of social support due to their close relationship with athletes during injury rehabilitation. For example, Bianco (2001) found SMPs as best suited to provide various types of emotional, informational, and tangible support (cf. Clement & Arvinen-Barrow, 2020a). Among professional rugby and association football players, those working with athletes on a daily basis were seen as important sources of emotional, informational, and motivational support (Arvinen-Barrow et al., 2014). The SMPs, for example, can provide listening support by allowing athletes to vent about their feelings and shared social reality support by relating to injury experiences (Arvinen-Barrow et al., 2017; Clement et al., 2015). The SMPs are an important source of informational support, enhancing understanding of the injury and the rehabilitation process (Carson & Polman, 2008; Rock & Jones, 2002) and educating and addressing misconceptions and doubts about injury and reha-bilitation (Essery et al., 2017; Podlog et al., 2013). Existing evidence also shows that not always does social support provided by SMPs meet the athletes perceived need, and that this can have a negative impact on the injury and rehabilitation experience (Arvinen-Barrow et al., 2019).

Sport Psychology Professionals

The SMPs are also in an ideal position to help athletes expand their social network, thereby increasing their amount of social support resources (Arvinen-Barrow et al., 2010). They may connect injured athletes with other injured athletes or with various other healthcare profession-als, such as SPPs. Other professionals might also be important sources of social support. Evans et al. (2000) found that when setbacks occurred during rehabilitation, the use of an SPP was par-ticularly important. A SPP can provide various forms of emotional support by letting the athletes speak about, and reflect upon on, the injury and rehabilitation experience, subsequently helping them manage their thoughts, emotions, and behavior (Arvinen-Barrow et al., 2017).

The Process of Using Social Support for Rehabilitation

A little research has examined how best to implement social support effectively within an injury context (Rees & Hardy, 2004). Based on evidence available, it appears that social support is provided in a number of ways (Freeman et al., 2011). Differing social support needs of athletes with injuries should be met through the corresponding types of support (Rees, 2007), provided at the right time and at the right level for effectiveness (Sarason et al., 1990; Udry, 2001). This is supported by Richman et al. (1989), who proposed that social support (a) is best provided by a network of individuals, (b) needs to be developed and nurtured, and (c) works best as part of an ongoing program rather than when employed purely as a reaction to a crisis.

One of the ways social support can be provided is via peer modelling, which Kolt (2004) describes as the process of pairing an athlete with injuries with a recovered (or nearly recovered) athlete who has undergone a similar rehabilitation process. Support for peer modelling has been found in research conducted with athletic trainers (Wiese et al., 1991) and injured athletes in the form of "buddy systems" (Walker, 2006). Other athletes with similar previous injury experiences have also been found to provide shared social reality support for male professional Irish rugby football players who sustained career-ending injuries (Arvinen-Barrow et al., 2017).

Another way to introduce social support is via injury support groups (Wiese et al., 1991) or performance enhancement groups (Clement et al., 2011). Often used with athletes undergoing lengthy rehabilitation, support groups can facilitate the establishment of important networks with other athletes and offer opportunities to discuss injury and rehabilitation experiences. Support groups have also been found to facilitate motivation (Weiss & Troxel, 1986), which can be a major factor in recovery. Being part of a performance enhancement group also exposes the athletes to important psychological skills to help them cope with the distress caused by injury (Clement et al., 2011). Since social support as a concept considers many social networks as potential sources of support, athletes with injuries have individual preferences for what sources they consider beneficial; it is likely that peer modelling and injury support groups may not suit all. An alternative approach is one-on-one intervention (Freeman & Rees, 2009), often resembling a typical counselling relationship, whereby the effectiveness of the social support intervention is highly dependent on the nature of the working alliance between the athlete and the support provider.

Critical Success Factors

In addition to considering the potential types, sources, processes, and mechanisms in which social support is best provided, those involved in social support provision should also consider (a) the characteristics of the support provider, (b) the concept of perceived versus received support, and (c) the negative effects of social support.

Characteristics of the Support Provider

Literature seems to suggest that individuals providing social support should possess certain intra- and interpersonal characteristics, skills, and techniques for social support provision to be effective. A person providing social support should be a good listener, can identify personal and gender differences in athletes receiving support, and be able to acknowledge both effort and mastery. With the help from systematic goal setting, the person should also be able to balance the use of technical appreciation and technical challenge during rehabilitation. They should also possess awareness of the role of social support as necessary yet not always available for rehabilitation with injury that requires surgery and lengthy rehabilitation, and to be able to identify correct social support interventions for individual athletes (see, for example, Everhart et al., 2015; Heil, 1993; Lisee et al., 2020; Rees, 2007; Richman et al., 1989; Udry, 2001).

Perceived Versus Received Support

An important critical success factor for social support is to differentiate between perceived and received support. The effectiveness of a support network is not necessarily associated with just the number of support providers available (Sarason et al., 1990; Thoits, 1995) but is related to the extent to which various individuals recognize the need to provide support and are willing and able to provide support when necessary (Bianco, 2001). There are likely to be differences in the type of support athletes require, expect to receive, and actually receive, resulting in variations in support needs. This is also dependent upon the support provider and their role in the injured athlete's life, as well as the actual stage of rehabilitation (Caron et al., 2021; Bianco, 2001; Clement & Arvinen-Barrow, 2020b; Handegard et al., 2006). The timing of the support, the injury type, and the injury severity can also influence an athlete's perception of required, provided, and received social support (Taylor & Taylor, 1997). Some scholars have suggested gender differences in perceptions and use of social support; female athletes have been perceived as having more emotional support available from their networks than male athletes (Hardy & Grace, 1991; Mitchell et al., 2007; Rock & Jones, 2002). Understanding the differences between perceived and received support is important, as it can influence cognitive appraisals and facilitate the development and use of effective coping skills. Increases in social integration, network size, and frequency of contact with others in the network are also associated with increases in positive outcomes (Rees, 2007). These positive outcomes of social support might be a result of an athlete simply being part of a network, leading to enhanced self-concept, self-worth, and personal control.

Negative Effects of Social Support

Although social support generally appears to have a positive influence on sport injury and rehabilitation, if provided insufficiently and inappropriately, it can have a negative effect on the athlete's overall health and well-being. Insufficient rehabilitation guidance, lack of sensitivity to the injury, and lack of concern from those surrounding the athlete have been perceived negatively by athletes with injuries (Arvinen-Barrow et al., 2017, 2019; Udry et al., 1997) and can be detrimental to the overall recovery process. If the provider is not adequately skilled to provide the support needed or is not aware of their role as a source of social support, this can also have a negative effect on the athlete and the overall rehabilitation. Those involved with athletes during injury and rehabilitation should (a) be aware of their possible role as a source of social support, (b) acknowledge their own competencies and limitations as potential providers of social support, and (c) possess an understanding of when and when not to provide support.

Recent Research on Social Support and Injuries

Over the past decade, research knowledge on the use of social support as a psychological intervention in response to injury and rehabilitation has highlighted a number of psychosocial, biological, and physiological benefits of social support. It has also focused on the impact satisfaction/lack of satisfaction with social support has on the athlete and identified some gender differences in how social support is perceived and provided.

Psychosocial Benefits of Social Support

A systematic review revealed that positive social support from family, friends, significant others, sport team members, and SMPs is a facilitator for numerous rehabilitation-related behaviors. These include increased exercise adherence among injured adults (Essery et al., 2017) and older adults after following a total knee arthroplasty (Bakaa et al., 2022), increased compliance with treatment (Everhart et al., 2015) and rehabilitation commitment (Podlog et al., 2013), increased motivation to return to participation following arthroscopic shoulder stabilization (Tjong et al., 2015), and commitment to return to sport (Iñigo et al., 2015).

Some of the cognitive-affective benefits of social support include more positive outlook on injury among adolescent Australian athletes (Podlog et al., 2013), professional Australian football players (Ruddock-Hudson et al., 2014), and previously injured athletes in the United States (Clement et al., 2015). University basketball coaches also believed social support increases confidence among athletes with injuries (Van Woezik et al., 2020) and among athletes who had had undergone anterior cruciate ligament reconstruction surgery and returned to participation (Burland et al., 2018). Social support has also been found to increase coping with injury (Burland et al., 2018), coping with anxiety (Tjong et al., 2015), and decrease fear of re-injury (Burland et al., 2019; Tjong et al., 2015). Additional psychosocial benefits include decreases in restlessness and feelings of isolation (Mitchell et al., 2014), protection from identity loss following an injury (Von Rosen et al., 2018), and overall boost of well-being and rehabilitation beliefs (Lu & Hsu, 2013). Social support has also been found to facilitate successful transitions out of sport among professional male cricket, rugby, and ice hockey players with career-ending injuries (Arvinen-Barrow et al., 2015, 2017, 2019).

Biological and Physiological Benefits of Social Support

While not commonly researched within sport injury, social support has also been found to decrease *pain severity* and *interference* (i.e., impact on daily functioning) following a total knee arthroplasty (Edwards et al., 2022). A scoping review of research examining social factors in recovery after hip fractures showed that social support improved physical functioning and decreased risk of mortality following surgery (Auais et al., 2019).

(Lack of) Satisfaction with Social Support

Satisfaction with social support from SMPs has also been found to decrease symptoms of anxiety and depression among collegiate athletes with injuries (Yang et al., 2014). The same research also found that of the athletes who did receive social support, approximately 50% felt that their SMP made them feel better when upset, and 20% of the sample did not receive social support at all. Recent research has also highlighted that not always do family members, friends, sport team members, and SMPs provide appropriate social support. For example, some Australian adolescent athletes with severe injuries reported feeling pressured to return to participation by family and friends (Podlog et al., 2013).

Other athletes have reported perceived lack of social support from their social networks (Arvinen-Barrow et al., 2017; Burland et al., 2018; Tjong et al., 2015). Caron et al. (2021) have identified differential perceptions of social support provision among athletes with injuries, their teammates, and their coaches. While coaches and teammates perceived providing sufficient support, the athletes perceived it to be insufficient for emotional and esteem support (Caron et al., 2021). Research has also highlighted some gender differences in social support needs. Lisee et al. (2020) found that following an anterior cruciate ligament reconstruction, female athletes may have higher social support needs than male athletes. In fact, male athletes in this research reported team involvement throughout the recovery process worsened their experience with injury rehabilitation.

Conclusion

Despite the lack of a distinct definition of *social support*, of all the psychological interventions available, social support appears to be one of the most used psychosocial strategies during sport injury rehabilitation. Athletes with injuries appear to benefit from a range of different types of social support, provided by several individuals they typically interact with on a day-to-day basis. This chapter has provided details of the mechanisms underlying the concept of social support, the different types and sources of social support that might be beneficial during rehabilitation, and discussed the range of potential sources of social support available during rehabilitation. Moreover, the chapter has outlined the process of utilizing social support during rehabilitation and highlighted critical success factors when implementing social support to sport injury and rehabilitation.

Case Study

Ethan is a 16-year-old high school baseball player. He lives with his parents and has two older sisters who both played collegiate basketball. Ethan's parents go to as many of his games as they can and are actively involved in his sport. Ethan's dad often compares Ethan to his sisters; they both were star players during high school and college, and it is obvious that Ethan's dad expects the same from him.

About five months ago, Ethan tore his anterior cruciate ligament (ACL) while playing basketball with his friends. He underwent ACL reconstruction surgery, which went well. Ethan's orthopedic surgeon and athletic trainer (AT) think it will be another four months before Ethan is fully fit to play again. Ethan's dad is not convinced of this timeline. With the baseball pre-season just around the corner, Ethan's dad thinks Ethan should "double his rehabilitation exercises, start running and jumping to help strengthen his leg." Ethan disagrees: "Dad, that's not what the surgeon or my AT says. Besides, remember what happened to Trey?"

"Trey who?" says Ethan's dad.

Ethan responds to his dad with frustration, "You don't remember, Dad? Trey is a junior on my team. He had an ACL reconstruction last year. He came back to baseball six months post-surgery and got re-injured almost immediately. I don't want that to happen to me. I'm worried that I will get injured again if I return back too early."

"Nonsense!" says Ethan's dad. "If you stick with the regimen I suggest, you can return to baseball in time for the regular season to begin."

Ethan felt unheard and confides to his AT about the pressure his dad puts on him to return to sport. Ethan also recently told his AT that he is bisexual but has not told his parents or sisters, as he is afraid his dad will be disappointed in him. Ethan said, "I'm already not good enough at baseball. And now I'm injured too. And I like boys and girls. Not wanting to follow his plan for my rehab will just be another reason for my dad to hate me."

Questions

1. Considering the mechanisms of social support, which (stress-buffering or direct) is likely to be effective for Ethan's rehabilitation and return to participation process?

2. What social support types are likely to be beneficial for Ethan, and why?
3. Who might be best suited to provide Ethan with the different types of social support, and why?
4. What factors do you think are important to consider for social support effectiveness?

References

Arvinen-Barrow, M., DeGrave, K., Pack, S. M., & Hemmings, B. (2019). Transitioning out of professional sport: The psychosocial impact of career-ending non-musculoskeletal injuries among male cricketers from England and Wales. *Journal of Clinical Sport Psychology, 13*(4), 629–644. https://doi.org/10.1123/jcsp.2017-0040

Arvinen-Barrow, M., Hurley, D., & Ruiz, M. C. (2017). Transitioning out of professional sport: The psychosocial impact of career-ending injuries among elite Irish rugby football union players. *Journal of Clinical Sport Psychology, 10*(1). https://doi.org/10.1123/jcsp.2016-0012

Arvinen-Barrow, M., Massey, W. V., & Hemmings, B. (2014). Role of sport medicine professionals in addressing psychosocial aspects of sport-injury rehabilitation: Professional athletes' views. *Journal of Athletic Training, 49*(6), 764–772. https://doi.org/10.4085/1062-6050-49.3.44

Arvinen-Barrow, M., Nässi, A., & Ruiz, M. C. (2015). Kun vamma päättää, milloin ura loppuu. [When injury determines when the career ends]. *Liikunta ja Tiede, 52*(6), 45–49.

Arvinen-Barrow, M., Penny, G., Hemmings, B., & Corr, S. (2010). UK chartered physiotherapists' personal experiences in using psychological interventions with injured athletes: An interpretative phenomenological analysis. *Psychology of Sport and Exercise, 11*(1), 58–66. https://doi.org/10.1016/j.psychsport.2009.05.004

Auais, M., Al-Zoubi, F., Matheson, A., Brown, K., Magaziner, J., & French, S. D. (2019). Understanding the role of social factors in recovery after hip fractures: A structured scoping review. *Health & Social Care in the Community, 27*(6), 1375–1387. https://doi.org/doi.org/10.1111/hsc.12830

Bakaa, N., Chen, L. H., Carlesso, L., Richardson, J., Shanthanna, H., & Macedo, L. (2022). Understanding barriers and facilitators of exercise adherence after total-knee arthroplasty. *Disability and Rehabilitation, 44*(21), 6348–6355. https://doi.org/10.1080/09638288.2021.1965232

Berkman, L. F. (1984). Assessing the physical health effects of social networks and social support. *Annual Review of Public Health, 5*, 413–432. https://doi.org/10.1146/annurev.pu.05.050184.002213

Bianco, T. M. (2001). Social support and recovery from sport injury: Elite skiers share their experiences. *Research Quarterly for Exercise and Sport, 72*(4), 376–388. https://doi.org/10.1080/02701367.2001.10608974

Bianco, T. M., & Eklund, R. C. (2001). Conceptual considerations for social support research in sport and exercise settings: The case of sport injury. *Journal of Sport & Exercise Psychology, 23*, 85–107. https://doi.org/10.1123/jsep.23.2.85

Burland, J. P., Toonstra, J. L., & Howard, J. S. (2019). Psychosocial barriers after anterior cruciate ligament reconstruction: A clinical review of factors influencing postoperative success. *Sports Health: A Multidisciplinary Approach, 11*(6), 528–534. https://doi.org/10.1177/1941738119869333

Burland, J. P., Toonstra, J., Werner, J. L., Mattacola, C. G., Howell, D. M., & Howard, J. S. (2018). Decision to return to sport after anterior cruciate ligament reconstruction, part I: A qualitative investigation of psychosocial factors. *Journal of Athletic Training, 53*(5), 452–463. https://doi.org/10.4085/1062-6050-313-16

Caron, J. G., Benson, A. J., Steins, R., McKenzie, L., & Bruner, M. W. (2021). The social dynamics involved in recovery and return to sport following a sport-related concussion: A study of three athlete-teammate-coach triads. *Psychology of Sport and Exercise, 52*, 101824. https://doi.org/10.1016/j.psychsport.2020.101824

Carson, F., & Polman, C. J. (2008). ACL injury rehabilitation: A psychological case study of a professional rugby union player. *Journal of Clinical Sport Psychology, 2*(1), 71–90. https://doi.org/10.1123/jcsp.2.1.71

Clement, D., & Arvinen-Barrow, M. (2020a). An investigation into former high school athletes' experiences of a multidisciplinary approach to sport injury rehabilitation. *Journal of Sport Rehabilitation, 30*(4), 619–624. https://doi.org/10.1123/jsr.2020-0094

Clement, D., & Arvinen-Barrow, M. (2020b). Psychosocial strategies for the different phases of sport injury rehabilitation. In A. Ivarsson & U. Johnson (Eds.), *Psychological bases of sport injuries* (4th ed., pp. 297–330). Fitness Information Technology.

Clement, D., Arvinen-Barrow, M., & Fetty, T. (2015). Psychosocial responses during different phases of sport injury rehabilitation: A qualitative study. *Journal of Athletic Training, 50*(1), 95–104. https://doi.org/10.4085/1062-6050-49.3.52

Clement, D., Shannon, V. R., & Connole, I. J. (2011). Performance enhancement groups for injured athletes. *International Journal of Athletic Therapy & Training, 16*(3), 34–36. https://doi.org/10.1123/ijatt.16.3.34

Cohen, S., & Wills, T. A. (1985). Stress, social support, and the buffering hypothesis. *Psychological Bulletin, 98*(2), 310–357. https://doi.org/10.1037/0033-2909.98.2.310

Cutrona, C. E., & Russell, D. (1990). Type of social support and specific stress: Toward a theory of optimal matching. In I. G. Sarason, B. R. Sarason, & G. R. Pierce (Eds.), *Social support: An interactional view* (pp. 319–366). Wiley.

Edwards, R. R., Campbell, C., Schreiber, K., Meints, S., Lazaridou, A., Martel, M. O., . . . Haythornthwaite, J. A. (2022). Multimodal prediction of pain and functional outcomes 6 months following total knee replacement: A prospective cohort study. *BMC Musculoskeletal Disorders, 23*, 302. https://doi.org/10.1186/s12891-022-05239-3

Essery, R., Geraghty, A. W. A., Kirby, S., & Yardley, L. (2017). Predictors of adherence to home-based physical therapies: A systematic review. *Disability Rehabilitation, 39*(6), 519–534. https://doi.org/10.3109/09638288.2016.1153160

Evans, L., Hardy, L., & Flemming, S. (2000). Intervention strategies with injured athletes: An action research study. *The Sport Psychologist, 14*(2), 188–206. https://doi.org/10.1123/tsp.14.2.188

Everhart, J. S., Best, T. M., & Flanigan, D. C. (2015). Psychological predictors of anterior cruciate ligament reconstruction outcomes: A systematic review. *Knee Surgery, Sports Traumatology, Arthroscopy, 23*(3), 752–762. https://doi.org/10.1007/s00167-013-2699-1

Freeman, P., Coffee, P., & Rees, T. (2011). The PASS-Q: The perceived available support in sport questionnaire. *Journal of Sport & Exercise Psychology, 33*(1), 54–74. https://doi.org/doi/10.1123/jsep.33.1.54

Freeman, P., & Rees, T. (2009). How does perceived support lead to better performance? An examination of potential mechanisms. *Journal of Applied Sport Psychology, 12*(4), 429–441. https://doi.org/10.1080/10413200903222913

Fromm, E. (1955). *The sane society.* Rinehart & Company, Inc.

Gould, D., Eklund, R. C., & Jackson, S. A. (1993). Coping strategies used by US Olympic wrestlers. *Research Quarterly for Exercise and Sport, 64*(1), 83–93. https://doi.org/10.1080/02701367.1993.10608782

Gould, D., Finch, L. M., & Jackson, S. A. (1993). Coping strategies used by national champion figure skaters. *Research Quarterly for Exercise and Sport, 64*(4), 453–468. https://doi.org/10.1080/02701367.1993.10607599

Handegard, L. A., Joyner, A. B., Burke, K. L., & Reimann, B. (2006). Relaxation and guided imagery in the sport rehabilitation context. *Journal of Excellence, 11*, 146–164. www.zoneofexcellence.ca/Journal/Issue11/RelaxationGuidedImagery.pdf

Hardy, C. J., & Grace, R. K. (1991). Social support within sport. *Sport Psychology Training Bulletin, 3*(1), 1–8.

Hardy, C. J., & Grace, R. K. (1993). The dimensions of social support when dealing with sport injuries. In D. Pargman (Ed.), *Psychological bases of sport injuries* (pp. 121–144). Fitness Information Technology.

Hardy, L., Jones, G., & Gould, D. (1996). *Understanding psychological preparation for sport: Theory and practice of elite performers*. John Wiley & Sons.

Heil, J. (1993). A comprehensive approach to injury management. In J. Heil (Ed.), *Psychology of sport injury* (pp. 137–149). Human Kinetics.

Iñigo, M. M., Podlog, L., & Hall, M. S. (2015). Why do athletes remain committed to sport after severe injury? An examination of the sport commitment model. *The Sport Psychologist, 29*(2), 143–155. https://doi.org/10.1123/tsp.2014-0086

Kamphoff, C., Thomae, J., & Hamson-Utley, J. J. (2013). Integrating the psychological and physiological aspects of sport injury rehabilitation: Rehabilitation profiling and phases of rehabilitation. In M. Arvinen-Barrow & N. Walker (Eds.), *Psychology of sport injury and rehabilitation* (pp. 134–155). Routledge.

Kolt, G. S. (2004). Injury from sport, exercise, and physical activity. In G. S. Kolt & M. B. Andersen (Eds.), *Psychology in the physical and manual therapies* (pp. 247–267). Churchill Livingstone.

Lisee, C. M., DiSanti, J. S., Chan, M., Ling, J., Erickson, K., Shingles, M., & Kuenze, C. M. (2020). Gender differences in psychological responses to recovery after anterior cruciate ligament reconstruction before return to sport. *Journal of Athletic Training, 55*(10), 1098–1105. https://doi.org/10.4085/1062-6050-558.19

Litwak, E., & Szelenyi, I. (1969). Primary group structures and their functions: Kin, neighbours and friends *American Sociological Review, 34*(4), 465–481. https://doi.org/10.2307/2091957

Lu, F. J. H., & Hsu, Y. (2013). Injured athletes' rehabilitation beliefs and subjective well-being: The contribution of hope and social support. *Journal of Athletic Training, 48*(1), 92–98. https://doi.org/10.4085/1062-6050-48.1.03

Maslow, A. H. (1954). *Motivation and personality*. Harper & Row.

Maslow, A. H. (1968). *Toward a psychology of being*. Van Nostrand.

Mitchell, I. D., Evans, L., Rees, T., & Hardy, L. (2014). Stressors, social support, and tests of the buffering hypothesis: Effects on psychological responses of injured athletes. *British Journal of Health Psychology, 19*(3), 486–508. https://doi.org/10.1111/bjhp.12046

Mitchell, I. D., Neil, R., Wadey, R., & Hanton, S. (2007). Gender differences in athletes' social support during injury rehabilitation. *Journal of Sport & Exercise Psychology, 29*(Suppl 1), S189–S190. https://doi.org/10.1123/jsep.29.s1.s144

Pines, A. M., Aronson, E., & Kafry, D. (1981). *Burnout*. Free Press.

Podlog, L., & Eklund, R. C. (2007). Professional coaches' perspectives on the return to sport following serious Injury. *Journal of Applied Sport Psychology, 19*(2), 207–225. https://doi.org/10.1080/10413200701188951

Podlog, L., Wadey, R., Stark, A., Lochbaum, M., Hannon, J., & Newton, M. (2013). An adolescent perspective on injury recovery and the return to sport. *Psychology of Sport and Exercise, 14*(4), 437–446. https://doi.org/10.1016/j.psychsport.2012.12.005

Rees, T. (2007). Influence of social support on athletes. In S. Jowett & D. Lavallee (Eds.), *Social psychology in sport* (pp. 223–232). Human Kinetics.

Rees, T., & Freeman, P. (2007). The effects of perceived and received support on self-confidence. *Journal of Sports Sciences, 25*(9), 1057–1065. https://doi.org/10.1080/02640410600982279

Rees, T., & Freeman, P. (2010). Social support and performance in a golf-putting experiment. *The Sport Psychologist, 24*(3), 333–348. https://doi.org/10.1123/tsp.24.3.333

Rees, T., & Hardy, L. (2000). An investigation of the social support experiences of high-level sports performers. *The Sport Psychologist, 14*(4), 327–347. https://doi.org/10.1123/tsp.14.4.327

Rees, T., & Hardy, L. (2004). Matching social support with stressors: Effects on factors underlying performance in tennis. *Psychology of Sport and Exercise, 5*(3), 319–337. https://doi.org/10.1016/S1469-0292(03)00018-9

Rees, T., Hardy, L., & Freeman, P. (2007). Stressors, social support, and effects upon performance in golf. *Journal of Sports Sciences, 25*(1), 33–42. https://doi.org/10.1080/02640410600702974

Richman, J. M., Hardy, C. J., Rosenfeld, L. B., & Callanan, R. A. E. (1989). Strategies for enhancing social support networks in sport: A brainstorming experience. *Journal of Applied Sport Psychology*, *1*(2), 150–159. https://doi.org/doi.org/10.1080/10413208908406411

Rock, J. A., & Jones, M. V. (2002). A preliminary investigation into the use of counseling skills in support of rehabilitation from sport injury. *Journal of Sport Rehabilitation*, *11*, 284–304.

Rotella, R. J., & Heyman, S. R. (1993). Stress, injury, and the psychological rehabilitation of athletes. In J. M. Williams (Ed.), *Applied sport psychology: Personal growth to peak performance* (2nd ed., pp. 338–355). Mayfield.

Ruddock-Hudson, M., O'Halloran, P., & Murphy, G. (2014). The psychological impact of long-term injury on Australian football league players. *Journal of Applied Sport Psychology*, *26*(4), 377–394. https://doi.org/10.1080/10413200.2014.897269

Sarason, B. R., Sarason, I. G., & Gurung, R. A. R. (1997). Close personal relationships and health outcomes: A key to the role of social support. In S. Duck (Ed.), *Handbook of personal relationships* (pp. 547–573). Wiley.

Sarason, B. R., Sarason, I. G., & Pierce, G. R. (1990). Social support, personality, and performance. *Journal of Applied Sport Psychology*, *2*(2), 117–127. https://doi.org/10.1080/10413209008406425

Taylor, J., & Taylor, S. (1997). *Psychological approaches to sports injury rehabilitation*. Aspen.

Thoits, P. A. (1995). Stress, coping and social support processes: Where are we? What next? *Journal of Health and Social Behaviour*, *Extra Issue*, 57–79. https://doi.org/10.2307/2626957

Tjong, V. K., Devitt, B. M., Murnaghan, M. L., Ogilvie-Harris, D. J., & Theodoropoulous, J. S. (2015). A qualitative investigation of return to sport after arthroscopic Bankart repair: Beyond stability. *American Journal of Sports Medicine*, *43*(8), 2005–2011. https://doi.org/doi.org/10.1177/0363546515590222

Udry, E. (2001). The role of significant others: Social support during injuries. In J. Crossman (Ed.), *Coping with sports injuries: Psychological strategies for rehabilitation* (pp. 148–161). University Press.

Udry, E. (2002). Staying connected: Optimizing social support for injured athletes. *Athletic Therapy Today*, *7*(3), 42–43. https://doi.org/10.1123/att.7.3.42

Udry, E., Gould, D., Bridges, D., & Tuffey, S. (1997). People helping people? Examining the social ties of athletes coping with burnout and injury stress. *Journal of Sport & Exercise Psychology*, *19*(4), 368–395. https://doi.org/10.1123/jsep.19.4.368

Van Woezik, R. A., Benson, A. J., & Bruner, M. W. (2020). Next one up! Exploring how coaches manage team dynamics following injury. *The Sport Psychologist*, *34*(3), 198–208. https://doi.org/10.1123/tsp.2019-0148

Von Rosen, P., Kottorp, A., Fridén, C., Frohm, A., & Heijne, A. (2018). Young, talented and injured: Injury perceptions experiences and consequences in adolescent elite athletes. *European Journal of Sport Science*, *18*(5), 713–740. https://doi.org/10.1080/17461391.2018.1440009

Walker, N. (2006). *The meaning of sports injury and re-injury anxiety assessment and intervention* University of Wales, Aberystwyth.

Weiss, M. R., & Troxel, R. K. (1986). Psychology of the injured athlete. *Athletic Training*, *21*, 104–110.

Wiese, D. M., Weiss, M. R., & Yukelson, D. P. (1991). Sport psychology in the training room: A survey of athletic trainers. *The Sport Psychologist*, *5*(1), 15–24. https://doi.org/10.1123/tsp.5.1.15

Wiese-Bjornstal, D. M., Smith, A. M., Shaffer, S. M., & Morrey, M. A. (1998). An integrated model of response to sport injury: Psychological and sociological dynamics. *Journal of Applied Sport Psychology*, *10*(1), 46–69. https://doi.org/10.1080/10413209808406377

Yang, J. Z., Shaefer, J. T., Zhang, N., Covassin, T., Ding, K., & Heiden, E. (2014). Social support from the athletic trainer and symptoms of depression and anxiety at return to play. *Journal of Athletic Training*, *49*(6), 773–779. https://doi.org/10.4085/1062-6050-49.3.65

Part 4

Return to Participation and Transition Out of Sport

19 Return to Sport Participation

Leslie Podlog, Ross Wadey, John Heil,
*and John J. Fraser**

Chapter Objectives

- To define *return to sport*.
- To describe the self-determination theory in the context of return to sport following an injury.
- To describe the psychological impact of return to participation from both the athlete's and other relevant stakeholders' perspective (e.g., sport coach, parents/caregivers, other athletes/teammates, and sport psychology professionals).

Introduction

Substantial research on the psychosocial implications of injury occurrence, rehabilitation, and return to sport (RTS) has focused on athletes with injuries (SDT; Podlog & Eklund, 2020; Tracey, 2003). Given that athletes with injuries are ultimately the ones experiencing a physical disruption and attempting to regain functional fitness, this focus is entirely logical. However, an exclusive emphasis on the impact of injury on athletes neglects the fact that injury occurs within a particular context and involves interactions with a variety of sport injury stakeholders (cf. Wadey, 2020). Recently, scholars have begun to adopt a relational perspective to injury, thus acknowledging that athletes with injuries may be impacted by multiple individuals and that athletes – including their behaviors, psychological states, and their return to sport outcomes – can have salient consequences for injury stakeholders (cf. Wadey et al., 2018).

The purpose of this chapter is to discuss the RTS participation literature by presenting both athlete and relational perspectives on the RTS following injury. In taking a relational perspective, we highlight the influence that returning athletes can have on several individuals and professionals who collectively represent a group of key injury stakeholders in athlete welfare and performance. The chapter will (a) define RTS, (b) provide an overview of self-determination theory (Ryan & Deci, 2000) that has been used to guide much of the research to date on the RTS, (c) describe research testing SDT contentions regarding athlete perspectives and RTS experiences, and (d) describe research findings pertaining to the psychological impact of athletes' RTS on relevant stakeholders, in particular, sport coaches, parents/caregivers, other athletes/teammates, and sport psychology professionals (SPPs).

DOI: 10.4324/9781003295709-23

Concept Definitions

Traditionally, an *RTS* has been defined in the sports medicine literature as a return to pre-injury sport performance levels (Doege et al., 2021). A RTS has usually been determined by functional (e.g., reactive balance, proprioception, neuromuscular function, endurance) or sport-specific measures of performance (e.g., goals, assists, performance times). In a recent systematic review, Doege et al. (2021) found that among the 29 research articles that provided a clear definition of RTS, *RTS* was defined differently depending upon the researcher in question. Twenty researchers (69.0%) defined *RTS* as an athlete competing in a game or other competitive play; three (10.3%) defined *RTS* as the athlete competing in a game or other competitive play and also included a particular competition-level modifier stipulating the athlete returning to his or her pre-injury level of competition; two articles (6.9%) included returning to training or practice; and the remaining four articles (13.8%) used terminology other than the standard RTS. In the present chapter, we define *RTS* as the time frame when athletes are transitioning from rehabilitation to sport-specific training and resumption of competitive activities, or, in the case of non-returning athletes, their segue out of sport (Podlog & Eklund, 2020).

Self-Determination Theory

Much of the research on the psychosocial aspects of RTS has been guided by self-determination theory (Ryan & Deci, 2000). It is a theory of motivation that examines the ways in which motivation is shaped and nourished by individuals' surrounding social environments (Ryan & Deci, 2000). From an SDT standpoint, *motivation* refers not only to the quantity of energy, drive, and persistence one puts forward in pursuit of goal-directed behaviors but also to the quality of the forces that energize them – that is, the reasons they engage in motivated behaviors. Ryan and Deci (2000) outlined a variety of motivational types, also referred to as behavioral regulations, existing on a continuum of self-determination. Autonomous forms of motivation exist on the one end of the continuum, that is, goals pursued for personally endorsed or valued reasons (Ryan & Deci, 2000). These include intrinsic motivation (activities that are inherently enjoyable, interesting, or satisfying for the individual), integrated regulation (actions performed for satisfying external imperatives that are fully assimilated into one's sense of self), and identified regulation (actions performed to fulfill consciously valued goals for reasons external to the self). On the other end of the continuum are more controlled (i.e., less autonomously controlled) forms of motivation. These forms of motivation underpin behaviors individuals feel compelled to do as a consequence of external or internal pressures. They include introjected regulation (behaviors engaged in to avoid internalized punishments, such as shame or guilt, or to attain internal rewards, such as pride or ego enhancements), external regulation (behaviors performed to obtain external rewards or avoid punishment), and amotivation (behaviors executed without goal intention or valuing of the activity, not feeling competent, or not believing effort will be rewarded by desired achievement).

Ryan and Deci (2000) also suggest that the degree to which an individual is guided by autonomous forms of motivation (intrinsic, identified, integrated) is a reflection of the extent to which one's psychological needs are satisfied by the surrounding environment. Three basic psychological needs for competence, autonomy, and relatedness have been espoused that are proposed to be invariant among individuals across cultures, genders, and social contexts (Ryan & Deci, 2000). The need for competence refers to the inherent imperative to view oneself as capable and efficacious in relation to the physical and social environments. The need for autonomy refers to the imperative experienced by individuals to perceive that their behavioral engagements involve a sense of agency, volition, and choice. The autonomous individual is one who acts in a manner

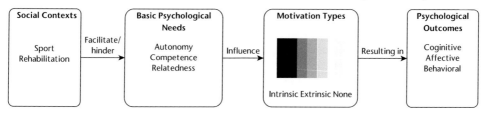

Figure 19.1 Self-determination theory adapted to sport injury rehabilitation.

Source: Adapted from *Concept Visualization: Self-Determination Theory*, Kevin Wee (2020). https://kevinwee. com/2020/10/self-determination-theory/

consistent with internalized beliefs about the value and personal benefits of their actions. Finally, the need for relatedness refers to the imperative for social interconnectedness and the perception of being enmeshed in a secure relational base. Relatedness involves feeling like one is cared for, connected to, and respected by others in the social environment.

Ryan and Deci (2000) contend that important behavioral consequences are fostered when all three basic psychological needs are satisfied. They further stipulate that social environments that thwart the basic psychological needs (e.g., feedback conveying a lack of skill/mastery, pressure and negative criticism, few opportunities for connection) result in ill-being, apathy, and a lack of persistence.

Athlete Perspectives and Experiences of RTS

Research has largely supported SDT contentions with autonomous motivations associated with more positive perceptions of RTS outcomes and a greater likelihood of RTS (versus non-return; Podlog & Eklund, 2020 for a detailed review). For instance, in a survey-based study with 180 competitive-level athletes from Canada, England, and Australia who RTS following injury, Podlog and Eklund (2005) found that intrinsic motivation (e.g., a love of the game, a desire to master skills) to resume sport participation was associated with "a renewed sport perspective," that is, positive perceptions of the RTS. Similarly, in an experimental study with 225 professional Australian footballers, Podlog and Eklund (2010) examined the effect of different motivational types to RTS on athletes' thoughts and emotions regarding a hypothetical return to competition. In line with SDT assumptions, greater self-determination in the return to competition resulted in more positive appraisals (increased desirability, reduced threat, unfairness, ego damage) and enhanced positive emotions (greater happiness and excitement).

Returning athletes may also experience doubts about their competence – namely, fears of re-injury, doubts about achieving pre-injury goals and performance levels, and a lack of psychological readiness to RTS (Podlog & Eklund, 2006; Podlog et al., 2012). Issues pertaining to athlete autonomy, such as returning to sport for controlled reasons (e.g., pressure or guilt) and a lack of control over the timing and circumstances of one's RTS, have also been reported (Bianco, 2001; Carson & Polman, 2017; Podlog & Eklund, 2006; Podlog et al., 2012). Further, relatedness concerns, such as isolation, inadequate social support, or perceptions of a lack of care from relevant others (e.g., sport coaches), may also be prevalent among returning athletes (Carson & Polman, 2017; Podlog & Eklund, 2006).

Evidence also suggests that injury stakeholders who support athletes' psychological needs can facilitate returning athletes' mental and physical health and post-injury performances (Podlog et al., 2010; Wadey et al., 2016). Scholars have shown that greater satisfaction of athlete's psychological needs predicts enhanced well-being (e.g., positive emotions during rehabilitation), positive return-to-sport outcomes (i.e., "renewed sport perspective"; Podlog et al., 2010), and a greater likelihood of stress-related growth (Wadey et al., 2016). Need satisfaction has also been positively related with post-traumatic growth among individuals with acquired disabilities (e.g., loss of a limb, lost vision, paralysis; Hammer et al., 2019).

Relational Perspectives and Experiences of RTS

A limited, albeit growing, body of research is beginning to highlight the influence of athletes' RTS following injury on relevant others, in particular on sport coaches, parents/caregivers, other athletes/teammates, and SPPs (Cavallerio et al., 2016; Day et al., 2013; Martinelli et al., 2017). We discuss each of these individuals in turn in the following sections.

Sport Coach

While there are several research articles that evidence how sport coaches can impact the onset and experience of athletes' injuries (e.g., Cavallerio et al., 2016; Roderick et al., 2000), this section extends and builds upon this body of literature to consider and problematize how athletes' returning to or away from sport can impact sport coaches. Reviewing the current evidence base, we consider this from two perspectives: (a) stress inducing and stress buffering and (b) vicarious trauma and vicarious growth. From a stress perspective, an athlete returning to sport can, on the one hand, induce strain on sport coaches. For example, it can lead to (a) administrative duties and communication tensions with the interprofessional care team to get medical clearance for the athlete's RTS; (b) team selection issues, role confusion, and interpersonal challenges within a team; (c) concerns about the safety of the returning athlete; (d) changes in the training environment and practices to accommodate the formerly injured athlete, and contractual issues if the athlete does not return; or (e) potentially helping the athlete navigate their transition away from sport (e.g., Olusoga et al., 2009; Thelwell et al., 2008). The resultant strain, in turn, can further impact the well-being and job performance of sport coaches. For example, Thelwell et al. (2017) identified that sport coaches perceive themselves to be less effective when stressed. Examples of this reduced effectiveness included talking down to players, forgetting about athletes' needs when instructing, and the creation of a negative atmosphere (Thelwell et al., 2017). On the one hand, an athlete returning to sport can buffer sport coaches' stress, as the returning athlete can strengthen a sporting team, give sport coaches more options in team selection, bolster and reinvigorate team atmosphere, and increase the likelihood of achieving key performance objectives (e.g., winning a game or league). The sport coach might also be joyful and happy for the athlete as they know what returning to sport and re-connecting with their teammates mean to them. Clearly, an athlete returning to sport can both be a stress-enhancing and stress-buffering experience for sport coaches.

Another perspective when considering how an athlete's RTS might impact sport coaches is by reflecting on the concepts of and research surrounding vicarious trauma and vicarious growth (Martinelli & Day, 2020). Vicarious trauma occurs when an individual is traumatized through a vicarious experience (i.e., witnessing trauma or listening to trauma accounts). Over the past decade, a growing body of research has evidenced that sport coaches can experience vicarious trauma from witnessing an athlete's injury. For example, Day et al. (2013) and Martinelli et al. (2017) identified that sport coaches experienced feelings of guilt, intrusive thoughts (e.g., involuntarily re-experiencing the event), and often avoided discussion of the injury event as well as interactions with the injured athlete. Day et al. also identified how sport coaches can involuntarily "re"-experience an athlete's injury upon "re"-entering the environment in which the incident took place, and from having direct contact with the injured athlete. Therefore, when the athlete returns to sport and re-enters the scene where the injury took place (e.g., training environment, competitive arena), it is possible that the sport coach could be re-traumatized and experience intrusions (e.g., involuntarily re-experiencing the event), a hallmark symptom of post-traumatic stress (Brewin & Holmes, 2003).

In addition to experiencing vicarious trauma upon an athlete's RTS, sport coaches might also experience the related and intertwined concept of vicarious growth, which refers to the development of positive changes because of vicarious exposure to trauma (Arnold et al., 2005). Outside of the sporting context, vicarious growth has been well-documented, particularly in healthcare professions and counsellors, who are often the main supporters of direct victims of trauma (cf. Manning-Jones et al., 2015). While there has been limited research on vicarious growth in sport injury, there are some indicators within the literature that sport coaches may experience this phenomenon. For example, Day et al. (2013) documented how one sport coach looked for reasons that the athlete's injury happened to consider possible benefits, develop new perspectives, and improve future coaching practices. Given that vicarious growth takes time to develop (Martinelli & Day, 2020), it is likely that by the time an athlete returns to sport following their rehabilitation, it might be possible for the sport coaches to harness something constructive from the sense of wrongdoing that underpinned their traumatic experience.

> It's that first one (observing an injury) that really sticks with you but then I felt that I learned a lot from it as well. . . . I know having looked back on it, that was one of the things that made me much better at dealing with parents. . . . If you don't think the pony is suitable for the child, as an instructor or coach you have to [pauses] you have to make your feelings clear. . . . If I'm not happy to teach that child on a pony, I as a professional, I have to be able to say, I have to be brave enough to say "I'm sorry that is a totally unsuitable pony."
>
> (Martinelli et al., 2017, p. 128)

Taken together, the experience of athletes returning to sport is a complex experience for sport coaches. It can bring them stress, and it can also bring them relief. It can be re-traumatizing, and it can also bring about lessons learned. The paradoxical nature of these experiences needs to be accounted for in future research and recognized by professional practitioners.

Significant Others

A population that has received limited research attention in the psychology of sport injury literature are significant others (e.g., parents/legal guardians of the athlete). This omission is surprising, given that athletes with injuries typically spend a significant time at home and that such individuals have been identified as a main support to athletes with injuries (Bianco, 2001). With respect to parents/legal guardians, drawing from the broader parenting in youth sport literature (see Harwood et al., 2019), most of the research has been one-directional in nature: How can parents help support their children? However, extending and building upon this literature, a few studies have started to give voice to parents' lived experiences of being a "sporting parent." Several studies have reported how injuries experienced by their children are a common stressor for parents and how they often feel unprepared to cope with their children's injuries (Cavallerio et al., 2020). Consequently, parents are often found searching for guidance and information pertaining to how best to support their children when they are injured (Knight et al., 2016). A lack of knowledge on the part of parents about how best to support their children may ultimately impact the athletes' psychological status as they attempt to RTS.

Extending the mainstream parenting in youth sport literature, a small handful of research articles have provided preliminary context-specific insights into how athletes' injuries impact parents generally and during their RTS specifically. The first researchers to give voice to parents' experiences of their children's injuries were Podlog et al. (2012). While much of the article explored parents' perspectives of their adolescents' injury rehabilitation and return to competitive experiences, one theme gave voice to parental concerns. Parents reported their fears of their children getting re-injured, apprehensions over having to cover medical expenses, and the implications of injury for interactions with other parents. To expand on this latter concern, just as injury impacted adolescents' social contact with teammates and training partners, it also exerted a parallel influence in minimizing parental interaction with parents of non-injured adolescents. For some, such interactions were an important source of connection and a significant contributor to their well-being. Given this finding, it could be inferred that athletes' RTS could be an uplifting experience for the well-being of parents, because they get to reconnect with other sporting parents. That said, researchers have also identified how returning to sport can bring stressors (e.g., communication issues with the sports medicine professionals and sport professionals) and strain (e.g., feeling helpless, guilt) for parents (Cavallerio et al., 2020; Cavallerio et al., 2022).

> I fear the combination of [my daughter's] desire to train and being pushed by the coaches to ignore the pain is going to drown out the voice of reason; I have no say in her training plan and know any interference will result in me being labeled a "difficult parent" and [my daughter] will bear the brunt of my actions in the training hall. . . . I leave the gym feeling as though I have failed my child: I have not demanded to watch the sessions, I have not stated we will be taking our business elsewhere if they do not conform to the medical advice, I have not asked them to treat my child with the respect she deserves. My parental instincts to protect my child from harm have been whittled away over the years. I have been conditioned to accept pain and injury as par for the course and accept the coaches are experts in their field. I have been pushed into the shadows of my daughter's life. Why have I let this happen?
>
> (Cavallerio et al., 2020, p. 136)

For athletes who retire from competitive sport following injury, however, research by Lally and Kerr (2008) illuminates the effects of gymnasts' retirement from sport on parents' lives. It was identified how the pain resulting from injuries remained prevalent in their children's lives "outside" the realms of sport, and how parents became increasingly concerned about the longer-term physical health of their children, given the damaging impact sport has had on them throughout their careers.

Other Athletes and Teammates

Injury may elicit a strong emotional impact on teammates or fellow athletes in one's sport. Consider the case of Nodar Kumaritashvili, who was on the threshold of becoming the first Georgian luger to participate in the Olympics, when he died in a training accident hours before the opening ceremony of the 2010 Vancouver Games. Kumaritashvili lost control of his sled, sailed off the track, and collided with a metal post. It is not hard to imagine how witnessing or having mere knowledge of such an event could exert a profound emotional impact on any athlete. A fairly significant body of research outside the sport domain has highlighted the vicarious impact of trauma experiences on those witnessing it (Maguen et al., 2009). However, very little parallel research has been undertaken within a sport injury context. Given this dearth, Day and Schubert (2012) utilized a qualitative approach to examine the impact of witnessing a catastrophic athletic injury requiring hospitalization among eight competitive female artistic gymnasts (aged 21–25). Initial injury responses included heightened fear, cognitive and somatic anxiety, sadness for and identification with one's teammates, and relief over non-injury to oneself. Participants also reported intrusive (non-voluntary) recurrent thoughts about their teammates' traumatic injuries, difficulties concentrating, heightened awareness of injury risk, and difficulty watching gymnastics. Gymnasts also engaged in avoidance coping strategies in the initial injury aftermath (fear and anxiety of completing certain skills, skill avoidance, avoidance of visual/verbal reminders of injury) and gradually engaged in more approach coping strategies (acceptance, self-talk, increased concentration), which diminished perceptions of injury vulnerability.

The deleterious impact of witnessing an injury on fellow athletes' psychological status was corroborated in a quantitative study by O'Neill (2008), who hypothesized that seeing a fellow competitor sustain a serious injury could illicit an emotional trauma that could, in turn, result in a change to one's performance tactics and subsequent injury – what O'Neill referred to as "injury contagion." In order to test this assumption, O'Neill examined 459 athletes (277 males and 182 females) from four ski academies. Over the three-year study period, 12 season-ending injuries were sustained. Results from psychological testing showed an increase in the use of fear words (e.g., "falling," "getting hurt," "crashing," "injuries," "scared," and "timid") and phrases after injury to a teammate (28.3% of athletes used words or expressions indicating a fear of injury compared with 10.4% of athletes from ski academies who did not witness a season-ending injury). While further research is needed to test whether an increase in fear words and phrases translated into actual injury occurrence among those observing severe injury, the findings suggest that merely witnessing an injury may leave a psychological imprint on non-injured athletes. Such responses merit attention from sport coaches, teammates, and SPPs with a vested interest in maintaining athlete mental and physical health and performance.

Sport Psychology Professionals

Limited research has examined the potential psychological impact of athletes' RTS following injury on SPPs. In one of the few exceptions, a licensed sport psychologist narrates her lived experience of the psychological impact of working with an elite athlete who, after being away from competition for two years due to injury, experienced another severe injury in the lead up to her first competition following RTS (Newcomer Appaneal, 2020).

In the narrative, the sport psychologist describes how her first meeting with the athlete took place during the final week of preparation for her first competition since the first injury occurrence two years prior. The sport psychologist also describes how she made efforts to normalize and validate athletes' feelings and fears of re-injury, by using metaphors and humor:

[H]ighly unlikely for the same thing to happen again. . . . As our conversation continued, we talked about her desire for control, and compared the situation to being a passenger on a plane during turbulence. We joked that the plane was not going to crash, and she was finding it really uncomfortable not to be flying the plane herself. We had a good laugh, and she seemed to relax a little. My sense at the time was that we had connected quite well and that our brief chat was helpful. As the days went on, we had a few more brief contact interventions again revisiting her fears and desire for control.

(Newcomer Appaneal, 2020, p. 219)

Upon MRI scan confirming everyone's worst fears, the athlete's response to her diagnosis reflected back to the metaphors and humor, as evidenced in the sport psychologist narrative: "she nervously laughed through tears and said: The plane is going down, again."

(Newcomer Appaneal, 2020, p. 219)

The narrative by Newcomer Appaneal (2020) also details numerous ways in which the injury affected the sport psychologist psychologically. In reflecting on her own state of mind and efforts to assist the athlete following the second injury, the sport psychologist remarked:

I don't recall too much about that evening, other than I felt completely incompetent. I beat myself up a good while for joking with [the athlete] about how it could not possibly happen again. Why did I try to predict the future, in attempt to reduce her discomfort about a re-injury? It's as if I was in control, the pilot in the cockpit in charge of the plane.

(Newcomer Appaneal, 2020, p. 219)

The sport psychologist also recalled feelings of "bitter sadness," "discomfort," and sleep problems:

I had trouble falling asleep that [injury] night and several subsequent nights, as my brain worked overtime trying to make sense of what had happened, my thoughts rewinding and replaying over and over our prior conversations, and future scenarios for how to support her and what to say.

(Newcomer Appaneal, 2020, pp. 220–221)

While research on understanding how injury may affect the sport psychology professionals involved in the care is limited, this case example illustrates how an "unsuccessful" RTS can place a significant emotional burden on the sport psychology professional working with the athlete. The impact can be significant, resulting in intensive self-reflection, questioning one's own skills as a practitioner, and potentially evoking insecurities and self-doubts:

Well after the tour ended, and through a lot of formal and informal supervision, I realized how preoccupied I was at the time with my "foot in mouth" failure. My insecure self and negative inner critic hijacked my attention, leaving little to give others such as [the athlete's] coach or other staff who were also struggling.

(Newcomer Appaneal, 2020, p. 221)

Conclusion

In this chapter, we discussed the return to sport (RTS) participation literature by presenting both athlete and relational perspectives on the RTS following injury. We defined the RTS time frame as the period when athletes are transitioning from sport-specific training to competitive play and/or segueing out of competitive sport. We highlighted the relevance of SDT as a framework for examining athletes' RTS experiences. First, we examined evidence indicating that the three basic psychological needs articulated in SDT – competence, autonomy, and relatedness – may be relevant factors for athletes' successful return to participation. We also described some of the ways in which returning athletes impact other injury stakeholders, such as sport coaches, parents, other athletes/teammates, and SPPs. Second, we highlighted a variety of positive (e.g., vicarious growth, an increased likelihood of achieving team performance objectives, reconnecting with other parents) and negative (e.g., stress, re-traumatization, feelings of professional incompetence and self-doubt) implications of athletes' RTS on various injury stakeholders.

Case Study

Upon entering his senior year of high school, Henri Suarez, aged 17, had already undergone two ACL knee reconstructions. Henri was a top soccer player in the state of Nevada. Despite not having had the opportunity to play or be seen by college coaches during his entire senior year, Henri wanted to play at the collegiate level. Approximately six months following his second ACL reconstruction, Henri started to work with a licensed sport psychology consultant (LSPP). The consultant had conflicting feelings about working with Henri. On one hand, the consultant wanted to help him resume a self-defining activity that gave Henri joy, purpose, and personal meaning. On the other hand, the consultant understood what Henri had been through – both physically and emotionally – and was aware that Henri might be vulnerable to further injury and the associated psychological sequalae.

During consultancy, Henri often referred to his mom, Sandy, who had raised him as a single parent and was a constant source of support and a confidant. As a mom who would do anything to support her sons' aspirations, Sandy was distressed after Henri's two injuries and worried that a return might result in further physical and psychological damage. Henri's surgeon shared these concerns; an RTS after two ACL was certainly possible, given surgical advances and numerous previous athletes who had RTS. Having Henri come back for a second ACL surgery was hard for the surgeon – as he "understood what Henri had gone through" and "was concerned that a pattern of injury might be developing for this young athlete."

At the start of his freshman year in college, Henri reached out to the soccer coach at his university. The coach informed him that he could try out for the team as a walk-on, but he would not be able to train with the team until he was selected to be on it. Henri decided to contact a few local soccer clubs and started playing in a competitive men's league. Over several months, he continued to improve his fitness and match skills, gaining a greater sense of competence in his abilities. He also felt a renewed sense of intrinsic motivation to continue improving and decided to reach out to the college coach again to see if he could watch him compete. After watching Henri, the coach was impressed with his skills and competitive spirit and saw Henri's potential to contribute to the team's success. The coach invited Henri to start training with the team as a walk-on. Henri quickly began integrating into the team – on a social and competitive level. His teammates commented that his relentless energy and positive attitude contributed to a positive team dynamic. Henri continued receiving support from his mom, who felt great pride in her son's efforts and was pleased he was once again experiencing the joy and pleasure that soccer brought him. Henri's on-field performances were of such high quality that by the end of the season, the coach offered him a scholarship and a regular spot on the team.

Questions

1. If you were acting as Henri's LSPP, how might you resolve the ambivalence about helping him return to soccer – knowing that he might be susceptible to further physical and psychological damage?
2. Using the self-determination theory framework, how could Henri's mom, Sandy, have supported his psychological needs for competence, autonomy, and relatedness?
3. How could Henry support his mom's psychological needs to feel competent, autonomous, and connected (related) to her son during injury recovery and/or return to participation?
4. Using the self-determination theory framework, if you were the coach of the university team, how could you help Henri's return to participation process?

Note

* **Disclaimer:** JJF is a military service member or employee of the US government. This work was prepared as part of his official duties. Title 17, USC §105, provides that copyright protection under this title is not available for any work of the US government. Title 17, USC §101, defines a US government work as work prepared by a military service member or employee of the US government as part of that person's official duties. The views expressed in this chapter are those of the authors and do not necessarily reflect the official policy or position of the Department of the Navy, Department of Defense, or the US government.

Disclosures of Interest: Dr. Fraser reports grants from Congressionally Directed Medical Research Programs and the Office of Naval Research outside of the submitted work. In addition, Dr. Fraser has a patent pending for an adaptive and variable stiffness ankle brace, US Provisional Patent Application No. 63254474.

References

Arnold, D., Calhoun, L. G., Tedeschi, R., & Cann, A. (2005). Vicarious posttraumatic growth in psychotherapy. *Journal of Humanistic Psychology*, *45*(2), 239–263. https://doi.org/10.1177/0022167805274729

Bianco, T. M. (2001). Social support and recovery from sport injury: Elite skiers share their experiences. *Research Quarterly for Exercise and Sport*, *72*(4), 376–388. https://doi.org/10.1080/02701367.2001.10608974

Brewin, C. R., & Holmes, E. A. (2003). Psychological theories of posttraumatic stress disorder. *Clinical Psychology Review*, *23*(3), 339–376. https://doi.org/10.1016/s0272-7358(03)00033-3

Carson, F., & Polman, R. C. J. (2017). Self-determined motivation in rehabilitating professional rugby union players. *BMC Sports Science, Medicine and Rehabilitation*, *9*(2), 1–11. https://doi.org/10.1186/s13102-016-0065-6

Cavallerio, F., Kimpton, N., & Knight, C. J. (2020). My daughter's injured again! I just don't know what to do anymore. In R. Wadey (Ed.), *Sport injury psychology: Cultural, relational, methodological, and applied considerations* (pp. 131–142). Routledge. https://doi.org/10.4324/9780367854997

Cavallerio, F., Wadey, R., & Wagstaff, C. R. D. (2016). Understanding overuse injuries in rhythmic gymnastics: A 12-month ethnographic study. *Psychology of Sport and Exercise*, *25*, 100–109. https://doi.org/10.1016/j.psychsport.2016.05.002

Cavallerio, F., Wadey, R., & Wagstaff, C. R. D. (2022). Impacting and being impacted by overuse injuries: An ethnodrama of parents' experiences. *Qualitative Research in Sport, Exercise and Health*, *14*(1), 19–36. https://doi.org/10.1080/2159676x.2021.1885480

Day, M. C., Bond, K., & Smith, B. (2013). Holding it together: Coping with vicarious trauma in sport. *Psychology of Sport and Exercise*, *14*(1), 1–11. https://doi.org/10.1016/j.psychsport.2012.06.001

Day, M. C., & Schubert, N. (2012). The impact of witnessing athletic injury: A qualitative examination of vicarious trauma in artistic gymnastics. *Journal of Sports Sciences*, *30*(8), 743–753. https://doi.org/10.1080/02640414.2012.671530

Doege, J., Ayres, J., Mackay, M., Tarakemeh, A., Brown, S., Vopat, B., & Mulcahey, M. K. (2021). Defining return to sport: A systematic review. *Orthopaedic Journal of Sports Medicine*, *9*(7). https://doi.org/10.1177/23259671211009589

Hammer, C., Podlog, L., Wadey, R., Galli, N., Forber-Pratt, A., & Newton, M. (2019). Cognitive processing following acquired disability for para sport athletes: A serial mediation model. *Disability and Rehabilitation*, *42*(17), 2492–2500. https://doi.org/10.1080/09638288.2018.1563639

Harwood, C. G., Thrower, S. N., Slater, M. J., Didymus, F. F., & Frearson, L. (2019). Advancing our understanding of psychological stress and coping among parents in organized youth sport. *Frontiers in Psychology*, 1600. https://doi.org/10.3389/fpsyg.2019.01600

Knight, C. J., Dorsch, T. E., Osai, K. V., Haderlie, K. L., & Sellars, P. A. (2016). Influences on parental involvement in youth sport. *Sport, Exercise, and Performance Psychology*, *5*(2), 161–178. https://doi.org/10.1037/spy0000053

Lally, P., & Kerr, G. (2008). The effects of athlete retirement on parents. *Journal of Applied Sport Psychology*, *20*(1), 42–56. https://doi.org/10.1080/10413200701788172

Maguen, S., Metzler, T. J., McCaslin, S. E., Inslicht, S. S., Henn-Haase, C., Neylan, T. C., & Marmar, C. R. (2009). Routine work environment stress and PTSD symptoms in police officers. *The Journal of Nervous and Mental Disease*, *197*(10), 754–760. https://doi.org/10.1097/NMD.0b013e3181b975f8

Manning-Jones, S., de Terte, I., & Stephens, C. (2015). Vicarious posttraumatic growth: A systematic literature review. *International Journal of Wellbeing*, *5*(2), 125–139. https://doi.org/10.5502/ijw.v5i2.8

Martinelli, L. A., & Day, M. C. (2020). "It's impacted me too" Where does vicarious growth fit in? In R. Wadey, M. Day, & K. Howells (Eds.), *Growth following adversity in sport* (pp. 47–58). Routledge.

Martinelli, L. A., Day, M. C., & Lowry, R. (2017). Sport coaches' experiences of athlete injury: The development and regulation of guilt. *Sports Coaching Review*, *6*(2), 162–178. https://doi.org/10.1080/21640629.2016

Newcomer Appaneal, R. (2020). Textbooks don't tell it like it is: Tales from working in the field with injured athletes. In R. Wadey (Ed.), *Sport injury psychology: Cultural, relational, methodological, and applied considerations* (pp. 217–231). Routledge. https://doi.org/10.4324/9780367854997

O'Neill, D. (2008). Injury contagion in alpine ski racing: The effect of injury on teammates' performance. *Journal of Clinical Sport Psychology*, *2*(3), 278–292. https://doi.org/10.1123/jcsp.2.3.278

Olusoga, P., Butt, J., Hays, K., & Maynard, I. (2009). Stress in elite sports coaching: Identifying stressors. *Journal of Applied Sport Psychology*, *21*(4), 442–459. https://doi.org/10.1080/10413200903222921

Podlog, L., & Eklund, R. C. (2005). Return to sport after serious injury: A retrospective examination of motivation and psychological outcomes. *Journal of Sport Rehabilitation*, *14*(1), 20–34. https://doi.org/10.1123/jsr.14.1.20

Podlog, L., & Eklund, R. C. (2006). A longitudinal investigation of competitive athletes' return to sport following serious injury. *Journal of Applied Sport Psychology*, *18*(1), 44–68. https://doi.org/10.1080/10413200500471319

Podlog, L., & Eklund, R. C. (2010). Returning to competition after a serious injury: The role of self-determination. *Journal of Sports Sciences*, *28*(8), 819–831. https://doi.org/10.1080/02640411003792729

Podlog, L., & Eklund, R. C. (2020). Psychosocial considerations of return to sport following injury. In A. Ivarsson & U. Johnson (Eds.), *Psychological bases of sport injuries* (4th ed.). Fitness Information Technology.

Podlog, L., Kleinert, J., Dimmock, J., Miller, J., & Shipherd, A. (2012). A parental perspective on adolescent injury rehabilitation and return to sport experiences. *Journal of Applied Sport Psychology*, *24*(2), 175–190. https://doi.org/10413200.2011.608102

Podlog, L., Lochbaum, M., & Stevens, T. (2010). Need satisfaction, well-being, and perceived return-to-sport outcomes among injured athletes. *Journal of Applied Sport Psychology*, *22*(2), 167–182. https://doi.org/10.1080/10413201003664665

Roderick, M., Waddington, I., & Parker, G. (2000). Playing hurt: Managing injuries in English professional football. *International Review for the Sociology of Sport*, *35*(2), 165–180. https://doi.org/10.1177/101269000035002003

Ryan, R. M., & Deci, E. L. (2000). Intrinsic and extrinsic motivations: Classic definitions and new directions. *Contemporary Educational Psychology*, *25*(1), 54–67. https://doi.org/10.1006/ceps.1999.1020

Thelwell, R. C., Wagstaff, C. R. D., Rayner, A., Chapman, M., & Barker, J. B. (2017). Exploring athletes' perceptions of coach stress in elite sport environments. *Journal of Sports Sciences*, *35*(1), 44–55. https://doi.org/10.1080/02640414.2016.1154979

Thelwell, R. C., Weston, N. J., Greenlees, I. A., & Hutchings, N. V. (2008). Stressors in elite sport: A coach perspective. *Journal of Sports Sciences*, *26*(9), 905–918. https://doi.org/10.1080/02640410801885933

Tracey, J. (2003). The emotional response to the injury and rehabilitation process. *Journal of Applied Sport Psychology*, *15*(4), 279–293. https://doi.org/10.1080/714044197

Wadey, R. (Ed.). (2020). *Sport injury psychology: Cultural, relational, methodological, and applied considerations*. Routledge.

Wadey, R., Day, M. C., Cavallerio, F., & Martinelli, L. A. (2018). Multilevel model of sport injury (MMSI): Can coaches impact and be impacted by injury? In R. C. Thelwell & M. Dicks (Eds.), *Professional advances in sports coaching: Research and practice* (pp. 336–357). Routledge. https://doi.org/10.4324/9781351210980

Wadey, R., Podlog, L., Galli, N., & Mellalieu, S. D. (2016). Stress-related growth following sport injury: Examining the applicability of the organismic valuing theory. *Scandinavian Journal of Medicine & Science in Sports*, *26*(10), 1132–1139. https://doi.org/10.1111/sms.12579

20 Transition Out of Sport

Derek M. Zike, Georgia K. Kundrat, and Monna Arvinen-Barrow

Chapter Objectives

- To summarize personal and sociocultural factors that have been found to influence the transition process due to sport injury.
- To summarize existing literature on adaptation to acquired disability associated with sport injury.
- To outline the role of sport psychology, sports medicine, and sports professionals in transition out of sport due to injury.

Introduction

Transition out of sport is a "turning phase in career development involving appraisals of, and coping with, transition demands leading to successful or less successful outcomes" (Stambulova et al., 2020, p. 4). The transition out of sport process is complex and multidimensional (Coakley, 2006), requiring athletes to manage many changes and make adjustments to how they view themselves and the world. Most athletes make a smooth transition out of sport, but how they respond to the process and its challenges can vary markedly (Stambulova et al., 2009). While it is fortunate that only a small number of athletes experience clinical levels of distress or depression in reaction to transition out of sport (Petitpas, 2009), findings from a systematic review (Park et al., 2013) revealed that some athletes experience difficulties or negative emotions, such as feelings of loss, identity crisis, and emotional distress, during the transition out of sport process. These challenges are likely to be amplified if the process happens before an athlete is psychologically "ready" to retire (Park et al., 2013) and/or able to achieve their sport goals (Petitpas, 2009). A major cause of forced or involuntary retirement from sport is career-ending injury (Moesch et al., 2012; Ristolainen et al., 2012), which, if not managed appropriately, can present unique challenges that can complicate and impede the transition out of sport process (Gilmore, 2008; Muscat, 2010).

The purpose of this chapter is to discuss the transition out of sport due to injury. The chapter will focus on two interconnected injury and rehabilitation outcome perspectives – injuries that result in a career termination and injuries that result in both a career termination and an acquired disability. This chapter will (a) provide an overview of the integrated career change and transition framework (Samuel et al., 2019), (b) summarize pertinent personal and sociocultural factors that have been found to influence the transition out of sport process, (c) outline relevant

DOI: 10.4324/9781003295709-24

theory and research on adaptation to acquired disability associated with sport injury, and (d) make recommendations for sport psychology (SPP), sports medicine (SMP), and sports professionals (SP) on how to support athletes during transition out of sport due to injury.

Integrated Career Change and Transition Framework

In an attempt to understand the process of sport career transition, a number of theoretical frameworks have been proposed in the literature (e.g., Samuel et al., 2019; Samuel & Tenenbaum, 2011b; Stambulova, 2003; Taylor & Ogilvie, 1994). At the core of the frameworks to date is an interplay of various personal and situational factors (e.g., demands, resources, barriers, coping strategies) and their influence on the different transition outcomes (e.g., successful, crisis, unsuccessful). In an attempt to create a comprehensive career change and transition framework accounting for multiple outcome pathways, Samuel et al. (2019) combined the existing conceptualizations (Samuel & Tenenbaum, 2011b; Stambulova, 2003) into an integrated career change and transition framework (ICCT). The ICCT considers transition out of sport as a career-change event (Samuel & Tenenbaum, 2011a, 2011b), which can be either a distinct event or a longitudinal process. According to the framework, the career-change event brings forth various demands that can create instability and provoke psycho-emotional imbalance in the athlete (Samuel & Tenenbaum, 2011a, 2011b).

In the ICCT, a career-change event (e.g., injury) compromises an athlete's status quo, subsequently initiating a pre-transition situation. The career-change event will present various transition demands related to different aspects of the athlete's life, including athletic, psychological, social, academic/vocational, financial, and cultural domains. Consistent with the transactional theory of stress and coping (Lazarus & Folkman, 1984), the primary appraisal following the career-change event is focused on transition demands, available resources to cope with the said demands, and potential barriers for successfully coping with these demands. These primary appraisals are influenced by (a) the significance of the career-change event on their future, (b) whether the transition is perceived as positive or negative, and (c) the athletes' perception of control over the career-change event. Following the primary appraisal, an athlete will make a strategic decision about the career-change event, which will result in one of three possible outcomes: (a) they will ignore/avoid the career-change event, (b) cope independently with the career-change event, or (c) consult with other individuals.

If an athlete decides to ignore/avoid the career-change event, they will either return to the status quo or move toward a crisis situation which would require an intervention. Depending on the effectiveness of the intervention (effective, ineffective, or no intervention), the transition outcome will either be positive or negative. If an athlete makes the strategic decision to cope independently with the career-change event or to consult with other people, a second cognitive appraisal of the transition demands, resources, and barriers will take place. The athlete will decide to either make a change (i.e., actively investing in coping) or to avoid change. Those who decide to avoid change will typically remain in a state of emotional instability, possibly leading to a crisis situation and to require intervention. Depending on the effectiveness of the intervention (effective, ineffective, or no intervention), the transition outcome will either be positive or negative. If an athlete makes the decision to change and actively invest in coping, they will implement various coping strategies (for more on coping, see Chapter 12) and/or psychosocial interventions (see Chapters 13–18), which can lead to a positive transition outcome.

Building on existing transition models (e.g., Samuel & Tenenbaum, 2011b; Stambulova, 2003; Taylor & Ogilvie, 1994), the ICCT model (Samuel et al., 2019) was first proposed and supported by research examining the cultural transition of the Israeli men's U18 national handball

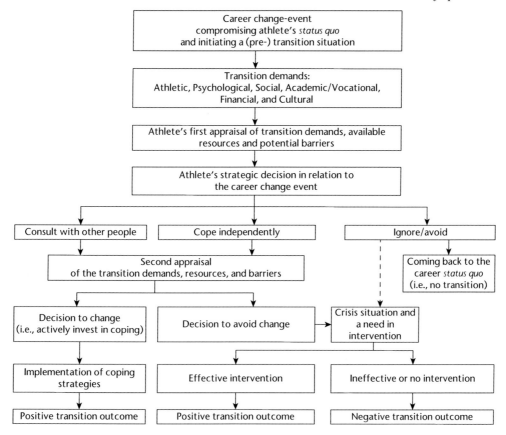

Figure 20.1 The integrated career change and transition framework.

Source: Adapted from Stambulova (2003) and Samuel and Tenenbaum (2011). Cultural transition of the Israeli men's U18 national handball team migrated to Germany: A case study. Roy S. Samuel, Natalia Stambulova, and Yaniv Ashkenazi. *Sport in Society*, 2022, Taylor & Francis Ltd. Reprinted by permission of the publisher (Taylor & Francis Ltd, http://www.tandfonline.com).

team. The data was collected when the team spent an entire competitive season in Germany as part of a specialized training program abroad. The results revealed that the cultural transition for the Israeli players support the ICCT model's pathways related to their primary and secondary appraisal of transition demands, barriers, and resources, decision-making, coping processes, and transition outcomes.

Psychosocial Factors in Transition Out of Sport Due to Injury

Research on understanding psychosocial factors in transition out of sport due to injury is sparse (Park et al., 2013). Consistent with the ICCT model (Samuel et al., 2019), the quality of sport career transition is dependent on the interplay of various factors, most notably those within the person (e.g., cognitive appraisals, emotional and behavioral responses) and those outside of the person (e.g., social and environmental factors). The transition out of sport process is also influenced by numerous psychosocial, developmental, and situational factors. These include the cause and voluntariness of retirement decision, short- and long-term effects on health, educational and financial status, time passed after retirement, sport career achievement, athletic identity and self-perceptions, personal coping and social resources, as well as perception of control of life (Knights et al., 2016; Kuettel et al., 2017; Park et al., 2013). What follows is a brief summary of pertinent psychosocial factors in transition out of sport due to injury: (a) psychosocial impact of career-ending injury, (b) athletic identity, (c) coping resources, (d) pre-retirement planning, and (e) social support.

Psychosocial Impact of Career-Ending Injury

Existing research confirms that transition out of sport elicits a myriad of psychosocial responses in athletes and that career-ending injuries have a negative impact on the athletes' biopsychosocial health during the transition out of sport process (Moore et al., 2022). The injury itself is often appraised in multiple ways. For example, Irish rugby football players appraised their career-ending injury as part of sport, a psychophysiological stressor, a life stressor, and a loss (Arvinen-Barrow et al., 2017). In a research study with Finnish professional ice hockey players, acceptance of the injury and its consequences was found to take some time (Arvinen-Barrow et al., 2015), whereas with professional Irish rugby football players, injury acceptance appeared to follow a cyclical yet stage-like process (Arvinen-Barrow et al., 2017). Following injury acceptance, athletes have also been able to appraise the injury as a positive experience. For example, professional cricket players in England have appraised their career-ending injuries as a blessing in disguise (Arvinen-Barrow et al., 2019), and collegiate athletes in the United States have discussed experiencing both gratitude and appreciation following injury (Stoltenburg et al., 2011).

Research has also found transition out of sport due to injury to evoke mixed emotions, mostly with negative valence. These include, but are not limited to, worries related to health and finances, anger, anxiety, bitterness, boredom, depression, disappointment, distress, emptiness, frustration, grief, helplessness, lack of purpose, loss, and stress (e.g., Alfermann et al., 2004; Arvinen-Barrow et al., 2019; Arvinen-Barrow et al., 2017; Arvinen-Barrow et al., 2015; Brown et al., 2017; Lavallee et al., 1997; Petitpas, 2009; Stoltenburg et al., 2011; Webb et al., 1998). Research has also found cultural differences in emotional responses – among a sample of elite French and Swedish athletes, Swedish athletes reported more positive emotional responses to their French counterparts (Stambulova et al., 2007). Some of the most pertinent behavioral responses to career-ending injury include maladaptive adjustment (Lavallee et al., 1997); sleep disturbances and alcohol misuse (Brown et al., 2017); use of profanities when discussing the emotions related to injury, rehabilitation, and recovery (Arvinen-Barrow et al., 2017); actively distancing from the sport environment (Arvinen-Barrow et al., 2015); and involvement in other activities outside of sport (Arvinen-Barrow et al., 2019; Stoltenburg et al., 2011).

Experiencing transition out of sport due to injury can also create occupational, financial, family, and social difficulties (Arvinen-Barrow et al., 2019; Arvinen-Barrow et al., 2017; Arvinen-Barrow et al., 2015; Cecić Erpič et al., 2004; Dimoula et al., 2013). Transition out of sport due to injury can also damage athletes' subjective system of meaning, consequently "disrupting the coherence of their life narrative" (Pitcho-Prelorentzos & Mahat-Shamir, 2019). Athletes with career-ending injuries have reported lower life satisfaction five to ten years following retirement (Kleiber & Brock, 1992). In general, athletes that have had physical problems after leaving sport have needed longer periods to adjust (e.g., Werthner & Orlick, 1986).

Athletic Identity

Athletic identity has been defined as "the degree to which an individual identifies with the athlete role" (Brewer et al., 1993, p. 237). Like other identities and roles in different social contexts (e.g., work, school, family, religion), athletic identity manifests in self-identity as part of a multidimensional self-concept (Marsh, 2008). Strong athletic identity is associated with self-worth, which is closely linked with participation and achievement in sport (Brewer et al., 1993); thus, transitioning out of sport can be perceived as threatening to one's sense of self and self-worth (Taylor & Ogilvie, 1994). Data from existing systematic reviews have concluded that athletic identity has a significant impact on the quality of transition out of sport (Knights et al., 2016; Park et al., 2013). Strong athletic identity is associated with maladaptive psychosocial responses to injury and difficulties related to adaptation into life beyond sport (Arvinen-Barrow et al., 2015, 2017, 2019; Ruiz et al., 2019; Stoltenburg et al., 2011).

It is possible that athletes with a strong athletic identity sometimes fail to develop the necessary coping skills to manage sport career transitions, making them potentially vulnerable to transition difficulties (Crook & Robertson, 1991). This could be due to athletes with a strong athletic identity being highly invested in their sport and thus being less likely to explore alternative careers, education advancement, and life activities while actively involved in sport (Brewer et al., 1993). In a study with Australian retired elite athletes, Grove et al. (1997) found a strong positive association between athletic identity and adjustment to retirement, coping with the transition out of sport process, and feelings of anxiety about career exploration/decision-making after retirement. Some athletes have also reported loss of identity as a consequence of transition out of sport (Lavallee et al., 1997). This is supported by research with former National Hockey League players who retired due to sport-related concussion (Caron et al., 2013), as many of the athletes had not known a life outside of hockey and subsequently experienced loss of identity, severe social withdrawal, depression, and suicidal ideation.

Coping Resources

Coping has been defined as "constantly changing cognitive and behavioral efforts to manage specific external and/or internal demands that are appraised as taxing or exceeding the resources of the person" (Lazarus & Folkman, 1984, p. 141). In general, coping has been divided into three main types: problem-focused coping, emotion-focused coping, and avoidance coping. According to Lazarus and Folkman (1984), problem-focused coping involves targeting the stressor directly by using plans or actions to change the situation causing distress. Emotion-focused coping, on the other hand, involves regulative efforts to manage the emotional distress caused by the situation, rather than the stressor itself. Avoidance coping involves actively trying to avoid stressors rather than dealing with them (American Psychological Association, 2022) and is considered a maladaptive form of coping that usually results in adding to the stress rather than alleviating it.

Existing research has identified coping and coping skills as critical to the transition out of sport (Clowes et al., 2015), influencing both the quality and outcome of the transition (Grove et al., 1997; Stambulova et al., 2007). Consistent with the ICCT model (Samuel et al., 2019) and the transactional theory of stress and coping (Lazarus & Folkman, 1984), how an athlete appraises their transition out of sport is likely to trigger different responses, subsequently leading to the utilization of diverse problem-focused, emotion-focused, or avoidance-focused strategies. Some of the coping strategies used by athletes who have sustained a career-ending injury include "taking control," "emotional avoidance," "using profanities," and "talking to someone" (Arvinen-Barrow et al., 2017), "keeping busy" (Arvinen-Barrow et al., 2019), "distancing from sport" (Arvinen-Barrow et al., 2015), "involvement in other activities" (Arvinen-Barrow et al., 2019; Stoltenburg et al., 2011), "alcohol misuse" (Brown et al., 2017), as well as various other emotion-focused and avoidance coping strategies (Stambulova et al., 2007).

Pre-Retirement Planning

Pre-retirement planning refers to the amount and quality of planning that an athlete engages in to prepare for the end of their sport career (Ruiz et al., 2019). Retirement planning may incorporate psychological, financial, educational, and/or vocational considerations before and after sport career transition in an effort to prepare for life after sport (Park et al., 2013). Pre-retirement planning has been found to be valuable by having a significant impact on the quality of transition out of sport (Alfermann et al., 2004; Arvinen-Barrow et al., 2015, 2017, 2019; Dimoula et al., 2013; Kuettel et al., 2017; Park et al., 2013; Stambulova et al., 2007). Pre-retirement planning is also associated with a successful transition out of sport, faster and easier adjustment to life outside of sport, and less emotional disruption (Alfermann et al., 2004; Lavallee, 2005; Roberts et al., 2015; Ryan, 2019; Stoltenburg et al., 2011). Athletes who plan for retirement in advance tend to exhibit higher cognitive, emotional, and behavioral readiness for transition than athletes who do not (Alfermann et al., 2004), and athletes with lower preparedness (Coakley, 2006) or lack of a "plan B" (Stoltenburg et al., 2011) report greater difficulty in sport career transition.

Social Support

Defined as "the provision of assistance or comfort to others, typically to help them cope with biological, psychological, and social stressors" (American Psychological Association, 2022), *social support* can have a positive influence on the process and quality of transition out of sport (Coakley, 2006; Knights et al., 2016; Park et al., 2013; Roberts et al., 2015). In particular, transition out of sport has been shown to be less difficult when athletes have a strong social support network (Schwendener-Holt, 1994). In contrast, when athletes report inadequate (or a lack of) social support, they are likely to also report psychological, emotional, and physical distress/difficulties in adjusting to the life outside of sport (Moore et al., 2022; Ruiz et al., 2019; Stoltenburg et al., 2011).

Research has highlighted that following retirement, many athletes miss aspects of their sport, such as competition and camaraderie with teammates and coaches (Andrijiw, 2011; Coakley, 2006; Roberts et al., 2015). The apparent change in social connections can lead to difficulties in sport career transition (Kane, 1991). Existing research has also found that athletes' perception of social support (or lack thereof), their satisfaction with social support, and the different sources of social support (family, coaches, teammates, and sport psychology professionals) have a significant impact on the process of transition out of sport due to injury (Arvinen-Barrow et al., 2015, 2017, 2019; Kaul, 2017; Moore et al., 2022; Ruiz et al., 2019; Stoltenburg et al., 2011; for more on social support, see Chapter 18).

Transition Out of Sport Due to Sport Injury Resulting in Acquired Disability

While most transitions out of sport due to injury result in transition difficulties (Moore et al., 2022), the experience of transition out of sport with acquired disability introduces unique demands that warrant further discussion. Many career-ending injuries result in a permanent disability, as evidenced in research with elite ($n = 574$) cross-country skiers, swimmers, long-distance runners, and soccer players in Finland (Ristolainen et al., 2012). The results of the survey found that, of the athletes who retired due to injury ($n = 27$), 70.4% reported that their "injury caused them mild or moderate permanent disability" (Ristolainen et al., 2012, p. 274). What follows next is a discussion of adaptation to acquired disability associated with sport injury.

Defining Acquired Disability

According to the World Health Organization and The World Bank (2011) report on disability, and consistent with the definition of disability put forth by Leonardi et al. (2006), the word *disability* is an "umbrella term for impairments, activity limitations and participation restrictions, referring to the negative aspects of the interaction between an individual (with a health condition) and that individual's contextual factors (environmental and personal factors)" (p. 4). Given that disability is "an evolving concept," and considering it is defined as an interaction, this means that disability is not an attribute of a person but rather a result of "the interaction between persons with impairments and attitudinal and environmental barriers that hinder their full and effective participation in society on an equal basis with others" (World Health Organization & The World Bank, 2011, p. 4). An acquired disability is a disability that originates after birth, is not caused by hereditary or developmental factors (Waldman et al., 2016), and its onset is often linked to traumatic injury or disease (Livneh & Antonak, 2005). Adaptation to acquired disability is a "process of responding to the functional, psychological, and social changes that occur with the onset and experience of living with a disability, chronic illness, or associated treatments" (Bishop, 2005, p. 6).

Psychosocial Adaptation to Chronic Illness and Disability Model

The psychosocial adaptation to chronic illness and disability model (Livneh, 2001, 2021) conceptualizes adaptation to acquired disability as a dynamic, complex process that involves numerous interacting factors (personal, acquired disability–related, external contextual) that lead to a multidimensional outcome. In the model, it is proposed that living with disability is a multidirectional interplay between a series of physical, psychological, social, and environmental processes that determine the trajectory of any experience that an individual with disability may encounter. The model includes three levels of factors: (a) antecedents, (b) process, and (c) outcomes.

The *antecedents* represent pre-acquired disability features that may have explicitly or implicitly caused the disabling condition or created the context where the disability occurred. These are divided into two interacting categories: triggering events (e.g., injury/accident, chronic disease/illness) and contextual status (i.e., biophysiological status, psychological/personality status, sociocultural status, and environmental conditions). The *process* represents three interacting psychological features associated with chronic illness and injury. The chronic illness– and disability-related medico-psychological status refers to numerous medical characteristics (e.g., functional restrictions, presence of pain) and psycho-medical influences (e.g., perceived uncertainty, uncontrollability, and perceived stigma). The chronic illness and disability-induced psychological reactions refer to cognitive-affective responses (e.g., anxiety, depression, anger, and denial). The generic chronic illness and disability-linked psychological approaches include cognitive-affective-behavioral strategies (e.g., appraisals and pre-coping approaches, coping strategies, and chronic illness and disability-impact perceptions). The *outcomes* represent various intra-, inter-, and extrapersonal functional quality of life–related domains that are likely outcomes of the adaptation process. The intrapersonal domain refers to health-biomedical and psychological objective symptoms, functional indicators, and subjective self-reports. The interpersonal functional domain refers to objective social indicators and subjective social experiences related to family/marriage and peers/social. The extrapersonal (community) functional domain refers to performance in various domains, including vocational/work, living/household, learning/school, and recreation/avocational.

The model depicts that pre–chronic illness and disability antecedents influence the adaptation *process*. During the process, three chronic illness and disability-related psychological processes interact bidirectionally with each other, ultimately influencing the adaptation *outcomes*. The model also considers successful adaptation to be both the process leading to, as well as a

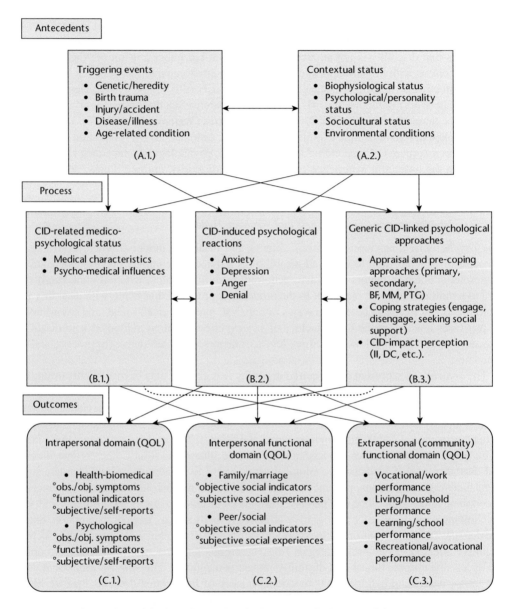

Figure 20.2 The psychosocial adaptation to chronic illness and disability model.

Note: A double-headed arrow (↔) represents a bi-directional relationship between two or more sets of variables (e.g., Triggering events and Contextual status [Antecedents]; CID-related medico-psychological status, and CID-induced psychological reactions [Process]). A single-headed arrow (→) represents a unidirectional relationship between a set of variables (presumed to be the cause) and a second set of variables (presumed to be the effect; e.g., Triggering events [Antecedents] and Generic CID-linked psychological approaches [Process]; CID-induced psychological reactions [Process]; and QOL intrapersonal domain [Outcomes]). CID = chronic illness and disability.

marker of, quality of life across life domains. The psychological process is also a moderator between the previous immutable life influences and chronic illness and disability onset–related elements represented in antecedents, and the person's current quality of life represented in outcomes. The model assumes that a successful adaptation outcome reflects an improved quality of life and having the ability to manage internal and external demands. As an adaptation outcome, quality of life represents an individual's efforts to re-establish psychosocial homeostasis and attain congruency between person and environment (Livneh, 2001).

Support for the psychosocial adaptation to chronic illness and disability model has been found in the literature. A research study with Portuguese patients who underwent lower-limb amputations due to diabetes mellitus type II (n = 86) found support for several elements of the model (Pedras et al., 2018). The results revealed negative associations between traumatic stress symptoms and adjustment, and adjustment and limitations. They also found perception of social support to have a mediating role between traumatic stress symptoms and adjustment, thus supporting the relationships between antecedents, process, and outcome as outlined in the psychosocial adaptation to chronic illness and disability model (Livneh, 2001, 2021). Bhattarai (2021) found both antecedents (e.g., self-efficacy) and the process (e.g., mindfulness and social support) to be significant predictors of higher quality of life among spinal cord–injured individuals (n = 231).

Psychosocial Factors in Adaptation to Acquired Disability due to Sport Injury

Research on understanding psychosocial factors in transition out of sport due to injury that result in acquired disability is sparse. In addition to the pertinent psychosocial factors outlined earlier in this chapter (i.e., psychosocial impact of career-ending injury, athletic identity, coping resources, pre-retirement planning, and social support), athletes who experience an acquired disability from career-ending sport injury have reported significant identity disruption (e.g., athletic, masculine, social, professional) post-injury (Crawford et al., 2014; Hawkins et al., 2014; Smith & Sparkes, 2008; Sparkes & Smith, 2002; Tangen & Kudlacek, 2014). Loss of identity has also been highlighted as a significant source of stress (Crawford et al., 2014), and athletes who attempt to hold on to their past athletic self have been found to experience increased identity dilemmas (Sparkes & Smith, 2002).

Research has also found that resuming similar athletic pursuits and reclaiming athletic identity can buffer the effects of loss and functional limitations, facilitate injury acceptance, provide a foundation for consistency in self-perception (Hawkins et al., 2014), and has the potential to foster self-confidence that may apply to other areas of life (Crawford et al., 2014). Sport involvement has also been found to provide an opportunity for re-establishment and continuity of athletic identity (Crawford et al., 2014; Hawkins et al., 2014), help athletes embrace their disability (Zurek et al., 2022), allow for behavioral independence, provide an environment for accomplishment, and promote positive emotions (Hawkins et al., 2014). Sport participation post-injury has also been found to provide social and therapeutic benefits (Tangen & Kudlacek, 2014). Receiving social support from family, friends, and teammates has the potential to ease the rehabilitation experience, reintegration into sport, and exit from the rehabilitation hospital (Crawford et al., 2014) and to enhance quality of life (Goraczko et al., 2020).

Recommendations for Sport Psychology, Sports Medicine, and Sports Professionals

Given the complexity and multidimensional nature of the transition out of sport (Coakley, 2006), each athlete will cope with the process in their own unique ways. Based on existing research, most prominent psychosocial responses to transition out of sport due to injury are, for the most part, negative and challenging to the athlete. Existing research also highlights athletic identity (and identity in general), coping skills, pre-retirement planning, and social support as being the most pertinent psychosocial factors influencing the transition out of sport process and outcomes. In what follows, recommendations are provided for sport psychology, sports medicine, and sports professionals to consider when working with athletes transitioning out of sport due to injury.

Sport Psychology Professionals

Depending on the severity of the psychosocial responses to the career-ending injury and its consequences (e.g., acquired disability), it is possible that ethically, SPPs who have clinical mental health competencies are best placed to treat injured athletes transitioning out of sport (for more on ethical considerations, see Chapter 8). Since returning to sport is not an option for the athlete, it might also be possible that not all athletes want to work with sport-trained psychology professionals but would prefer a professional who has competency in addressing mental health and/or sport career transition concerns. It is important to note that any psychology-trained professional who works with athletes transitioning out of sport due to injury should have thorough theoretical and empirical understanding of all the unique domains presented in this athlete population. These include (a) psychosocial aspects of sport injuries, (b) sport career transition processes, (c) clinical mental health symptoms, (d) mental health referral, (e) psychosocial aspects of acquired disability, and (f) use of counseling skills and psychosocial strategies deemed appropriate for the athlete.

Sports Medicine Professionals

Treating and rehabilitating athletes with career-ending injury presents numerous psychosocial challenges to sports medicine professionals (SMPs). First, the SMP should ensure the athlete has adequate psychosocial support in place and, if necessary, make a mental health referral (for more on assessment and referral, see Chapter 10). Typically, the goal of sport injury rehabilitation is to return to pre-injury level of performance; with career-ending injury, such a goal is usually unrealistic. The SMPs should therefore be mindful of possible incongruence between athletes' desired rehabilitation goals and rehabilitation goals that are realistic. Since the injury acceptance process can take time (Arvinen-Barrow et al., 2017), not all athletes are ready for rehabilitation but rather engage in maladaptive behaviors, such as over- or under-adherence and substance and/or prescription drug misuse, which can create further complications for the rehabilitation process. One possible effective strategy to help athletes with rehabilitation is setting short-term goals *with* the athlete (for more on goal setting, see Chapter 14) and by showing positive regard and actively listening to their concerns without judgment (for more on counseling skills, see Chapter 9).

Sports Professionals

Recognizing the importance of pre-retirement planning and social support in coping with transition out of sport, sport professionals (e.g., coaches and administrators) can be instrumental in facilitating both strategies before and after career-ending injury. Connecting athletes with career development professionals and retired athletes (e.g., peer mentors; Clowes et al., 2015; Gilmore, 2008) early on in their career to develop a "plan B" is integral for successful transition out of sport. Equally, ensuring the athlete has access to social support within and outside of the sport setting after injury is an important part of sport professionals' role (for more on social support, see Chapter 18).

Conclusion

There has been limited research conducted on the psychosocial impact of transition out of sport due to injury. What does exist, however, extends across different sports and cultures and presents a consensus that the process of transition out of sport due to injury is complex and multidimensional. Successful sport career transition outcomes are dependent on athletes' cognitive appraisals, their ability to cope with a myriad of emotions, and their engagement in behaviors that facilitate the transition out of sport process. Equally, the transition out of sport process and outcome is influenced by athletic identity, coping resources, pre-retirement planning, and social support.

Case Study

Sophie, aged 20, is a disabled young woman living with quadriplegia. She was a talented first-year ice hockey player on a collegiate team with championship ambitions. She incurred a spinal cord injury in the first game of the conference tournament and underwent surgery to stabilize her neck. Despite the best efforts by her medical team, Sophie did not regain physical function to pre-injury levels.

Sophie's injury happened 11 months ago. Reflecting on the early weeks after the injury, Sophie recalls her initial reactions to the injury: "I remember, when the doctors told me that my college hockey career was over, I just crashed inside. It is like they ripped my heart out. I refused to believe them. I was determined to play hockey again, regardless of what the doctors said. I guess you could call it denial . . . but for months I devoted myself and all my time and energy to rehabilitation. I mean . . . as a hockey player, I knew what hard work was, and this was no different."

Sophie's parents watched on helplessly as she continued efforts to regain her function. "It was a heartbreaking time," Sophie's dad recalls. "We knew she wanted nothing more than to lace her skates up again and play the sport she loves. Ice hockey was her whole world. She knew who she was because of hockey. The rink was where she met and interacted with her closest friends – all on the hockey team. It was also where she spent the majority of her time, at practice, games, in the training room." Sophie's mother added, "Yes, it was so hard to watch her spend months figuring out how to use her body again. Some of the simplest taken-for-granted tasks – for example, using food utensils, bathing, clothing – were now extremely difficult to do on her own. We tried to help, but . . . it was hard. There were days when she did not want our help, but because of her limited physical function, we had to help her. This would upset her. And us."

Sophie nods and continues, "I know I grew increasingly frustrated with the lack of progress in returning to the physical function I had before my injury. I was devastated. And angry. The injury stole my life away from me. My friends, my purpose, my identity. I didn't know who I was without hockey. And now, looking back, I think I was deeply depressed, sad, and hopeless." Sophie recalls while holding back her tears, "It was so hard . . . I hated being with my friends, as I kept evaluating myself in comparison to them and others. I could somehow always find something negative about myself. My parents tried to encourage me to join these support groups for disabled youth, but I didn't want to. I did not want to be disabled. I wanted to regain the function I had lost. I wanted to be me again."

In the months that followed, Sophie struggled to accept her disability. She disliked how apparent her bodily differences were as she navigated society in a wheelchair and thought that having a disability meant she could not consider herself an athlete or elite performer. She found it hard to assume other roles outside of sport. Her hockey-related friendships suffered, and as an introvert, she struggled to be proactive in developing new relationships.

To cope with her new normal, Sophie focused on her schoolwork. "Excelling in school was my coping strategy. Whenever I felt stuck and dissatisfied by the lack of progress in recovery, I just hit the books. I took all that energy I used to pour into hockey and used it for school. That was my getaway," Sophie recalls. "It gave me a sense of normalcy, a feeling of being not so different from my peers despite my disability. I also think my family and closest friends were amazing. They definitely played a huge role in helping me feel comfortable, whether we were at home, at school, at sporting events, at concerts, or in other social situations."

Today, Sophie (and her parents) is meeting with a licensed sport psychology professional (LSPP) for the first time. When asked about what prompted Sophie to reach out to a mental health provider, she responds, "I think it's time. I mean, I have been unhappy for a long time, and I'm tired of feeling that way. I'm not getting better either, and that frustrates me. I think I need help."

Questions

1. What factors, transition demands, and available resources outlined in the case study appear to be affecting Sophie's transition out of sport?
2. What are Sophie's appraisals of her injury, rehabilitation, and transition out of sport?
3. How are Sophie's appraisals affecting her emotional and behavioral responses to injury and disability?
4. How are Sophie's thoughts about disability affecting her response to transition out of sport, and how might her responses be different if the career-ending injury did not result in a disability?

References

Alfermann, D., Stambulova, N., & Zemaityte, A. (2004). Reactions to sport career termination: A cross-national comparison of German, Lithuanian, and Russian athletes. *Psychology of Sport & Exercise*, *5*(1), 61–75. https://doi.org/10.1016/S1469-0292(02)00050-X

American Psychological Association. (2022). APA dictionary of psychology. In *APA dictionary of psychology*. https://dictionary.apa.org/

Andrijiw, A. M. (2011). *Life after hockey: An examination of athletic career transition and the National Hockey League's career transition program* (Unpublished Masters Thesis). Brock University.

Arvinen-Barrow, M., DeGrave, K., Pack, S. M., & Hemmings, B. (2019). Transitioning out of professional sport: The psychosocial impact of career-ending non-musculoskeletal injuries among male cricketers from England and Wales. *Journal of Clinical Sport Psychology*, *13*(4), 629–644. https://doi.org/10.1123/jcsp.2017-0040

Arvinen-Barrow, M., Hurley, D., & Ruiz, M. C. (2017). Transitioning out of professional sport: The psychosocial impact of career-ending injuries among elite Irish rugby football union players. *Journal of Clinical Sport Psychology*, *10*(1). https://doi.org/10.1123/jcsp.2016-0012

Arvinen-Barrow, M., Nässi, A., & Ruiz, M. C. (2015). Kun vamma päättää, milloin ura loppuu. [When injury determines when the career ends]. *Liikunta ja Tiede, 52*(6), 45–49.

Bhattarai, M. (2021). *Contextual influences, acceptance of disability, and quality of life in persons with spinal cord injury: Utilization of Livneh's psychosocial adaptation model* (Publication Number 28715518) (Doctoral dissertation). The University of Wisconsin-Madison. Madison ProQuest Dissertations Publishing.

Bishop, M. (2005). Quality of life and psychosocial adaptation to chronic illness and disability: Preliminary analysis of a conceptual and theoretical synthesis. *Rehabilitation Counseling Bulletin, 48*(4), 219–231. https://doi.org/10.1177/00343552050480040301

Brewer, B. W., Van Raalte, J. L., & Linder, D. E. (1993). Athletic identity: Hercules' muscles or Achilles' heel? *International Journal of Sport Psychology, 24*(2), 237–254.

Brown, J. C., Kerkhoffs, G., Lambert, M. I., & Gouttebarge, V. (2017). Forced retirement from professional rugby union is associated with symptoms of distress. *International Journal of Sports Medicine, 38*(8), 582–587. https://doi.org/10.1055/s-0043-103959

Caron, J. G., Bloom, G. A., Johnston, K. M., & Sabiston, C. M. (2013). Effects of multiple concussions on retired national hockey league players. *Journal of Sport & Exercise Psychology, 35*(2), 168–179. https://doi.org/10.1123/jsep.35.2.168

Cecić Erpič, S., Wylleman, P., & Zupančič, M. (2004). The effect of athletic and non-athletic factors on the sports career termination process. *Psychology of Sport & Exercise, 5*(1), 45–59. https://doi.org/10.1016/S1469-0292(02)00046-8

Clowes, H., Lindsay, P., Fawcett, L., & Knowles, Z. R. (2015). Experiences of the pre and post retirement period of female elite artistic gymnasts: An exploratory study. *Sport and Exercise Psychology Review, 11*(2). https://doi.org/10.53841/bpssepr.2015.11.2.4

Coakley, S. C. (2006). *A phenomenological exploration of the sport-career transition experiences that affect subjective well-being of former national football league players* (Unpublished doctoral dissertation). University of North Carolina-Greensboro.

Crawford, J. J., Gayman, A. M., & Tracey, J. (2014). An examination of post-traumatic growth in Canadian and American Parasport athletes with acquired spinal cord injury. *Psychology of Sport & Exercise, 15*(4), 399–406. https://doi.org/10.1016/j.psychsport.2014.03.008

Crook, J. M., & Robertson, S. E. (1991). Transitions out of elite sport. *International Journal of Sport Psychology, 22*(2), 115–127.

Dimoula, F., Torregrosa, M., Psychountaki, M., & Fernandez, M. D. G. (2013). Retiring from elite sports in Greece and Spain. *The Spanish Journal of Psychology, 16.*

Gilmore, O. (2008). *Leaving competitive sport: Scottish female athletes' experiences of sport career transitions* (Unpublished doctoral dissertation). University of Stirling.

Goraczko, A., Zurek, G., Lachowicz, M., Kujawa, K., Blach, W., & Zurek, A. (2020). Quality of life after spinal cord injury: A multiple case study examination of elite athletes. *International Journal of Environmental Research and Public Health, 17*(20).

Grove, R., Lavallee, D., & Gordon, S. (1997). Coping with retirement from sport: The influence of athletic identity. *Journal of Applied Sport Psychology, 9*(2), 191–203. https://doi.org/10.1080/10413209708406481

Hawkins, C., Coffee, P., & Soundy, A. (2014). Considering how athletic identity assists adjustment to spinal cord injury: A qualitative study. *Physiotherapy, 100*(3), 268–274. https://doi.org/10.1016/j.physio.2013.09.006

Kane, M. A. (1991). *The metagonic transition: A study of career transition, marital stress and identity transformation in former professional athletes* (Publication Number 746446081) (Doctoral dissertation). ProQuest Dissertations and Theses Database.

Kaul, N. (2017). Involuntary retirement due to injury in elite athletes from competitive sport: A qualitative approach. *Journal of the Indian Academy of Applied Psychology, 43*(2), 305–315.

Kleiber, D. A., & Brock, S. C. (1992). The effect of career-ending injuries on the subsequent well-being of elite college athletes. *Sociology of Sport Journal, 9*(1), 70–75. https://doi.org/10.1123/ssj.9.1.70

Knights, S., Sherry, E., & Ruddock-Hudson, M. (2016). Investigating elite end-of-athletic-career transition: A systematic review. *Journal of Applied Sport Psychology, 28*(3), 291–308. https://doi.org/10.1080/10413200.2015.1128992

300 *Derek M. Zike, Georgia K. Kundrat, and Monna Arvinen-Barrow*

Kuettel, A., Boyle, E., & Schmid, J. (2017). Factors contributing to the quality of the transition out of elite sports in Swiss, Danish, and Polish athletes. *Psychology of Sport & Exercise, 29*, 27–39. https://doi.org/10.1016/j.psychsport.2016.11.008

Lavallee, D. (2005). The effect of a life development intervention on sports career transition adjustment. *The Sport Psychologist, 19*(2), 193–202. https://doi.org/10.1123/tsp.19.2.193

Lavallee, D., Grove, R. J., & Gordon, S. (1997). The causes of career termination from sport and their relationship to post-retirement adjustment among elite-amateur athletes in Australia. *Australian Psychologist, 32*(2), 131–135. https://doi.org/10.1080/00050069708257366

Lazarus, R., & Folkman, S. (1984). *Stress, appraisal, and coping.* Springer.

Leonardi, M., Bickenbach, J., Ustun, T. B., Kostanjsek, N., Chatterji, S., & MHADIE Consortium. (2006). The definition of disability: What is in a name? *Lancet, 368*, 1219–1221. https://doi.org/10.1016/S0140-6736(06)69498-1

Livneh, H. (2001). Psychosocial adaptation to chronic illness and disability: A conceptual framework. *Rehabilitation Counseling Bulletin, 44*(3), 151–160. https://doi.org/10.1177/003435520104400305

Livneh, H. (2021). Psychosocial adaptation to chronic illness and disability: An updated and expanded conceptual framework. *Rehabilitation Counseling Bulletin, 65*(3), 171–184. https://doi.org/10.1177/00343552211034819

Livneh, H., & Antonak, R. F. (2005). Psychosocial adaptation to chronic illness and disability: A primer for counselors. *Journal of Counseling & Development, 83*(1), 12–20. https://doi.org/10.1002/j.1556-6678.2005.tb00575.x

Marsh, H. W. (2008). A multidimensional, hierarchical model of self-concept: An important facet of personality. In G. J. Boyle, G. Matthews, & D. H. Saklofske (Eds.), *The Sage handbook of personality theory and assessment, vol. 1: Personality theories and models* (pp. 447–469). Sage Publishing.

Moesch, K., Mayer, C., & Elbe, A. M. (2012). Reasons for career termination in Spanish elite athletes: Investigating gender differences and the time-point as potential correlates. *Sport Science Review, 21*(5), 49–69. https://doi.org/10.2478/v10237-012-0018-2

Moore, H. S., Walton, S. R., Eckenrod, M. R., & Kossman, M. K. (2022). Biopsychosocial experiences of elite athletes retiring from sport for career-ending injuries: A critically appraised topic. *Journal of Sport Rehabilitation, 31*(8), 1095–1099. https://doi.org/10.1123/jsr.2021-0434

Muscat, A. C. (2010). *Elite athletes' experience of identity changes during a career-ending injury: An interpretative description* (Unpublished doctoral dissertation). University of British Columbia.

Park, S., Lavallee, D., & Tod, D. (2013). Athletes' career transition out of sport: A systematic review. *International Review of Sport and Exercise Psychology, 6*(1), 22–53. https://doi.org/10.1080/1750984X.2012.687053

Pedras, S., Vilhena, E., Carvalho, R., & Pereira, M. G. (2018). Psychosocial adjustment to a lower limb amputation ten months after surgery. *Rehabilitation Psychology, 63*(3), 418–430. https://doi.org/10.1037/rep0000189

Petitpas, A. J. (2009). Sport career termination. In B. W. Brewer (Ed.), *Handbook of sports medicine and science: Sport psychology* (pp. 113–120). John Wiley & Sons. https://doi.org/10.1002/9781444303650.ch11

Pitcho-Prelorentzos, S., & Mahat-Shamir, M. (2019). A shattered dream: Meaning construction in response to retirement from professional sport due to career-ending injury. *The Sport Psychologist, 33*(2), 110–118. https://doi.org/10.1123/tsp.2018-0069

Ristolainen, L., Kettunen, J. A., Kujala, U. M., & Heinonen, A. (2012). Sport injuries as the main cause of sport career termination among Finnish top-level athletes. *European Journal of Sport Science, 12*(3), 274–282. https://doi.org/10.1080/17461391.2011.566365

Roberts, C. M., Mullen, R., Evans, L., & Hall, R. (2015). An in-depth appraisal of career termination experiences in professional cricket. *Journal of Sports Sciences, 33*(9), 935–944. https://doi.org/10.1080/02640414.2014.977936

Ruiz, M. C., Kaski, S., Frantsi, P., & Robazza, C. (2019). Reactions to a career-ending sport injury: Pekka Hirvonen, a professional ice hockey player. In M. Arvinen-Barrow & D. Clement (Eds.), *The psychology of sport and performance injury: An interprofessional case-based approach* (pp. 148–164). Routledge. https://doi.org/10.4324/9781351111591

Ryan, L. (2019). *Flourishing after retirement: Understanding the sport career transition of New Zealand's elite athletes* (Unpublished doctoral dissertation). The University of Waikato.

Samuel, R. D., Stambulova, N., & Ashkenazi, Y. (2019). Cultural transition of the Israeli men's U18 national handball team migrated to Germany: A case study. *Sport in Society*, *23*(4), 697–716. https://doi.org/10.1080/17430437.2019.1565706

Samuel, R. D., & Tenenbaum, G. (2011a). How do athletes perceive and respond to change events: An exploratory measurement tool. *Psychology of Sport & Exercise*, *12*(4), 392–406. https://doi.org/10.1016/j.psychsport.2011.03.002

Samuel, R. D., & Tenenbaum, G. (2011b). The role of change in athletes' careers: A scheme of change for sport psychology practice. *The Sport Psychologist*, *25*(2), 233–252. https://doi.org/10.1123/tsp.25.2.233

Schwendener-Holt, M. J. (1994). *The process of sport retirement: A longitudinal study of college athletes* (Publication Number 740933881) (Doctoral dissertation). ProQuest Dissertations and Theses Database.

Smith, B., & Sparkes, A. C. (2008). Changing bodies, changing narratives and the consequences of tellability: A case study of becoming disabled through sport. *Sociology of Health & Illness*, *30*(2), 217–236. https://doi.org/10.1111/j.1467-9566.2007.01033.x

Sparkes, A. C., & Smith, B. (2002). Sport, spinal cord injury, embodied masculinities, and the dilemmas of narrative identity. *Men and Masculinities*, *4*(3), 258–285. https://doi.org/10.1177/1097184X02004003003

Stambulova, N. B. (2003). Symptoms of a crisis-transition: A grounded theory study. In N. Hassmén (Ed.), *Yearbook: Swedish Sport Psychology Association [Årsbok: Svensk idrottspsykologisk förening]* (pp. 97–109). Orebro University.

Stambulova, N. B., Alfermann, D., Statler, T., & Côté, J. (2009). ISSP position stand: Career development and transitions of athletes. *International Journal of Sport and Exercise Psychology*, *7*(4), 395–412. https://doi.org/10.1080/1612197X.2009.9671916

Stambulova, N. B., Ryba, T. V., & Henriksen, K. (2020). Career development and transitions of athletes: The international society of sport psychology position stand revisited. *International Journal of Sport and Exercise Psychology*, *19*(4), 524–550. https://doi.org/10.1080/1612197X.2020.1737836

Stambulova, N. B., Stephan, Y., & Jäphag, U. (2007). Athletic retirement: A cross-national comparison of elite French and Swedish athletes. *Psychology of Sport & Exercise*, *8*(1), 101–118. https://doi.org/10.1016/j.psychsport.2006.05.002

Stoltenburg, A. L., Kamphoff, C. S., & Lindstrom Bremer, K. (2011). Transitioning out of sport: The psychosocial effects of collegiate athletes' career-ending injuries. *Athletic Insight*, *11*(2), 1–11.

Tangen, S., & Kudlacek, M. (2014). Extreme sport and reconstruction of identity in persons with spinal cord injuries (SCI). *European Journal of Adapted Physical Activity*, *7*(2), 3–12. https://doi.org/10.5507/EUJ.2014.006

Taylor, J., & Ogilvie, B. (1994). A conceptual model of adaptation to retirement among athletes. *Journal of Applied Sport Psychology*, *6*(1), 1–20. https://doi.org/10.1080/10413209408406462

Waldman, H. B., Rader, R., Perlman, S. P., & Garey, M. (2016). *Children with acquired disabilities*. Retrieved September 29, from www.eparent.com/wellness/children-with-acquired-disabilities/

Webb, W. M., Nasco, S. A., Riley, S., & Headrick, B. (1998). Athlete identity and reactions to retirement from sport. *Journal of Sport Behavior*, *21*(3), 338–362.

Werthner, P., & Orlick, T. (1986). Retirement experiences of successful Olympic athletes. *International Journal of Sport Psychology*, *17*, 337–363.

World Health Organization, & The World Bank. (2011). *World report on disability 2011*. World Health Organization, & The World Bank.

Zurek, G., Goraczko, A., Żurek, A., Lachowicz, M., & Kujawa, K. (2022). Restored life of elite athletes after spinal cord injury. *International Journal of Environmental Research and Public Health*, *19*(14).

21 From Present to Future

Calls for New Paths in Sport Injury Psychology Research

Monna Arvinen-Barrow and Amanda J. Visek

Chapter Objectives

- To synthesize key themes and limitations that define sport injury psychology at present.
- To propose new paths to propel sport injury psychology forward.

This book extends the first edition of *The Psychology of Sport Injury and Rehabilitation* by demonstrating the importance of adopting a holistic, athlete-centered, and socioculturally situated interprofessional approach to sport injury risk and rehabilitation management. This book was divided into four interdependent parts: "Biopsychosocial Approach to Sport Injury," "Professional Practice in Sport Injury," "Psychosocial Strategies in Sport Injury," and "Return to Participation and Transition Out of Sport." Collectively, these sections made the case for sport injuries being a biological phenomenon, both affecting and being affected by, psychological and sociocultural factors (Arvinen-Barrow & Clement, 2019; Brewer & Redmond, 2017; Wadey, 2021). By incorporating the latest theoretical and research evidence from sport psychology and sports medicine, this book, the second edition of *The Psychology of Sport Injury and Rehabilitation*, reflects what sport injury psychology currently is and provides a vision for what it can become in years to come.

The Present

The content of the book augments key themes that define sport injury psychology at present. First, the book highlights the importance of, and evidence in support for, a robust theoretical understanding of sport injury psychology. Within the "Biopsychosocial Approach to Sport Injury" section, Chapter 1 outlined the three phases of rehabilitation as a plausible conceptual framework for understanding the interrelationships between physical and psychosocial rehabilitation phases. Chapter 2 introduced four independent yet overlapping conceptual models aimed to explain sport injury risk. Collectively, Chapters 3–6 focused on providing an understanding of (bio)psychological and sociocultural responses to acute, chronic overuse injury, and sport concussion injury.

The "Professional Practice in Sport Injury" section of the book also presented several theoretical frameworks. Chapter 7 explained how interprofessional practice can be conceptualized within sport injury management. Chapters 8 and 10 discussed how ethical decision-making and mental health referral processes can be navigated in a systematic, step-by-step manner, respectively. Chapter 9 introduced selected key theoretical and applied counseling models that can be used to navigate interpersonal counseling relationships within sport injury. Chapter 11 emphasized the importance of both multicultural psychology paradigm and intersectionality as important guiding frameworks, with individuals representing multiple multicultural identities within sport injury management.

The "Psychosocial Strategies in Sport Injury" section of the book, including Chapters 12–18, underscored the importance of theory in guiding the selection, development, and implementation of various interventions. Depending on the desired outcome of the intervention (e.g., stress management, arousal and anxiety regulation, confidence), theories such as transactional theory of stress and coping, self-efficacy theory, and self-determination theory were proposed as appropriate frameworks to conceptualize a myriad of signs and symptoms during sport injury rehabilitation. Chapters 14–18 also presented several theoretical frameworks and step-by-step processes to explain the mechanisms of, and guide the development and implementation for, goal setting, self-talk, relaxation strategies, imagery, and social support. The final section of the book, "Return to Participation and Transition Out of Sport," framed resuming sport participation, and the move out of sport, within appropriate theoretical frameworks that explained the motivations, processes, and adaptions that occur with injury, chronic illness, or disability.

Second, the book presents existing empirical research evidence while simultaneously exposing the apparent research–practice gaps (see also Evans & Brewer, 2022) that exist in the current literature. Albeit limited in parts, existing research findings provide strong support for the stress and injury incidence relationship. Evidence also confirms the presence of numerous cognitive, emotional, and behavioral responses to sport injuries and the importance of considering psychological factors when making return to participation decisions. Much of the research to date has been athlete-centered, with little to no emphasis on the impact of injury on those around the athlete (e.g., family, significant others, sport coach, teammates, sport psychology, or sports medicine professionals).

Sport injury psychology research has also included recreational, collegiate, national, international, and Olympic athletes from numerous nations (e.g., Australia, Canada, Finland, Ireland, Israel, Norway, Sweden, United Kingdom, and United States) participating in a wide variety of sports. This is somewhat unsurprising, given the true pioneers of sport injury psychology are from numerous countries of origin. While there appears to be convenient heterogeneity in the samples used, what research to date has not yet intentionally considered is possible multicultural athlete and practitioner factors that may influence the sport injury rehabilitation experience.

Despite the book making a compelling case for the role of psychological and sociocultural factors in sport injury, much research is needed to close the research–practice gap. Collectively, the book highlights how research continues to be limited in understanding the intricacies of adopting an interprofessional practice approach to sport injury rehabilitation (see Hess et al., 2019). There is also an apparent theory-research-practice gap in understanding the *how to*, *the accuracy of*, and *the benefits of* using psychological assessments during sport injury and making mental health referrals. Research investigating the use of psychosocial interventions for injury prevention, rehabilitation, return to participation, and transition out of sport also appears predominantly foundational, early stage, exploratory, or design and development focused (for more details on research types, see Institute of Education Sciences & Foundation, 2013, August). In short, sport injury psychology – while theoretically strong – lacks efficacy, efficiency, and effectiveness research, particularly as it relates to psychosocial interventions (see Evans & Brewer, 2022).

The Future

Recently, Evans and Brewer (2022) reflected on what is required of sport injury psychology to reach or cross its "valleys of death" (p. 1012), where "policy and practice lag behind research evidence" (Reis et al., 2008; cited in Evans & Brewer, 2022, p. 1012). They called for *intentionality*, *diligence*, and *patience* in conducting translational research that bridges this gap and best serves athletes and professionals in mitigating the harmful psychological and sociocultural effects of sport injury. Based on the present state of sport injury psychology, we intersect Evans and Brewer's call for intentionality, diligence, and patience with six areas for further inquiry to advance the science and practice of sport injury psychology.

First, while sport injury psychology has a strong theoretical foundation, all too often, when psychological variables are investigated in conjunction with biomechanical sport injury variables, research study designs (a) lack construct clarity for psychological variables, (b) fail to ground the study in appropriate biopsychological theory, or (c) both. This is problematic, given empirically based theory is one of the main elements of the scientific method and provides research a framework for testing its hypotheses (Briner & Rousseau, 2011). Theoretically grounded research can also help researchers in being purposeful when selecting the study design and developing and choosing data collection tools, instruments, and measures, which will yield scientific rigor and, as a result, more robust research findings (Stewart & Klein, 2016). As such, we call for well-designed, theoretically grounded sport injury psychology research that extends beyond current traditional disciplinary boundaries and aims to systematically address the existing research–practice gap with *intentionality*.

Second, the content presented in this book highlights the importance of authentic representation of research participants that fosters diversity, equity, inclusion, and justice. Much of the health-, illness-, and injury-related clinical trials, at least in the United States, are underrepresented by minority participants, resulting in "compounding health disparities, with serious consequences for underrepresented groups and for the nation" (National Academies of Sciences, 2022, p. excerpt). The social responsibility to study all athletes and the consequent effects of not fulfilling this responsibility was also recently discussed by Voelker et al. (2022). Inclusion of a more diverse sample of research participants, in any area of study, may elucidate new findings that would otherwise not be discovered. That said, there are numerous personal, community, research design, and process-related barriers to research participation among underrepresented and excluded participants in health-related research that have been identified. These include, though are not limited to, (mis)trust, (un)willingness to participate, health and research literacy, research site selection, consent and research processes, sampling and recruitment methods, and investigator bias (National Academies of Sciences, Engineering, and Medicine, 2022; Yates et al., 2020). To extend sport injury psychology, we call for research to deliver on the obligation it has to represent all populations afflicted equitably. Such research will require a balance of (a) *intentionality* in inclusive research design, (b) *diligence* to reduce barriers for underrepresented groups to engage as research participants, such as through information and resource supports, along with (c) *patience*, given the sociocultural barriers faced by underrepresented groups.

Third, the content presented in this book highlights the importance of exploring and understanding the psychology of sport injury experience from multiple relational perspectives (see Wadey, 2020; Wadey & Day, 2022). It also emphasizes the importance of gaining further insight into understanding how athletes *cope* with their injury, which warrants further exploration. This is particularly important, given how culture, values, and beliefs can affect common and idiosyncratic psychosocial responses (see Chapter 11) and how a myriad of coping strategies (see Chapter 12) can benefit athletes during sport injury rehabilitation, return to participation, and transition out of sport. As such, we call for *intentional* research study designs that identify multicultural athlete and practitioner factors that influence the sport injury rehabilitation experience. Such research should also include studies that explore humor, profanity, metaphor, spirituality, and religion as coping strategies, the biopsychosocial effects they have, and how to use them as effective interventions during sport injury rehabilitation, return to participation, and transition out of sport.

Fourth, though much attention has been paid to understanding factors that promote positive sport experiences during training and competition (e.g., Bailey et al., 2013), along with a specific focus on fun (e.g., Visek et al., 2015, 2020) and enjoyment (e.g., Jones et al., 2021), there is a striking dearth of research aimed at identifying factors that make sport injury rehabilitation a more positive, if not fun, experience. This is somewhat surprising, given that injury, and, by consequence, rehabilitation, are natural and expected parts of sport participation. Perhaps this is because the injury rehabilitation experience has been broad stroked as one of boring monotony (e.g., repetitive treatment modalities), pain and discomfort (e.g., inflammation and swelling), and drudgery (e.g., laborious agony to be avoided), rather than of pleasure, satisfaction, and joy.

Research has shown, though, when treatment modalities such as active video gaming (Arvinen-Barrow et al., 2020) are designed to make rehabilitative exercises a fun and generally enjoyable experience, it can result in better psychological rehabilitation outcomes while maintaining comparable functional outcomes. Further, within addiction recovery, fun has been suggested to facilitate better rehabilitation experiences and outcomes (e.g., Avalon Malibu, 2019; Casa Nuevo Vida, 2017; Linney, 2021; Melemis, 2015). Kawabata and Mallett (2022) recommended investigating mechanisms for making the "uninteresting, boring, or stressful . . . joyful or fun," in concert with established theoretical frameworks. In sport, the fun integration theory (Visek et al., 2015, 2023) offers an umbrella framework, grounded in established theories of motivation and achievement, for studying the hedonic and eudemonic qualities of positive sport injury rehabilitation experiences. To advance the science and practice of sport injury psychology, with an *intentionality* to improve the quality of rehabilitation experiences and outcomes, we call for innovative research designs that discover the precise determinants and mechanisms of influence that make the injury rehabilitation experience dubbed boring and mundane instead fun.

Fifth, there has also been a dearth of research studying the impact of injury on those surrounding, and supporting, the athlete. These include family, significant others, sport coach, teammates, sport psychology, or sports medicine professionals. While athlete-centered research is vitally important to understanding sport injury psychology, so too is the need to understand sport injury psychology through the worldviews of those around and caring for the athlete. Doing so would provide a more holistic conceptualization of sport injury psychology than currently exists. One method of doing this is through the ecological systems theory (Bronfenbrenner, 1977, 1995), or the multilevel model of sport injury (Wadey et al., 2018), where, consistent with the approach adopted by Voelker et al. (2022), the referent other to the athlete (e.g., sport coach), rather than the athlete, would be placed at the center of the model. Such allows for the study of the individual at the center of the model, while accounting for multiple systems of influence and interaction, on how they care and support the injured athlete. As such, we call for new multi-methodological research approaches to provide a more complete and, importantly, nuanced understanding of sport injury psychology from the perspective of reference others that would open new paths of research and discovery that could improve sport injury rehabilitation, return to participation, and transition out of sport. This will require patience, because, as Voelker et al. (2022) noted, such outcomes cannot be achieved through a single study and thus will require intentionality and diligence, through multiple research designs that establish a body of research evidence to come to common and nuanced conclusions, in sport injury psychology.

Sixth, and lastly, the collective content of this book also highlights a pertinent theme: sport injury, while generally negative and undesired in nature, does not always result in negative cognitive appraisals (Brewer, 2017; Brewer & Redmond, 2017) and can be an opportunity for personal growth (Wadey et al., 2016) and the pursuit of new personal and career trajectories (e.g., Arvinen-Barrow et al., 2019; Arvinen-Barrow et al., 2015). Without empirical study of these cases, sport injury psychology will remain incomplete. Therefore, we call for more qualitative research to capture the rich, layered positive experiences sport injury can have on athletes. We also call for more quantitative research to capture positive outcomes resulting in injury or rehabilitation, particularly as it relates to efficacy, efficiency, and effectiveness of psychosocial interventions in sport injury.

Conclusion

This, the final chapter of the second edition of *The Psychology of Sport Injury and Rehabilitation*, has synthesized key knowledge themes, and the limits of the current body of knowledge, that currently define sport injury psychology. While much has been learned, there is still much to be discovered. Accordingly, the chapter proposed new paths with specific calls to propel sport injury psychology forward in research. Of which, the findings would significantly advance sport injury psychology beyond what it is today, by narrowing the theory-research-practice gap through holistic, athlete-centered, and sociocultural interprofessional approaches to sport injury risk and rehabilitation management.

Reflective Questions

1. What themes in "The Present" section of this chapter resonate most with you, and why?
2. What are three of the six calls to advance sport injury psychology in research? Why are these significant toward offering a more complete understanding of sport injury psychology?
3. What are the roles of intentionality, diligence, and patience in advancing sport injury psychology?
4. Among the six calls to advance sport injury psychology, which would you be most interested in conducting research, and why?

References

Arvinen-Barrow, M., & Clement, D. (Eds.). (2019). *The psychology of sport and performance injury: An interprofessional case-based approach*. Routledge. https://doi.org/10.4324/9781351111591.

Arvinen-Barrow, M., DeGrave, K., Pack, S. M., & Hemmings, B. (2019). Transitioning out of professional sport: The psychosocial impact of career-ending non-musculoskeletal injuries among male cricketers from England and Wales. *Journal of Clinical Sport Psychology*, *13*(4), 629–644. https://doi.org/10.1123/jcsp.2017-0040

Arvinen-Barrow, M., Maresh, N., & Earl-Boehm, J. E. (2020). Functional outcomes and psychological benefits of active video games in the rehabilitation of lateral ankle sprains: A case report. *Journal of Sport Rehabilitation*, *29*(2), 213–224. https://doi.org/10.1123/jsr.2017-0135

Arvinen-Barrow, M., Nässi, A., & Ruiz, M. C. (2015). Kun vamma päättää, milloin ura loppuu. [When injury determines when the career ends]. *Liikunta ja Tiede*, *52*(6), 45–49.

Avalon Malibu. (2019). *Redefining "fun" in recovery.* www.avalonmalibu.com/blog/redefining-fun-in-recovery/#:~:text=Redefining%20%E2%80%9CFun%E2%80%9D%20in%20Recovery%201%20Go%20Your%20Own,Group%20Thing%20 . . . %205%20It%E2%80%99s%20a%20Journey%20

Bailey, R., Hillman, C., Arent, S., & Petitpas, A. J. (2013). Physical activity: An underestimated investment in human capital? *Journal of Physical Activity & Health, 10*(3), 289–308. https://doi.org/10.1123/jpah.10.3.289

Brewer, B. W. (2017). Psychological responses to injury. In *Oxford research encyclopedia of psychology.* Oxford University Press.

Brewer, B. W., & Redmond, C. J. (2017). *Psychology of sport injury.* Human Kinetics.

Briner, R. B., & Rousseau, D. M. (2011). Evidence-based I – O psychology: Not there yet. *Industrial and Organizational Psychology, 4*(1), 3–22. https://doi.org/10.1111/j.1754-9434.2010.01287.x

Bronfenbrenner, U. (1977). Toward an experimental ecology of human development. *American Psychologist, 32*(7), 513–531. https://doi.org/10.1037/0003-066X.32.7.513

Bronfenbrenner, U. (1995). Developmental ecology through space and time: A future perspective. In P. Moen, G. H. Elder Jr, & K. Lüscher (Eds.), *Examining lives in context: Perspectives on the ecology of human development* (pp. 619–647). American Psychological Association.

Casa Nuevo Vida. (2017). *Self-care: The importance of having fun in recovery.* https://casanuevovida.com/having-fun-in-recovery/

Evans, L., & Brewer, B. W. (2022). Applied psychology of sport injury: Getting to – and moving across – The valley of death. *Journal of Applied Sport Psychology, 34*(5), 1011–1028. https://doi.org/10.1080/10413200.2021.2015480

Hess, C. W., Grnacinski, S., & Meyer, B. B. (2019). A review of the sport-injury and -rehabilitation literature: From abstraction to application. *The Sport Psychologist, 33*(3), 232–243. https://doi.org/10.1123/tsp.2018-0043

Institute of Education Sciences, U. S. D. O. E., & Foundation, T. N. S. (2013, August). *Common Guidelines for Education Research and Development.* U. S. D. O. E. A. T. N. S. F. Institute of Education Sciences. https://ies.ed.gov/pdf/CommonGuidelines.pdf

Jones, B., Hope, E., Hammond, A., Moran, J., Leeder, T., Mills, J., & Sandercock, G. (2021). Play more, enjoy more keep playing: Rugby is a simple game. *International Journal of Sports Science & Coaching, 16*(3), 636–645. https://doi.org/10.1177/1747954121991444

Kawabata, M., & Mallett, C. J. (2022). Progressing the construct of enjoyment: Conceptualizing enjoyment as a proactive process. *Discover Psychology, 2.*

Linney, S. (2021). *Redefining fun in recovery.* https://americanaddictioncenters.org/blog/redefining-fun-in-recovery

Melemis, S. M. (2015). Relapse prevention and the five rules of recovery. *The Yale Journal of Biology and Medicine, 88*(3), 325–332. www.ncbi.nlm.nih.gov/pmc/articles/PMC4553654/pdf/yjbm_88_3_325.pdf

National Academies of Sciences, Engineering, and Medicine. (2022). *Improving representation in clinical trials and research: Building research equity for women and underrepresented groups.* National Academies Press. https://doi.org/10.17226/26479

Stewart, D., & Klein, S. (2016). The use of theory in research. *International Journal of Clinical Pharmacy, 38*(3), 615–619. https://doi.org/10.1007/s11096-015-0216-y

Visek, A. J., Achrati, S. M., Mannix, H., McDonnell, K., Harris, B. S., & DiPietro, L. (2015). The fun integration theory: Towards sustaining children and adolescents sport participation. *Journal of Physical Activity & Health, 12*(3), 424–433. https://doi.org/10.1123/jpah.2013-0180

Visek, A. J., Ivarsson, A., Putt, G., & Learner, J. L. (2023). To have fun: What it means and its significance in sport. In M. Toms & R. Jeanes (Eds.), *Routledge handbook of coaching children in sport* (pp. 51–61). Routledge. https://doi.org/10.4324/9781003199359

Visek, A. J., Mannix, H., Chandran, A., Clearly, S., McDonnell, K., & DiPietro, L. (2020). Toward understanding youth athletes' fun priorities: An investigation of sex, age, and levels of play. *Women in Sport & Physical Activity Journal, 28*(1), 34–49. https://doi.org/10.1123/wspaj.2018-0004

Voelker, D. K., Visek, A. J., Learner, J. L., & Dibasio, M. (2022). Toward understanding the role of coaches in athletes' eating pathology: A systematic review and ecological application to advance research. *Psychology of Sport & Exercise, 58.*

Wadey, R. (Ed.). (2020). *Sport injury psychology: Cultural, relational, methodological, and applied considerations*. Routledge.

Wadey, R. (Ed.). (2021). *Sport injury psychology: Cultural, relational, methodological, and applied considerations*. Routledge.

Wadey, R., & Day, M. C. (2022). Challenging the status quo of sport injury psychology to advance theory, research, and applied practice: An epilogue to a special issue. *Journal of Applied Sport Psychology*, *34*(4), 1029–1036. https://doi.org/10.1080/10413200.2022.2100006

Wadey, R., Day, M. C., Cavallerio, F., & Martinelli, L. A. (2018). Multilevel model of sport injury (MMSI): Can coaches impact and be impacted by injury? In R. C. Thelwell & M. Dicks (Eds.), *Professional advances in sports coaching: Research and practice* (pp. 336–357). Routledge. https://doi.org/10.4324/9781351210980

Wadey, R., Podlog, L., Galli, N., & Mellalieu, S. D. (2016). Stress-related growth following sport injury: Examining the applicability of the organismic valuing theory. *Scandinavian Journal of Medicine & Science in Sports*, *26*(10), 1132–1139. https://doi.org/10.1111/sms.12579

Yates, I., Byrne, J., Donahue, S., McCarty, L., & Mathews, A. (2020). Representation in clinical trials: A review on reaching underrepresented populations in research. *Clinical Researcher*, *34*(7).

Index

Note: Page numbers in *italics* indicate a figure